Atherogenesis

Progress in Biochemical Pharmacology

Vol. 13

Series Editor: R. Paoletti, Milan

S. Karger · Basel · München · Paris · London · New York · Sydney

Atherogenesis

Morphology, Metabolism and Function
of the Arterial Wall

Volume Editors
H. SINZINGER, Vienna; W. AUERSWALD, Vienna;
H. JELLINEK, Budapest, and W. Feigl, Vienna

Collaborators
B. BINDER, Vienna; M.D. HAUST, London, Ont.; Ch. LEITNER, Vienna;
J. LINDNER, Hamburg; H.C. STARY, New Orleans, La., and G. WEBER, Siena

143 figures and 29 tables, 1977

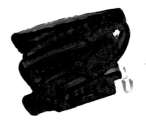

S. Karger · Basel · München · Paris · London · New York · Sydney

Progress in Biochemical Pharmacology

Vol. 11: Biological Basis of Clinical Effect of Bleomycin. Editor: CAPUTO, A. (Rome).
X + 230 p., 74 fig., 69 tab., 1976
ISBN 3-8055-2338-6

Vol. 12: Drugs Affecting the Renin-Angiotensin-Aldosterone System. Use of Angio-
tensin Inhibitors. Editors: STOKES, G.S. (Sydney), and EDWARDS, K.D.G. (New
York). XIV + 258 p., 98 fig., 18 tab., 1976
ISBN 3-8055-2410-2

Cataloging in Publication

International Atherosclerosis Conference, Vienna, 1977
Atherogenesis: morphology, metabolism, and function of the arterial wall
International Atherosclerosis Conference, Vienna, 1977
Volume editors, H.F. Sinzinger et al.; collaborators, B. Binder et al. – Basel,
New York, Karger, 1977
(Progress in biochemical pharmacology, v. 13)
1. Atherosclerosis – congresses I. Binder, Bernd, ed. II. Sinzinger, H.F., ed. III.
Title IV. Series
W1 PR66H v. 13/WG 550 I603 1977a

ISBN 3-8055-2761-6

© Copyright 1977 by S. Karger AG, 4011 Basel (Switzerland), Arnold-Böcklin-Str. 25
Printed in Switzerland by Graphische Anstalt Schüler AG, Biel
ISBN 3-8055-2761-6

Contents

Contents

Smooth Muscle Cell in Atherosclerosis

Permeabiliti

Contents

Scanning Electron Microscopy and Surface Coat

Arterial Cell Injury

Contents

Experimental Atherosclerosis

Platelets, Thrombosis and Atherosclerosis

Preface

The Proceedings of the First International Atherosclerosis Conference, comprising Introductory Lectures, Special Sessions, and Workshops, held in Vienna from the 12th to the 16th of April, 1977 under the auspices of the Austrian Association for Morphological and Functional Research in Atherosclerosis (AMFA), are recorded in this volume. The aim of this conference was to obtain an overall view of the basic events in atherosclerosis – beginning with the first lesions of the vessel wall, following with their interaction with platelets, and, especially, dealing with the role of the cellular constituents of the arteries in the genesis of atherosclerotic lesions.

The several topics were effectively reviewed by appropriate leading experts who acted not only as moderators but also summarized the most recent findings in their field. The simultaneous presence of contributing distinguished representatives of world-recognized teams engaged in atherosclerosis research provided a welcome occasion to record and compare results obtained from a variety of investigative assumptions and experimental methods and to indicate for the future better integrated approaches towards our understanding and successful therapy of atherosclerosis in man.

The publication of these Proceedings of the First International Atherosclerosis Conference makes the material of this meeting available to a broad group of interested scientists. It contributes to a better appreciation of the key events in early atherosclerosis and should stimulate further basic research in a field so important for the establishment of preventive and therapeutic measures against cardiovascular diseases.

H. SINZINGER, W. AUERSWALD, H. JELLINEK, W. FEIGL

Progress in Biochemical Pharmacology, Vol. 13: Atherogenesis

Dear Reader,
Please note that an unfortunate mistake occurred during the final production stage. On short notice the volume number of the book was changed to 13. While this was done in the title and in all other means of documentation, we failed to change it in the citation title. When referring to any article in this book, please use the following citation title:

Prog. biochem. Pharmacol., **vol. 13**, pp. ...–... (Karger, Basel 1977)

Thanking you for your understanding,
S. Karger AG, Basel

Prog. biochem. Pharmacol., vol. 14, pp. 1–8 (Karger, Basel 1977)

Morphological Functional Changes of Aortic Endothelium During Different Types of Hypertension[1]

G. Gabbiani, G. Elemer, M.C. Badonnel and I. Hüttner

Department of Pathology, University of Geneva, Geneva, and
Department of Pathology, McGill University, Montreal, Que.

Introduction

The response of the vascular wall to various types of damage leads to complex changes among which atherosclerotic lesions with proliferation of smooth muscle cells, accumulation of lipids and connective tissue are the most characteristic [1]. It is widely accepted that hypertension is one of the most important if not the most important predisposing factor for atherosclerotic lesions. However, the mechanisms of this noxious action are not clear. Lipid deposition, which generally precedes the formation of the atherosclerotic plaque, could be mediated through (1) endothelial injury (which would partially deendothelialize the luminal surface of arteries) or (2) increased endothelial permeability. The purpose of this paper is to discuss the variations of endothelial morphology and permeability during different types of hypertension [2, 3].

Material and Methods

A total of 50 male Wistar rats weighing 170–250 g were used for the experiments. A group of 10 animals was left as untreated controls. In the other rats, the aorta was completely ligated between the two renal arteries below the superior mesenteric artery. The resulting low perfusion of the left kidney is known to produce hypertension associated with stimu-

[1] Supported by the Swiss Medical Research Foundation (Grant No 3.692-0.76) and the Medical Research Council of Canada (Grant MA-5958).

lation of the renin angiotensin system [4]. Blood pressure was recorded through the right carotid artery using a Hewlett Packard 77028 recorder (Hewlett Packard, Geneva, Switzerland). During periods of continuous blood pressure recordings, control animals, early hypertensive (6–7 days) animals, and late hypertensive (30–40 days) animals were given horseradish peroxidase (HRP) Sigma type II intravenously in a dose of 5 mg in 0.5 ml of saline per 100 g body weight. Perfusion of glutaraldehyde started 5 min after HRP injection and was carried out *via* the left ventricle of the heart. Segments of the thoracic aorta were processed for electron microscopy as described previously [2]. Unstained thick sections were prepared from all Epon-embedded aortic segments and were reviewed by light microscopy. From selected blocks, thin sections were cut on LKBIII ultrotomes (LSB Produckter AB, Stockholm, Sweden) or Reichert ultramicrotomes (C. Reichert, AG, Vienna, Austria) and examined either unstained or following lead citrate and uranyl acetate staining with Philips EM300 electron microscopes. *En face* preparations of endothelial cells were made from thoracic aortae of 5 control rats as well as 5 from the 6- to 7-day and 5 from the 30- to 40-day hypertensive groups. The preparations were treated either with normal human serum or with anti-actin antibodies (AAA) containing sera from patients with chronic aggressive hepatitis [5, 6] and were then stained with fluorescein conjugated IgG fraction of goat antiserum to human IgG (code 64.070 Miles Seravac, Lausanne, Switzerland) according tot the technique previously described [5]. The specificity of the sera was assessed as previously described [5, 6].

Results

Systolic and diastolic blood pressure of control rats at 6–7 and 30–40 days was 84/59 und 117/86 mm Hg, respectively. In rats with aortic ligation the blood pressure above the ligature was 179/142 mm Hg

---

Fig. 1. Aortic endothelial cell of an hypertensive rat 7 days after ligature of the aorta. Note the bundles of microfilaments; dense areas similar to 'attachment sites' are regularly distributed throughout the microfilaments. × 14,500.

Fig. 2. Unstained section of aortic endothelium from an hypertensive rat 7 days after ligature of the aorta. The rat has received intravenously 5 mg HRP/100 g body weight during 5 min. The endothelial cell contains a bundle of microfilaments (arrows) and the subendothelial space is filled with HRP revelation product. × 12,000.

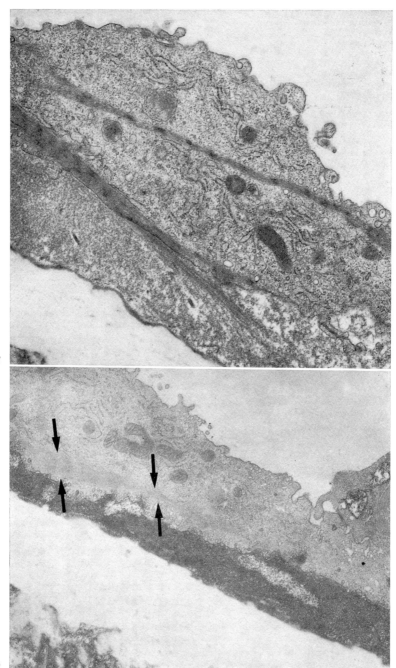

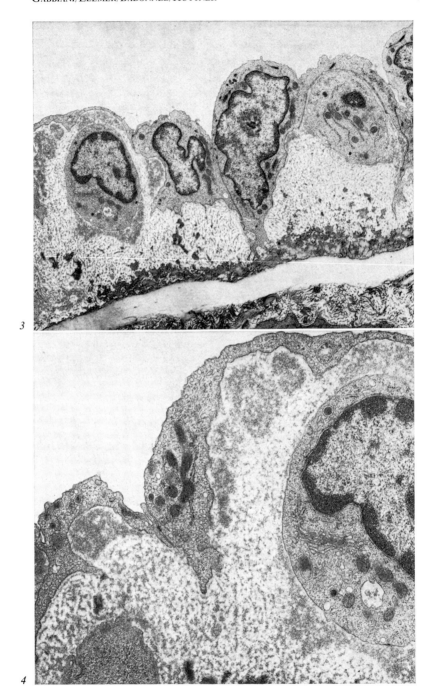

in the 6–7 day group and 192/135 mm Hg in the 30–40 day group. On fixed sections, the endothelium of control thoracic aortae was identified as a flat cell layer lying on the external elastic lamina. As compared with controls, the aortic segments at 6–7 days after operation had a widened subendothelial space and a thickened endothelial cell layer. At 30–40 days after operation the aortic endothelium formed an undulated layer lying above an expanded subendothelium. However, the size of endothelial cells in most segments examined was comparable to that of control rats.

In normotensive animals, the aortic subendothelium was negative for HRP reaction product. At 6–7 days, the subendothelial HRP reaction was found to be very intense; at 30–40 days after operation most aortic segments examined were negative for HRP.

No fluorescence was seen in any *en face* preparations after treatment with normal serum. After incubation with AAA serum a week fluorescence was detected at the periphery of the endothelial cells of control animals. Intense fluorescence was visible in the cytoplasm of the majority of endothelial cells prepared from thoracic aortae, 6–7 days after operation [2]. In endothelial cells of the 30- to 40-day group, fluorescence was much less intense than at 6–7 days and was comparable to that of controls [3]. In preparations treated with AAA serum, previously incubated with skeletal muscle actin, no fluorescence was present. On electron microscopic examination, the aortic intima of normotensive controls was as previously described [2, 7]. At 6–7 days after aortic ligation, endothelial cells of thoracic aortae from hypertensive rats bulged into the lumen and showed many microvillous and/or flat-like cytoplasmic projections [2]. The endothelial cell cytoplasm exhibited general organellar hyperplasia. In addition, an extensive microfilamentous apparatus was localized mainly through the cell periphery [2] (fig. 1). HRP reaction product was evident along the entire length of the intercellular clefts in plasmalemmal vesicles and also in the subendothelial space (fig. 2). At 30–40 days aortic endothelial cells had irregular contours but were much

---

Fig. 3. Aortic endothelial layer from an hypertensive rat 40 days after ligature of the aorta. Endothelial cells are seen and the subendothelial layer is thickened and contains large amounts of basement membrane-like material but not HRP. $\times$ 5,500.

Fig. 4. A detail of figure 3 showing that the cytoplasm of endothelial cells does not contain microfilaments. In the subendothelial space a lymphocyte is present. $\times$ 14,000.

smaller than those of the 6- to 7-day group (fig. 3, 4). Cytoplasmic micro-filaments were exceptionally seen. The endothelial cell layer was separated from the internal elastic lamina by markedly increased amounts of a cellular connective tissue matrix presenting as a complex network of multi-layered basement laminae associated with collagen and elastic fibers [3]. HRP reaction product was present only in occasional endothelial vesicles. Few macrophages and lymphocytes located in the subendothelial layer contained HRP in dense bodies.

Discussion

Ligature of the aorta between the renal arteries results within a few days in hypertension associated with stimulation of the renin angiotensin system [4]. This is evident by the high plasma renin activity recorded in such animals during the first 2 weeks of hypertension [8, 9]. After the third week however, plasma renin activity declines to normal or low levels while high blood pressure persists [10]. Our results show an increased permeability of the thoracic aortic endothelium to HRP in hypertensive animals on the 6–7 days whereas at 30–40 days after aortic ligation, increased permeability of aortic endothelium was no longer evident despite the presence of elevated blood pressure. Variations in permeability to HRP paralleled the changes in the endothelial cell layer and subendothelium. In the 6- to 7-day group, aortic endothelial cells were markedly hypertrophic and contained a prominent cytoplasmic contractile apparatus. In the 30- to 40-day group, aortic segments showed much smaller endothelial cells with much less prominent cytoplasmic microfilaments than those found at the early stage of hypertension. In addition, there was an increased amount of connective tissue matrix in the subendothelium. The changes of endothelial morphology and permeability could be ascribed to the different types of hypertension, which at the early stage is mediated through different mechanisms than at the late stage. In recent years several reports have suggested a higher incidence of cardiovascular complications in hypertensive patients with high plasma renin levels than in those with low renin levels [11, 12]. Although the validity of statistical evidence for this suggestion has recently been challenged [10], this strong contrast between endothelial cell changes observed parallel with high and low renin levels in the hypertensive model utilized herein indicates the necessity of further studies along this line.

Summary

In rats, ligature of the aorta between the renal arteries produces hypertension which in the early phase (6–7 days) is associated with elevated plasma renin content, and later (40 days) is associated with low plasma renin. During the early phase, the endothelium of the aorta shows elevated permeability to HRP, endothelial cells are hypertrophic and contain bundles of actin microfilaments. During the late phase, permeability to HRP is normal, the endothelial cells are flat and do not contain bundles of microfilaments. Probably the endothelial cells of aorta react in different ways to various hypertensive stimuli and/or adapt to high levels of blood pressure.

References

1 ROSS, R. and HARKER, L.: Hyperlipidemia and atherosclerosis. Science *193:* 1094–1100 (1976).

2 GABBIANI, G.; BADONNEL, M.C., and RONA, G.: Cytoplasmic contractile apparatus in aortic endothelial cells of hypertensive rats. Lab. Invest. *32:* 227–234 (1975).

3 HÜTTNER, I.; BADONNEL, M.C.; ELEMER, G., and GABBIANI, G.: The aortic endothelium during different stages of hypertension. Lab. Invest. (submitted for publication).

4 ROJO-ORTEGA, J.M. and GENEST, J.: A method for production of experimental hypertension in rats. Can. J. Physiol. Pharmacol. *46:* 883–885 (1968).

5 GABBIANI, G.; RYAN, G.B.; LAMELIN, J.P.; VASSALLI, P.; MAJNO, G.; BOUVIER, C.A.; CRUCHAUD, A., and LÜSCHER, E.F.: Human smooth muscle autoantibody. Its identification as antiactin antibody and a study of its binding to 'non-muscular' cells. Am. J. Path. *72:* 473–488 (1973).

6 CHAPONNIER, C.; KOHLER, L., and GABBIANI, G.: Fixation of human antiactin autoantibodies on skeletal muscle fibers. Clin. exp. Immunol. *27:* 278–284 (1977).

7 SCHWARTZ, S.M. and BENDITT, E.P.: Studies on aortic intima. I. Structure and permeability of rat thoracic aortic intima. Am. J. Path. *66:* 241–264 (1972).

8 ROJO-ORTEGA, J.M.; BOUCHER, R., and GENEST, J.: Experimental hypertension in rats. Abstract. Clin. Res. *16:* 394 (1968).

9 ROJO-ORTEGA, J.M. and GENEST, J.: Experimental hypertension in rats; in Abstr. 3rd Int. Congr. Endocrinol., p. 132, Mexico 1968.

10 ROJO-ORTEGA, J.M.; CASADO, S.; BOUCHER, R., and GENEST, J.: Renal renin content does not always represent renin secretion; in Abstr. 4th Int. Congr. Nephrol., vol. 1, p. 265, Stockholm 1969.

11 BRUNNER, H.R.; LARAGH, J.H.; BAER, L.; NEWTON, M.A.; GOODWIN, F.T.; KRAKOFF, L.R.; BARD, R.H., and BUHLER, F.R.: Essential hypertension: renin

and aldosterone, heart attack and stroke. New Engl. J. Med. *286:* 441–449 (1972).

12 BRUNNER, H.R.; SEALEY, J.E., and LARAGH, J.H.: Renin as a risk factor in essential hypertension: more evidence. Am. J. Med. *55:* 295–302 (1973).

G. GABBIANI, MD, PhD, Department of Pathology, University of Geneva, Boulevard de la Cluse 40, *CH-1211 Geneva 4* (Switzerland)

Prog. biochem. Pharmacol., vol. 14, pp. 9–14 (Karger, Basel 1977)

Nature of the Endothelial Cement and the Connections between Endothelial Cells and Smooth Muscle Cells

R. GOTTLOB and H.F. HOFF

Department of Experimental Surgery, Ist Surgical University Clinic, Vienna, and Department of Neurology and Pathology, Baylor Medical College, Houston, Tex.

The Nature of the Intercellular Cement and the Mechanics of Silver Staining

The silver nitrate procedure has been suggested to stain a cement substance the existence of which has been doubted because of the inability to visualize such a structure with the electron microscope [see, however, LUFT, 6]. The cement or silver lines can be stained with metal stains such as silver nitrate, which requires the presence of chloride ions in the tissue as well as exposure to light. Other staining procedures are iron, or osmium ions plus hematoxylin [2, 7], polyanions plus basic dyes [2, 7], colloids plus colloidal iron [7], and finally cationic detergents plus bromocresol-green [4].

Silver staining can be prevented by prior dechlorination of the tissue, by omitting exposure to light, and by treating with organic solvents [4, 8], cationic detergents [4, 5], or free iodide ions [4, 5].

We assume that cationic detergents prevent silver staining by blocking the polyanionic groups of the substance. The presence of the cationic detergents themselves is proven by the staining with bromocresol-green, a specific stain for quaternary ammonium bases.

It is suggested that tissue chloride ions play an important role in the staining reaction by forming silver chloride throughout the tissue [1]. Silver ions bound to polyanionic structures are reduced to metallic silver. However, since these are too small to be visualized by light microscopy, the presence of silver chloride is necessary, together with exposure to light, to trigger further reduction of silver around the original foci of silver deposits [3, 4].

Silver staining can, however, be achieved after tissue dechlorination by any of the following: rechlorination [1, 8], treatment with heparin, gold chloride or a dilute solution of silver nitrate [3, 4]. It is suggested that the action of heparin results from its binding to the intercellular junctions, thereby increasing the concentration of polyanionic material and inducing greater and more visible deposits of reduced silver. Gold chloride is suggested to bind to the minute foci of reduced silver leading to microscopically visible silver lines.

Photographic developers can take the place of light exposure in reducing the silver chloride around foci of metallic deposits on polyanionic material [4]. This can also be achieved by longer treatments with dilute silver nitrate or gold chloride.

Silver staining has many parallels to the steps in photography. Silver bromide is present in a photographic emulsion. In photography light reduces silver ions producing silver grains; while in silver staining a cement substance, presumed to represent polyanionic material, reduces silver ions, thereby producing silver grains. Finally in photography a developer reduces the silver ions around the silver foci, while in silver staining this is performed by light.

The Fixation of Endothelia to Basal Structures

In figure 2 (vena cava) we see the network of silver lines surrounding endothelial cells of a large vein. Small spurs can also be seen extending from the silver lines. When the time of staining is extended these spurs get longer and longer until they are found to belong to the network of silver lines between medial smooth muscle cells running perpendicular to the endothelial silver lines (fig. 1).

In the preparation (fig. 2) of a vein we see that the endothelial silver lines are pulled out of shape presumably due to the contraction of medial smooth muscle cells. In other preparations of the aorta it is the perpendicular network of lines that is pulled out of shape. These results suggest a connection between the two networks of cement substances, possibly due to the presence of endothelial smooth muscle cell junctions [9]. Further evidence for this possibility came from studying the morphology of silver-stained preparations of veins in sectioned material.

In figure 3 we see in cross-section the presence of silver lines from both networks of silver-stained cement lines on both sides of the internal

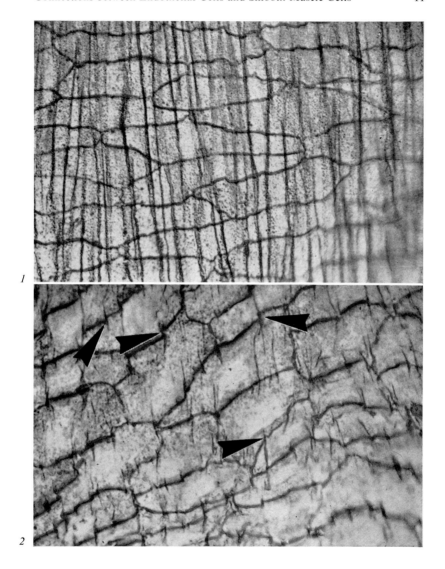

Fig. 1. Normal vein, en face preparation. Staining of endothelial silver lines (running horizontally) and transverse lines of the media.

Fig. 2. Endothelial silver lines displaying the 'spurs' and distortions of the endothelial silver lines (arrows).

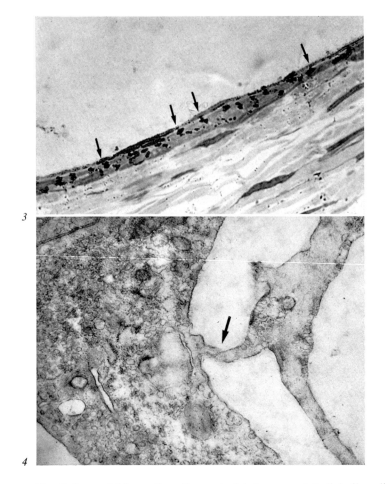

Fig. 3. In semi-thin sections the contact between endothelial silver lines and transverse lines is seen to occur in the fenestrae of the elastic membrane (arrows).

Fig. 4. Processes of endothelial cell and smooth muscle cell meeting in a fenestra of the elastic membrane (arrow), ultrathin section.

elastic membrane. It is clearly seen how endothelial silver lines meet muscle silver lines.

On the electron microscope level we can see the medial silver lines in cross-section. Here we see the connection of an endothelial silver line presumably staining the junction between overlapping endothelial cells, and the silver line staining a junction between two smooth muscle cells.

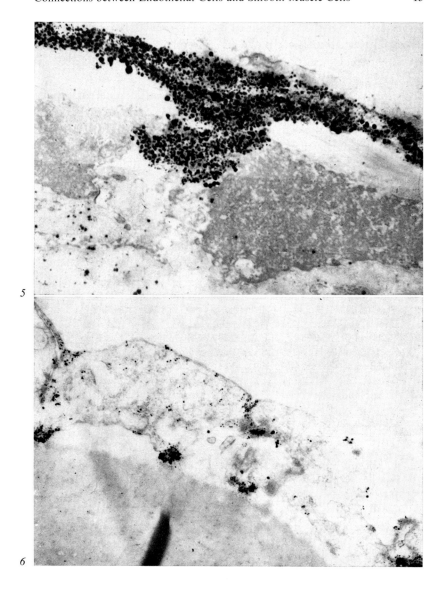

Fig. 5. An endothelial silver line and its contact with a transverse line in an ultrathin section. Endothelial damage due to silver staining.

Fig. 6. A damaged endothelium is partially detached from the elastic membrane. Note that the points of adhesion are silver stained.

Tissue preservation is very poor since perfusion with silver nitrate destroys tissue ultrastructure (fig. 5). We have frequently observed junctions between endothelial cells and underlining medial smooth muscle cells which meet in a fenestra of the elastic membrane (fig. 4).

Finally, we have observed that the attachment plates which appear to connect foot processes of the endothelium to underlining structures such as the internal elastic membrane of this rabbit aorta, also stain positively following silver nitrate treatment (fig. 6). These results suggest that a cement substance, presumably of polyanionic nature, not only holds endothelial cells onto a single sheet, but also binds endothelial cells to the remaining vessel wall.

References

1   ACHARD, C. et AYNAUD, M.: Recherches sur l'imprégnation histologique de l'endothelium. Archs Méd. exp. Anat. path. *19:* 437–458 (1907).
2   FLOREY, H.W.; POOLE, J.C.F., and MEEK, G.A.: Endothelial cells and 'cement' lines. J. Path. Bact. *77:* 625–636 (1959).
3   GOTTLOB, R. and HOFF, H.F.: A study of the relation between endothelial silver lines, medial transversal silver lines and the ultrastructural morphology of blood vessels. Vasc. Surg. *1:* 92–100 (1967).
4   GOTTLOB, R. and HOFF, H.F.: Histochemical investigations on the nature of large blood vessel endothelial and medial argyrophilic lines and on the mechanims of silver staining. Histochemie *13:* 70–83 (1968).
5   GOTTLOB, R. und SCHLOBIES, M.: Über die Einwirkung von Verödungsmitteln auf die Endothelien. Medsche Welt *17:* 1225–1227 (1966).
6   LUFT, J.H.: Fine structure of capillary and endocapillary layer as revealed by ruthenium red. Fed. Proc. *25:* 1773–1783 (1966).
7   SAMUELS, P.B. and WEBSTER, D.R.: The role of venous endothelium in the inception of thrombosis. Ann. Surg. *136:* 422–438 (1952).
8   SINAPIUS, D.: Über Grundlagen und Bedeutung der Vorversilberung und verwandter Methoden nach Untersuchungen am Aortenendothel. Z. Zellforsch. mikrosk. Anat. *44:* 27–56 (1956).
9   ZINNER, G. und GOTTLOB, R.: Weitere Beobachtungen zur pathologischen Histologie der Venenendothelien. Virchows Arch. path. Anat. Physiol. *334:* 337–341 (1961).

R. GOTTLOB, MD, Department of Experimental Surgery, Ist Surgical Clinic, Vienna University, Alserstrasse 4, *A-1097 Vienna* (Austria)

Prog. biochem. Pharmacol., vol. 14, pp. 15–18 (Karger, Basel 1977)

Effects of Different Serum Components on the Cultured Endothelial and Smooth Muscle Cells

E. Csonka and L. Romics

2nd Department of Pathology and 3rd Department of Medicine, Semmelweis Medical University, Budapest

Introduction

In a previous study [2], the effect of cholesterol suspended in the medium was studied on the morphology of cultured endothelial or smooth muscle cells. In the present series of examinations we studied the effect of patients' sera with high cholesterol content on the growth of endothelial or smooth muscle cells *in vitro*.

Material and Methods

Sera from a total of 20 patients with high hypercholesterolemia and/or diabetes were used. In table I we summarized the main clinical and laboratory data of the patients involved. The cell cultures were primarily explants of the aortas of individual mini pigs. The method of the preparation of explants was the same as that used in our department since 1973 [1]. Each individual piece of tissue was explanted separately into a well of a flat-bottom microtest plate, as seen in figure 1.

Results

The effect of each serum on the explants was expressed as percent of growth area as referred to the control. Since this method permitted reasonable estimation rather than exact quantitative evaluation, the sera were finally grouped as highly stimulatory, ineffective and inhibitory.

Table I. Clinical and laboratory data of the patients

No.	Age years	Sex	Diagnosis	Cholesterin mg^0/$_0$	Triglyceride mg^0/$_0$	Glucose mg^0/$_0$	Therapy
1	57	male	diabetes mellitus	195	115	100	insulin
2	63	male	diabetes mellitus retinopathia	220	348	100	insulin
3	42	male	diabetes mellitus	320	173	300	insulin
4 X	77	female	diabetes mellitus pyelonephritis chr.	260	210	100	glibenclamide
5 O	75	female	diabetes mellitus	290	329	100	glibenclamide
6	56	female	diabetes mellitus hyperlipoproteinemia	345	960	325	–
7 O	52	female	diabetes mellitus	270	355	228	biquanid clofibrate
8 X	61	female	diabetes mellitus retinopathia Kimmelstiel-Wilson syndrome azotemia	195	136	116	insulin anabolic hormone
9	54	female	diabetes mellitus	240	187	265	insulin
10 O	30	male	hypercholest. famil.	405	150	93	–
11	73	female	hypercholesterolemia	385	302	94	–
12	55	female	hypercholesterolemia	340	215	100	clofibrate
13	43	female	hypercholesterolemia	322	141	96	–
14	51	female	hypercholesterolemia	359	272	100	–
15	24	female	essential. hypercholest.	660	140	100	–
16	73	male	coronariasclerosis	295	194	96	–
17 X	52	female	cerebrosclerosis gravis	307	201	112	
18	39	female	xanthoma periorbitale	275	179	100	–
19	52	female	decomp. artis Card. min. grad.	310	194	98	–
20	35	female	ulcus	312	125	96	–
21		Control human serum		150	54	92	–
22		Control calf serum		89	77	41	–

X = Highly stimulatory sera; O = inhibitory sera.

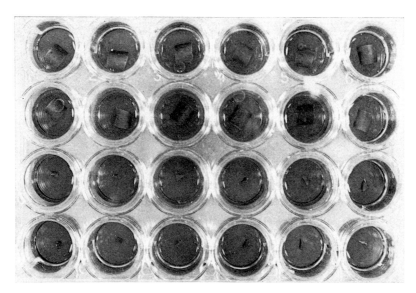

Fig. 1. Explants for endothelium or smooth muscle cell culturing in microtest plates.

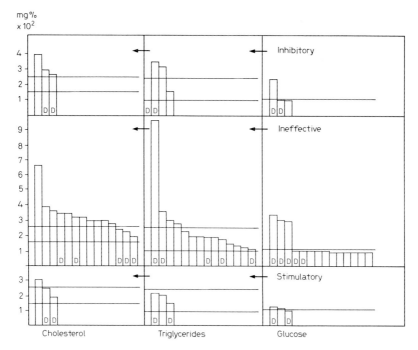

Fig. 2. Diagrammatic presentation of the effects of patients sera on the growth of explants. D = Diabetic sera.

As demonstrated in figure 2 by the diagram presented, no conspicuous correlation was seen between the cholesterol, triglycerides, or glucose content of sera and their effect on the tissue culture.

In conclusion we may state that we were not able to reveal any conspicuous correlation between the effect on the growth of mini pig aortic explants and the cholesterol, triglyceride or glucose content of the sera tested. As to the effect of diabetic sera we refer to the works of LEDET et al. [3]. They produced diabetes in rabbits and found the sera of these animals to induce growth of cultured smooth muscle cells in the stationary phase. Also LEDET [4] obtained similar results with sera of patients with juvenile diabetes. None of the authors quoted was, however, able to correlate the stimulatory effect with any known components of the sera studied. In our experiments diabetes itself did not seem to be responsible for the inhibitory, ineffective or stimulatory character of the patients' serum on the growth of aortic explants.

References

1   CSONKA, E.; KERENYI, T.; KOCH, A.S., and JELLINEK, H.: *In vitro* cultivation and identification of aortic endothelium from miniature pig. Arterial Wall *3:* 31–37 (1975).
2   CSONKA, E.; BERNOLÁK, B.; KOCH, A.S., and JELLINEK, H.: Studies of the influence of membrane active substances on cell surface morphology in cultured aortic endothelial cells (in press).
3   LEDET, T.; FISCHER-DZOGA, K., and WISSLER, R.W.: Growth of rabbit aortic smooth-muscle cells cultured in media containing diabetic and hyperlipemic serum. Diabetes *25:* 207–215 (1976).
4   LEDET, T.: Growth of rabbit aortic smooth muscle cells in serum from patients with juvenile diabetes. Acta path. microbiol. scand., Sect. A *84:* 508–516 (1976).

Dr. EVA CSONKA, 2nd Department of Pathology, University Medical School, *Budapest* (Hungary)

Prog. biochem. Pharmacol., vol. 14, pp. 19–25 (Karger, Basel 1977)

Studies on the Pinocytosis of Hyaluronate and Proteoglycans

Hans Kresse and Wolfgang Truppe

Institute of Medical Chemistry, University of Graz, Graz

Mammalian arterial tissues are known to synthesize hyaluronate and different types of proteoglycans containing predominantly copolymeric chondroitin and dermatan sulfate, and heparan sulfate as glycosamino-glycan moieties [1, 2]. As one of the earliest biochemical events in the development of arteriosclerosis an altered rate of synthesis and/or turnover rates of sulfated glycosaminoglycans have been reported [3, 4]. Furthermore, in intact normal arterial tissue the individual glycosamino-glycan types can be characterized by different metabolic activities [5, 6].

Such metabolic differences might be explained by a different labelling of the immediate radioactive precursors [7], or by different rates of synthesis and degradation. Divergent degradation rates could be either the result of different activities of metabolizing enzymes or the consequence of the existence of topographically distinct glycosaminoglycan pools differing in their accessibility for degradative processes or a combination of both. In an attempt to distinguish between the latter possibilities cells were cultured from the intima of bovine thoracic aorta and the formation, composition and metabolic fate of various glycosaminoglycan pools were investigated.

The experimental details of initiation and maintenance of tissue culture and of isolation and characterization of different glycosamino-glycan pools have been described previously [8, 9]. As in the case of cultured human skin fibroblasts [10] the glycosaminoglycans newly synthesized by bovine intimal cells can be isolated from three principal pools. Glycosaminoglycans present in the culture medium represent the homogenous extracellular pool. Material which can be solubilized from the cell periphery by mild trypsin treatment has been considered as pericellular pool, the remaining cellular glycosaminoglycans were designated as intracellular pool.

After incubation of confluent cultures in the presence of 2 μCi/ml [1-^{14}C]glucosamine for 48 h, 74 % of the glycosaminoglycan-associated radioactivity was found in the extracellular pool, 20 % in the pericellular pool and 6 % in the intracellular pool. Each pool exhibited a characteristic distribution pattern of the individual glycosaminoglycan types which did not change within the labelling period. The extracellular pool had a similar composition as intact arterial tissue – 41 % chondroitin sulfate (CS), 13 % dermatan sulfate (DS), 7 % heparan sulfate (HS), and 39 % hyaluronate (HA). The pericellular pool contained 54 % CS, 10 % DS, 7 % HS and 29 % HA, whereas intracellularly 27 % CS, 21 % DS, 22 % HS and 30 % HA were found.

Using [^{35}S]sulfate as a metabolic precursor of sulfated glycosaminoglycans the following results were obtained: (1) 42 % of the synthesized sulfated glycosaminoglycans enters primarily the extracellular, 32 % the pericellular and 26 % the intracellular pool. On the basis of the distribution pattern and under the assumptions that the various glycosaminoglycan types have an equimolar degree of sulfation and that [^{35}S]PAPS has a uniform specific radioactivity, one can therefore calculate that 49 % of the HS remains in the intracellular pool, 26 % reaches the pericellular pool, and 25 % the extracellular pool. In contrast, 38 and 44 % of the CS and 18 and 48 % of the DS are transferred to the pericellular and extracellular pools, respectively. (2) The polymer-bound [^{35}S]radioactivity of the intracellular and pericellular pool increases with time in a hyperbolic manner and reaches a constant level, which reflects an equilibrium between the entry of labelled macromolecules into the pool and their disappearance from it, after about 10 h (intracellular pool) and 24 h (pericellular pool), respectively.

Pulse chase experiments revealed that the bulk of sulfated glycosaminoglycans inside the cells disappears with a half-life of 7 h. The rate of decay of CS, DS and HS was rather similar for each glycosaminoglycan type. Pericellular glycosaminoglycans disappear with a half-life of 12–14 h. About 60 % of the membrane-bound material is shedded off into the medium, 40 % is found inside the cells and as inorganic sulfate in the culture medium. Detailed investigations revealed furthermore, that pericellular glycosaminoglycans destined for uptake by the cells have a more rapid turnover than the macromolecules which are reaching the extracellular pool.

During an experimental period of up to 6 days no equilibrium was reached between the secretion of glycosaminoglycans into the culture medium and their disappearance from it by pinocytosis and/or degradation. No experimental evidence for a degradation of proteoglycans by enzymes present in the culture medium could be obtained. On addition of [35S]sulfate-labelled proteoglycans partially purified from arterial cell cultures, up to 12 % of the material was taken up by arterial cells within 24 h. Pinocytosed proteoglycans were rapidly degraded, followed by the release of inorganic [35S]sulfate into the culture medium. Knowing the initial rate of pinocytosis and the concentration of internalized proteoglycans, it was calculated that the half-life of internalized proteoglycans is in the order of 3 h. Pinocytosed proteoglycans were therefore considered as being catabolized more rapidly than those proteoglycans which remain within the cell after their biosynthesis.

From the amount of internalized proteoglycans, from the temperature dependence and from the dose dependence of uptake (fig. 1) the conclusion can be drawn that the uptake of proteoglycans is brought about by

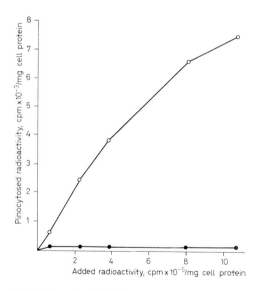

Fig. 1. Uptake of [35S]proteoglycans by bovine arterial intima cells. The amount of pinocytosed radioactivity after incubation for 24 h at 37° C (○) or at 4° C (●) was determined as described [9].

Table I. Adsorption, pinocytosis and degradation of $^{35}SO_4$-labelled proteo-glycans rich in HS, CS or DS by cultured bovine intima cells.

	Arterial fibroblast secretions		Skin fibroblast secretions	
	HS-rich proteo-glycans	CS-rich proteo-glycans	HS-rich proteo-glycans	CS-rich proteo-glycans
Adsorption, % of added amount	1.9	2.1	1.7	1.8
Pinocytosis, % of added amount	2.3	4.2	2.0	16.8
Degradation, % of pinocytosed amount	75	75	69	73

50,000 cpm of the particular preparation was added per plate. After 24 h of incubation, the cultures were worked up as described [9].

adsorptive pinocytosis. Thus, an interaction of recognition site(s) of the molecule to be pinocytosed with a cell membrane receptor is required.

Individual proteoglycans seem to be recognized by different receptors on the cell surface. As shown in table I intimal cells internalize best a DS-rich protein from human skin fibroblast secretions. From arterial cell secretions a CS-rich protein is pinocytosed better than a HS-rich protein. No competition for uptake occurred when a [^{35}S]-labelled HS-rich protein was simultaneously added with unlabelled DS-rich protein to the culture medium (table II). This finding suggests that different receptors might be present on the cell membrane which interact with specific proteoglycan types.

As a couterpart for surface receptors, the molecule to be pinocytosed has to possess recognition sites for binding to the surface receptor. Recognition sites for the uptake of proteoglycans could principally be located on the protein moiety and/or on the carbohydrate moieties of the molecules. For a comparison of the uptake of proteoglycans and carbo-hydrate chains [^{35}S]glycosaminoglycans were prepared from skin fibro-blast secretions when the cells were grown in the presence of 1 mM p-nitrophenyl-β-D-xyloside or 22 mM D-xylose, respectively [11]. As in the case of proteoglycans the internalization by skin fibroblasts of protein-free glycosaminoglycan chains follows saturation kinetics. By converting the curves according to Lineweaver-Burk, the graphic analysis reveals that maximally 10,600 cpm of proteoglycans, 2,600 cpm of p-nitrophenyl-β-D-xyloside-induced glycosaminoglycans, and 3,300 cpm of xylose-

Table II. Pinocytosis of [35S] HS-rich protein by bovine intima cells in the presence of unlabelled DS-rich protein

Ratio [35S]HS:DS	Pinocytosis, % of added radioactivity
1:0	1.11
1:1	1.03
1:5	1.07
1:10	1.08

47,000 cpm of a HS-rich protein were added per plate. Unlabelled DS-rich protein was prepared from parallel cultures and eluted from the anion exchange resin at the same conductivity as labelled DS-rich protein. On the basis of the radioactivity of the labelled material the amount of unlabelled DS was calculated. After 24 h of incubation the experiment was terminated, and the cultures were worked up as described [9].

induced glycosaminoglycans can be internalized within 8 h per 0.3 mg cell protein. On a molar basis the maximal uptake rate for proteoglycans is one order of magnitude lower than for free glycosaminoglycan chains, but proteoglycans have a higher affinity than chains for the proposed receptors.

Competition experiments were performed by adding [35S]proteoglycans together with the induced carbohydrate chains or with unlabelled proteoglycan chains which were prepared by a β-elimination reaction. Doses of [35S]proteoglycan approaching saturation conditions were employed. The competitors should have contained roughly the same amount of disaccharide units as the labelled material. Free carbohydrate chains do not compete for the uptake of native proteoglycans at the doses used. By the addition of unlabelled proteoglycans, however, the amount of pinocytosed radioactivity was reduced.

Unexpected results were obtained when the uptake of labelled HA was investigated. Hyaluronic acid was obtained by ion exchange chromatography from the media of skin fibroblasts cultured in the presence of [1-14C]glucosamine. The purity of the preparation was established by cellulose acetate electrophoresis and digestion with hyaluronidase and pronase, respectively [5]. Neither bovine intima cells nor human skin fibroblasts were able to incorporate significant amounts of added [14C]HA. Cultured rat liver parenchymal cells, however, pinocytosed efficiently the material by a process, which followed again saturation kinetics.

Competition experiments revealed that the internalization of [^{14}C]HA can be reduced by the simultaneous addition of unlabelled even numbered HA oligosaccharides. [^{14}C]-labelled HA oligosaccharides, however, cannot be taken up by adsorptive pinocytosis, but are able to bind weakly to the cell membrane of cultured hepatocytes. The conclusion can be drawn that for adsorptive pinocytosis of hyaluronate an interaction of the molecule with at least two membrane receptors is required. The distance between the receptors should be longer than the length of a hyaluronate decasaccharide. Whether the inability of skin fibroblasts and intima cells to internalize HA is a peculiarity of the tissue culture system cannot be decided at the present time.

In summary, our results indicate that the analysis of radioactive glycosaminoglycans extracted from whole tissue might lead to over-simplified or erroneous interpretations when the localization within topographically distinct pools is not considered. Furthermore, for the uptake of proteoglycans and glycosaminoglycan chains, different cell membrane receptors with different specificities should be postulated. The pathophysiological significance of possible alterations of the rates of pinocytosis in disorders of connective tissue remains to be investigated.

Acknowledgement

This work was supported in part by a grant from the 'Fonds zur Förderung der wissenschaftlichen Forschung in Österreich'. We are indebted to Dr. L.E. GERSCHENSON (University of California, Los Angeles) for kindly providing us with cultured rat hepatocytes.

References

1   ANTONOPOULOS, C.A.; GARDELL, S., and HAMNSTRÖM, B.: J. Atheroscler. Res. 5: 9–15 (1965).
2   KLYNSTRA, F.B.; BÖTTCHER, C.J.F.; MELSEN, J.A. VAN, and LAAN, J. VAN DER. J. Atheroscler. Res. 7: 301–309 (1967).
3   HAUSS, W.H.; JUNGE-HÜLSING, G. und GERLACH, U.: Die unspezifische Mesenchymreaktion (Thieme, Stuttgart 1968).
4   SANWALD, R.; RITZ, E., and WIESE, G.: Atherosclerosis 13: 247–254 (1971).
5   KRESSE, H. and BUDDECKE, E.: Hoppe-Seyler's Z. physiol. Chem. 351: 151–156 (1970).

6 PICARD, J. and LEVY, P.: C.r. hebd. Séanc. Acad. Sci., Paris, Ser. D *277:* 373–376 (1973).
7 FIGURA, K. VON; KIOWSKI, W., and BUDDECKE, E.: Eur. J. Biochem. *40:* 89–94 (1973).
8 KRESSE, H.; FIGURA, K. VON; BUDDECKE, E., and FROMME, H.G.: Hoppe-Seyler's Z. physiol. Chem. *356:* 929–941 (1975).
9 KRESSE, H.; TEKOLF, W.; FIGURA, K. VON, and BUDDECKE, E.: Hoppe-Seyler's Z. physiol. Chem. *356:* 943–952 (1975).
10 NEUFELD, E.F. and CANTZ, M.: The mucopolysaccharidoses studied in cell culture; in HERS and VAN HOOF Lysosomes and storage disease, pp. 261–275 (Academic Press, New York 1973).
11 GALLIGANI, L.; HOPWOOD, J.; SCHWARTZ, N.B., and DORFMAN, A.: J. biol. Chem. *250:* 5400–5406 (1975).
12 KRESSE, H.; HEIDEL, H., and BUDDECKE, E.: Eur. J. Biochem. *22:* 557–562 (1971).

HANS KRESSE, Institute of Medical Chemistry, University of Graz, *Graz* (Austria)

Prog. biochem. Pharmacol., vol. 14, pp. 26–30 (Karger, Basel 1977)

Quo vadis, Cholesterol?

O.J. POLLAK

Dover Medical Research Center, Dover, Del.

Where are you headed, cholesterol? And how do you get there?

The origin of lipoid-laden cells, usually referred to as 'boam cells', has been debated ever since these cells were first seen in tissue sections of human and of experimental atherosclerotic lesions. At one time it had been suggested that they are Kupffer cells. Now, their arterial origin has been established. Intimal endothelial cells, smooth muscle cells, fibrocytes, macrophages, tissue mast cells and, in the rabbit, eosinophiles have been implicated. All these cells can undergo transformation into 'foam cells', though not at an equal rate or to equal degrees.

These cells do not have uniform origin, size, shape, and chemical makeup. Equal attention should be paid to all components of the 'lipoid spectrum'. But, let me single out cholesterol and some compounds interacting with cholesterol.

The question concerning the mode by which lipoid matter appears in the arterial cells and accumulates therein has not been answered to universal satisfaction. Several cell types could participate in more than one mechanism, either simultaneously or in sequence [5].

Whereas all cell types seem capable of lipoid biosynthesis – though not to equal degrees – it seems unlikely that synthesis accounts for much of the intracellular cholesterol, especially in the early phase of atherogenesis. Muscle cells probably contribute more phospholipid than cholesterol to the evolving plaque. This is interpreted as a defensive mechanism which leads to the bonding of cholesterol by these phospholipids.

Fatty degeneration occurs rapidly in aging cells in culture, especially in fibrocytes. *In vivo,* this process is slow and accumulation of lipoids, mainly triglycerides, is not as marked as *in vitro*. Fatty degeneration may play a role when it is caused by cytotoxins, such as nicotine.

Endocytosis may be the prevalent mode of lipoid uptake by smooth muscle cells. They have more pinocytotic vesicles than other cell types. Not that the number of pinosomes is constant for any one cell type or population. Their numbers are not the same at all surfaces. In endothelial cells pinocytic vesicles are less prominent at the luminal than at the basal surface. There is a transition between pinosomes and phagosomes.

Phagocytosis has been observed *in vitro* and *in vivo*. In cultures, it decreases with cellular aging. The phagocytic index is highest for macrophages, lower for endothelial cells, lowest for fibrocytes and myocytes. The process could play some role for endothelial cells, hardly for others.

The concept of phanerosis, mediated by lipfanogens and regulated by antilipfanogens, is based on study of fibroblasts in cultures. It has lost significance with the disclosure that arterial cells are capable of lipoid biosynthesis.

The value of tissue cultures for research in atherosclerosis cannot be disputed. However, we must not assume that all the phenomena observed *in vitro* have validity for *in vivo* events. 'In vivo veritas'.

Influx of blood plasma into the arterial wall is a prerequisite for the nutrition of the inner layer, the intima. Lipoid-laden cells which have the morphologic characteristics of endothelial cells are seen above or between intact endothelial cells within minutes after intravascular injection of colloidal cholesterol in the arteries of rabbits. In man, similar cells are seen at or just beneath the row of intact endothelial cells in only microscopically visible fatty streaks. Even the most ardent advocates of the concept that smooth muscle cells are the principal precursors of 'foam cells' admit that myocytes have to migrate to the area of initial intimal alteration. The endothelial cells are in the front line, exposed to the blood stream and to plasma insudate.

The insudate can enter the arterial wall either through intercellular gaps or by passage through the endothelial cells. Normally, the gap-route seems to predominate. With injury, the situation is reversed. The earliest damage is characterized by edema, and cellular edema precedes interstitial edema. The degree of insudation increases with injury to the cells and also widening of old or opening of new gaps. Injury is a sine qua non for atherogenesis. The term 'injury' is broad and ill-defined. Injury can cause focal loss of endothelial cells: Such defect will be repaired through interaction of thrombocytes and myocytes (in analogy of the organization of a thrombus), and this may or may not be followed by endothelial cell proliferation. More often, injury, especially chemical injury, does not cause loss of endothelial cells but leads to morphologic and functional alteration of these cells.

Arterial edema, seen as histamine reaction to shock, is patchy and reminiscent of urticaria. Its topographic distribution corresponds to the location of early atherosclerotic plaques. The events support the concept of episodic atherogenesis.

Edema of either the outer layer or of both layers of a bilayer membrane facilitates the bonding of cholesterol, of its H from the OH-group, with carbonyl oxygen of phosphoglyceride esters and amide groups of sphingolipids. The concomitant loss of calcium ions – from the acknowledged membrane stabilizer calcium chloride – in the outer polar zone where the electrostatic bonding takes place lowers the resistance of the cell membrane. The external membrane layer can also be viewed as an unstirred water layer which acts as a diffusion barrier. It is considerably stirred in edema. Water molecules more downward, through the cell membrane, into the cytosol, causing cellular edema, and readying for interaction with cholesterol and phospholipids [2, 3].

If we take a contemporary look at the cell membrane phospholipids we find a pool of phosphatidic acid, phosphatidyl-choline, -serine, -taurine, -ethanolamine, -N-methyl-ethanolamine, -N-dimethyl-ethanolamine, myo-inositol-4-monophosphate, -4,5-diphosphate, -diamannoside, and many others. If we single out the phospholipids and phosphoglycerides it is because of their leading role in bonding cholesterol. This role is supported by sphingolipids, sphingosine, amino acids, water, and electrolytes. Proteins and cholesterol compete for the phospholipid $C=O$ groups. The participation of carbohydrates is hardly known, that of lipoproteins is disputed. The partition between phospholipids, phosphoglycerides, sphingolipids, sphingosine, triglycerides, glucolipids, glucoproteins and, of course, cholesterol determines the quality of the asymmetric bilayer membrane. Models of such membranes are constantly being revised as new knowledge makes them more and more complex [1, 4].

Considering the transmembrane kinetics of lipoproteins one asks whether they actively penetrate the cell membrane or whether their movement is one of passive diffusion. Both processes are influenced by similar factors. Membrane permeability depends heavily on the cholesterol content and it is regulated by the density of hydrogen bonding in the hydrogen belts.

In cells with lipoid bilayer membranes there is an interaction between phosphate and carboxyl groups of cholesterol and amide of phosphatidyl serine with positive charges from Ca, Mg and the amino groups of amino acids. The permeability depends not only on qualitative and quantitative distribution of organic compounds and of electrolytes. Total thickness and that of the two layers, pressure gradients and topical temperature changes play a role. The constellation of the plasma challengers – and VLDL and LDL are not the only ones seeking entry into the cells – such as size and stereochemical structure, the physical state of lipoproteins and sterols, the length of side chains, the number and position of double bonds of fatty acids, the type of apoproteins present important factors.

The transmembrane passage is influenced by the membrane dynamics, by bending and stretching vibrations, lateral movements and flexing of side chains caused by ionic exchange within the cell membrane. The constant activity of membrane lipoids also plays a role in the 'gel to liquid crystal' transition, with cholesterol acting as an intermediary fluid state for other lipoids.

What is the fate of the lipoproteins? In the case of entry through gaps the LP molecule may be broken down in the ground substance and cholesterol could enter the cells in free or esterified form. In the case of transmembrane passage from the luminal surface, the LP molecule could be broken up within the membrane or after transit – in the cytosol. It has been proven that some labeled LDL cholesterol becomes entrapped in the membrane, replacing some of the membrane cholesterol. However, most of the lipoprotein is degraded by enzymes released by the Golgi apparatus. Over half of the liberated cholesterol appears in microsomes and in mito-chondria. Here, cholesterol encounters the locally synthesized phospho-lipids. Water molecules from the cytosol participate in the new bonding process. The phenomenon can be interpreted as chemotaxis involving the insudated cholesterol and the phosphatides of the target organelles.

References

1   BROCKENHOFF, H.: Model of interaction of polar lipids, cholesterol, and proteins in biologic membranes. Lipids *9:* 645–650 (1974).

2   CHAPMAN, D.: Biologic membranes, vol. I (Academic Press, London 1968).

3   CHAPMAN, D. and WALLACH, F.F.H.: Biological membranes, vol. II (Academic Press, London 1973).

4   POLLAK, O.J.: Recent advances in the metabolism of arteries. Prog. biochem. Pharmacol., vol. 4, pp. 265–269 (Karger, Basel 1968).

5   Pollak, O.J.: The arterial foam cell – *in vitro* and *in vivo* studies' in Peeters
     Protides in the biologic fluids, vol. 19, pp. 209–215 (Pergamon Press, Oxford
     1972).

Dr. O.J. Pollak, Dover Medical Research Center Inc., 9 Kings Highway E.,
P.O.B. 724, *Dover, DE 19901* (USA)

Morphology, Metabolism and Function of the Arterial Smooth Muscle Cell

Prog. biochem. Pharmacol., vol. 14, pp. 31–34 (Karger, Basel 1977)

Smooth Muscle Cell Changes of Media Underlying Experimental Arterial Thrombosis

Robert H. More, Avrum Gotleib and Bernard Weigensberg

Department of Pathology, McGill University, Montreal, Canada

In the past two decades studies of atherosclerosis have shifted emphasis on a number of occasions. This has included a shift from lipids to connective tissue, from lipids in the plasma to lipids in the arterial wall, and the smooth muscle cell [1, 2] has become the center of interest in much of this. The role of the smooth muscle cell was emphasized first in relation to the fibrous cap of atherosclerosis [3]. Soon it became apparent that it was involved in the accumulation of lipid in the experimental atherosclerotic lesion [4] and in man [5]. For some time many considered that there was something unique about the smooth muscle cell of the arterial wall in relation to lipid metabolism but recently it has been shown that lipid may accumulate in the smooth muscle cells of the uterine wall in human toxemia of pregnancy [6]. It was therefore of interest to note the accumulation of lipid in the smooth muscle cells of the aortic media beneath the experimental organizing thrombus of a normocholesterolemic rabbit. The following reports some details of these observations and their relation to the events occurring in the overlying thrombus.

The observations were made on catheter-induced thrombi of the aorta of normocholesterolemic rabbits [7] studied by light and EM microscopy and by autoradiography of tritium-labelled cells at serial time intervals from day 1 to 26 weeks.

Tritium-labelled cells were found throughout the thrombus and in the media beneath the thrombus. The percentage of labelled cells was determined in these areas. Polymorphonuclear leukocytes and macrophages were not counted. Labelled cells were present in the thrombus within 24 h and reached a peak at 3–4 days which was maintained at a high level for 28 days and then slowly declined. In the media labelled cells did not appear until the third day reaching a peak between day 4 and 5. A high level of labelled cells was maintained for only 14 days and then gradually declined. By electron microscopy an attempt was made to identify the proliferating cells in the organizing thrombus and underlying media.

In the thrombus by day 2 small numbers of unusual appearing cells were present which could not be identified with respect to cell type. These cells had scanty cytoplasm containing sparsely scattered ribosomes and a few mitochondria which constituted the only cell organelles. The nucleus had no clumping of chromatin and consisted of a diffuse finely granular structure. This type of cell was not seen in the media. After day 3 a variety of cells were present in the thrombus. In succeeding days there were increased amounts of cytoplasm and an increasing complexity of cell organelles with much dilated rough surfaced endoplasmic reticulum and prominent Golgi. By day 5 some features of smooth muscle cells were present and by day 9 these were well developed. Also by this time many cells were in the active process of producing abundant extracellular microfibrils and recognizable elastic tissue. In the media adjacent to the overlying thrombus a small number of cells had a considerable amount of dilated endoplasmic reticulum but the cells were always recognizable as smooth muscle cells. None of the peculiar cells previously described in the organizing thrombus were seen in the media. In the thrombus some macrophages were present but these were not seen in the media. After the 10th day an increasing number of cells contained lipid droplets. Many of these were smooth muscle cells and some progressed to foam cells to constitute the myogenic foam cell. In addition there were some macrophages with lipid droplets in the cytoplasm. At the foam cell stage it was not always possible to determine whether the foam cell was derived from a smooth muscle cell or a macrophage.

In the media beneath the thrombus some lipid droplets appeared in smooth muscle cells but this occurred later than the appearance of intracellular lipid droplets in the organizing thrombus. There was a gradual development of lipid droplets in many of the smooth muscle cells of this part of the media. These droplets varied in number from a few to a foam cell stage. As long as these lipid-laden cells could be defined with respect to their cell type they were all smooth muscle cells. Although in the thrombus some cells containing lipid could be distinguished as macrophages there were no cells in the media that could be identified as macrophages with intracellular lipid. Some very advanced foam cells could not be identified as either smooth muscle cells or macrophages and at this stage some lipid droplets were being shed into the intercellular connective tissue of the media. Many of the smooth muscle cells did not contain visible lipid.

Discussion

The presence of proliferating cells in the thrombus before they occurred in the media indicates that some of the proliferating cells of the organizing thrombus were derived from pre-existing cells of the intima. The nature of the pre-existing cells could not be established with certainty. However, the presence of an unusual cell of very primitive character suggests the possibility of some undifferentiated stem cells either present in the intima or being deposited in the thrombus from the blood. This strange cell may represent some phase of activity of a smooth muscle cell but failure to see similar cells in the media where smooth muscle cells were in the process of active metabolism is against this possibility.

The presence of intracellular lipid in the media is of interest from a number of points of view. It was found in medial cells only in the area beneath the organizing thrombus. Also of interest is the fact that the rabbits were normocholesterolemic. An understanding of the pathogenesis of this lipid accumulation would be of importance in our understanding of the factors that determine the lipid accumulation in smooth muscle cells in the atherosclerotic lesion. One possible explanation of the lipids in the media may be that there is increased transport of lipid through the media from those trapped in the thrombus. Alternatively the thrombus overlying the media may injure the smooth muscle cells of the media. There is much evidence that platelet thrombi release many factors which can alter endothelial permeability and may alter other cell membrane permeability. A large thrombus could also interfere with the diffusion of oxygen to the inner media. In either case injury of the medial cells may affect their ability to metabolize lipid.

Summary

There is much evidence that platelet thrombi release many factors which can alter endothelial permeability and may alter other cell membrane permeability. A large thrombus could also interfere with the diffusion of oxygen to the inner media. In either case injury of the medial cells may affect their ability to metabolize lipid.

References

1   GEER, J.C. and HAUST, M.D.: Smooth muscle cells in atherosclerosis (Karger, Basel 1972).
2   ROSS, R. and GLOMSET, J.A.: The pathogenesis of atherosclerosis. New Engl. J. Med. 295: 369–376 (1976).
3   HAUST, M.D. and MORE, R.H.: New functional aspects of smooth muscle cells. Abstract. Fed. Proc. Fed. Am. Socs exp. Biol. 17: 440 (1958).
4   HAUST, M.D.; BAYLES, J.U., and MORE, R.H.: Electron microscropic study of intimal lipid accumulation in human aorta and their pathogenesis. Abstract. Circulation 26: 656 (1962).
5   PARKER, F.: An electron microscopic study of experimental atherosclerosis. Am. J. Path. 36: 19 (1960).
6   HAUST, M.D.; HERAS, G.L., and HARDING, P.G.: Fat containing uterine smooth muscle cells in 'toxemia'. Possible relevance to atherosclerosis. Sciene 195: 1353 (1977).
7   SUMIYOSHI, A.; MORE, R.H., and WEIGENSBERG, B.I.: Aortic fibrofatty type atherosclerosis from thrombus in normolipidemic rabbits. Atherosclerosis 18: 43 (1973).

Dr. R.H. MORE, Department of Pathology, McGill University, *Montreal, Que.* (Canada)

Prog. biochem. Pharmacol., vol. 14, pp. 35–38 (Karger, Basel 1977)

Role of Smooth Muscle Cells in the Organization of Experimental Thrombi

Z. JURUKOVA

Institute of Cardiovascular Diseases, Medical Academy, Sofia

Thrombosis is essentially a reparative process, since thrombi cover endothelial defects following vascular injury and the cellular reaction of the vessel wall provides a lasting repair and restoration of functional and structural integrity. In the present electron microscopic study of experimental thrombi in rat carotid artery we were able to demonstrate that arterial medial smooth muscle cells (SMC) are entirely responsible for the organization of thrombi.

Material and Methods

Experimental thrombosis of the common carotid artery of Wistar rats was induced by clamping the artery for 15 min with a plastic-covered Kocher clamp. The injured arteries were removed from the living animals under Nembutal narcosis at intervals ranging from 5 to 30 days after injury. They were fixed in 2.5 % glutaraldehyde and 2 % OsO_4 and embedded in Epon 712. Ultrathin sections were stained with uranyl acetate and lead oxide and examined in an RCA EMU 3G electron microscope.

Results and Discussion

Electron microscopic examination of 5-day-old thrombi revealed platelet-fibrin accumulations, invaded by blood monocytes and polymorphonuclear leukocytes, adherent to the denuded internal elastic membrane. At this early stage signs of a beginning organization are already established – large, elongated cells grow into the thrombotic mass, displaying the characteristics of SMC. Two ultrastructural forms are distinguished among them. The first one includes fibroblast-like cells, fusiform in shape, with ovoid, smooth-surfaced nuclei. The cytoplasm is scanty, showing abundant granular endoplasmic reticulum with dilated cisternae and scattered mitochondria. Microfilaments are observed in the cytoplasm which correspond to myofilaments, but are very scarce, concentrated in the cell periphery. Very few micropinocytotic vesicles are present along the plasma membrane. A limiting basement membrane is absent in most cells or small portions of it are revealed on the cell surface. The second ultrastructural form of SMC penetrating the thrombotic mass varies considerably in shape and organelle content but still more resembles the typical medial SMC than does the first cell type. They are rich in myofilaments, sometimes dense areas are seen, identical to the attachment bodies in SMC. The plasma membrane contains a variable number of micropinocytotic vesicles and is partly or completely surrounded by a basement membrane. The nucleus is chromatin poor, with folded surface.

The examination of thrombi 10–12 days old showed an increased number of SMC invading the thrombotic mass. Their cytoplasm contains bundles of myofilaments and relatively abundant organelles. Collagen fibrils are encountered between the cells and residual cellular debris and altered platelets are still present. The surface of the thrombus is covered with endothelial cells.

The ultrastructural pattern of 20- and 30-day-old thrombi are closely similar to each other. The final result of the organization of mural thrombi is an intimal thickening, made of SMC arranged in layers, surrounded by abundant extracellular matrix.

The cellular elements organizing an experimental thrombus display considerable variations in their ultrastructure, but we consider the wide range of appearances representing a single cell type – SMC, of differing degrees of maturation or of diverse functional state. The SMC invading the organizing thrombi have the general characteristics of this cell type, differing from the typical medial SMC by their greater richness in cytoplasmic organelles and reduced number of myofilaments. This ultrastructure testifies that the cells are engaged in intense synthesis and secretion of connective tissue matrix components and this synthetizing function highly dominates over the contractile one. They produce the

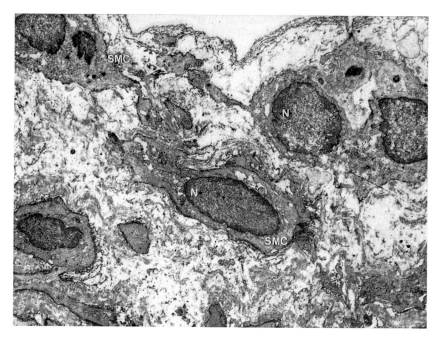

Fig. 1. Electron micrograph of an organized thrombus (20 days old), made of smooth muscle cells (SMC); between the cells there is abundant connective tissue matrix. N = Nucleus. × 6,200.

proteins and mucopolysaccharides of the abundant connective tissue matrix surrounding them. The fibroblast-like cells, seen in the early stages of thrombus organization, are morphologically considerably divergent from the SMC described above. Their distinction from fibroblasts is rather difficult. However, the absence of nonmuscular connective tissue cells in mammalian arteries [1[and the lack of evidence about a possible hematogenic origin of fibroblasts [2] make it likely that this cell type has also to do with SMC. They probably represent immature SMC.

The organization of arterial thrombi by proliferating SMC is a manifestation of the general tendency of the arterial wall to react uniformly to injuries of various nature, by growth of SMC, invading and replacing the lesion. The thrombus organizing tissue, as a repair tissue, is composed of the same cellular elements as those involved in reparative processes following various arterial aggressions. In the arterial wall diverse pathogenesis does not imply a different morphology. This reveals a limited tissue reaction in response to injury, ending in focal accumulations of SMC in the intima in disorders so diverse as nonspecific arterial injuries, hypertensive arteriopathy and atherosclerosis.

References

1   BUCK, R.C.: Histogenesis and morphology of arterial tissue; in SANDLED and BOURNE Atherosclerosis and its origin, pp 1–38 (Academic Press, New York 1963).
2   ROSS, R.; EVERETT, N.B., and TYLER, R.: Wound healing and collagen formation. VI. The origin of the wound fibroblast studied in parabiosis. J. Cell Biol. *44:* 645–654 (1970).

Dr. Z. JURUKOVA, Institute of Cardiovascular Diseases, Medical Academy, *Sofia* (Bulgaria)

Prog. biochem. Pharmacol., vol. 14, pp. 39–45 (Karger, Basel 1977)

Births of Smooth Muscle Cells in Atherogenesis[1]

W.A. Thomas, J.M. Reiner, K. Janakidevi and R.A. Florentin

Albany Medical College, Albany, N.Y.

Atherosclerosis in man is characterized in the early stages by excessive focal proliferation of smooth muscle cells (SMC) in the arterial intima and adjacent inner media. In the advanced stages necrosis in the masses of proliferated SMC becomes a prominent feature, with focal accumulation of lipid-rich necrotic debris. However, excessive SMC births are not limited to the early stage of atherogenesis; nor are excessive SMC deaths limited to the late stage. Excessive arterial SMC births and deaths appear to be prominent features of all stages of atherogenesis; and the state of balance (or imbalance) between them is a major determinant of the rate of progression or regression of a lesion.

This presentation will be limited to a discussion of arterial SMC births. We first present some studies in experimental animals and later some human autopsy studies.

McMillan and Duff [1948] demonstrated in 1948 that the SMC of atherosclerotic lesions induced in rabbits by hyperlipidemic (HL) diets showed far more cells in mitosis than were found in normal media. We demonstrated in swine in 1969 [Florentin et al., 1969] increases in the numbers of mitoses of both arterial SMC and endothelial cells (EC) within 3 days after beginning an HL diet, which is long before overt lesions appear. However, mitotic indices are exceedingly low in arteries, even in proliferating lesions, making counting a laborious procedure.

[³H]-thymidine labelling indices provide a more practical approach, since a pulse label identifies an entire DNA synthesis period's 'worth', and the time for synthesis is much longe than that for mitosis. We have

1 Supported by USPHS NHLBI.

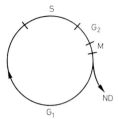

Fig. 1. Cell cycle. M = mitosis, ND = nondividers, G_1 = the gap between M and S, S = DNA synthesis, G_2 = the gap between S and M, G_0 is ignored.

shown [THOMAS *et al.,* 1968] the [³H]-thymidine indices to increase about 50 % in aortic SMC of swine within 3 days after beginning HL diets and to increase 3 to 10-fold further in overt lesions when they appear 30–60 days later. Other investigators have shown similarly high indices in athero-sclerotic lesions in experimental animals [McMILLAN and STARY, 1968; STARY and McMILLAN, 1970].

However, the [³H]-thymidine pulse labelling index only gives the proportion of cells in the DNA synthesis portion of the cell cycle (fig. 1) at one point in time. These cells may become arrested in G_2 (which is the gap between completion of synthesis and beginning of mitosis during which the proteins of the mitotic apparatus are synthesized); they may die in synthesis, G_2, or mitosis; or they may proceed through mitosis to 'give birth' to two daughter cells. The latter is the criterion that must be met if labelling indices are to be used to study cell births. We have dem-onstrated in aortic SMC of young swine *prior* to development of overt lesions that nearly all labelled cells proceed through mitosis; here the [³H]-thymidine labelling index can be used to measure births (THOMAS *et al.,* 1971]. However, we have some preliminary evidence from studies of aortas of somewhat older HL diet-fed swine suggesting that many cells are arrested in G_2.

Another approach to the study of cell birth is by the dilution-of-label technique. When cells that have been labelled with [³H]-thymidine pass through mitosis approximately half the label goes to each daughter cell. This will be reflected in autoradiographs by a halving of the number of developed grains in the overlaying emulsion. In practice animals given [³H]-thymidine at a common time are sacrificed in two groups. A 'base-line' group is sacrificed first and a 'test' group at a later time point. By

Table I. Cell births in initiation of early progression of atherosclerotic lesions in HL diet-fed swine.

Groups	Number of divisions						Total
	0	1	2	3	4	5	0–5
HL diet only (7), %	28	10	41	12	9	0	100
HL diet + int. trauma (4), %	8	27	7	26	24	8	100

Division pattern of ancestors of atherosclerotic lesion cells expressed as percent of cells labelled at 0 HL diet time that divided 0–5 times in 60 days.

determining grain number distributions over nuclei in each of the two groups and using appropriate mathematical procedures, the number of divisions (if any) made by various subsets among the labelled cells during the interval (from the time of sacrifice of the baseline group to that for the test group), can be calculated, along with other useful information.

Using the above method with swine, we have sacrificed a baseline group with the [³H]-thymidine label prior to giving an HL diet; the test group, which had been given [³H]-thymidine at the same time as the baseline group, was then started on an HL diet and sacrificed 60 days latter, by which time small overt lesions had developed (THOMAS *et al.,* 1976a]. The results of the grain number analyses are shown in the first part of table I. These data show that multiple SMC were involved in initiation and progression of these lesions; i.e., these lesions were *not* monoclonal in origin. They also show a marked heterogeneity of division patterns with some SMC not dividing at all while other subsets have gone through 1, 2, 3, or 4 divisions. If this heterogeneity persisted for many generations, with constant selection of cells with greatest division potential, we might eventually find that some regions of a lesion are oligoclonal or even monoclonal in origin (while the lesion as a whole was of multicellular origin).

In the second part of table I [THOMAS *et al.,* 1976b] are shown results in which the atherosclerotic process was accelerated by subjecting the swine to balloon-catheter-EC-denudation prior to giving the HL diets. These data show a larger proportion of lesion SMC going through multiple divisions than in the swine fed HL diet alone.

In the remainder of this presentation we shall discuss data from studies of postmortem human aortas from black women with glucose-6-phosphate dehydrogenase (G-6-PD) mosaicism. In a common form of G-6-PD mosaicism in black women the body consists of a mixture of two cel types wiith respect to G-6-PD. One cell type has the 'A' variant of G-6-PD and the other the 'B' variant. These two variants can be distinguished by electrophoresis of extracts from normal tissue, including aorta.

BENDITT and BENDITT [1973] reported that thick atherosclerotic lesions ('fibrous plaques') from the aortas of black females with G-6-PD mosaicism frequently showed monotypism. That is, some of the thick lesions showed either the A or the B variant but not both, while normal aorta had the mixture of A and B. One of several possible explanations for the monotypism is that each lesion originated from a single cell, i.e., each was monoclonal in origin. The observation of monotypism was confirmed by PEARSON et al. [1975], and in our laboratory at Albany [THOMAS et al., 1976c]. However, the interpretation remains in dispute.

From our experimental animal studies, described earlier, we had developed a strong bias in favor of a multicellular origin of atherosclerotic lesions accompanied by heterogeneity of division potential among the SMC involved in the birth of the lesion. We postulated that the heterogeneity of division potential might account for the eventual development of monotypism in advanced lesions.

If our hypothesis was correct, the presence of monotypism should be related to the stage of development (reflecting the number of SMC generations) and the thickness of the atherosclerotic lesions might be used as an index of the stage. In table II are shown results from two subjects from which numerous lesions of different thicknesses were sampled. It is apparent that there is a close relationship with thickness, thus supporting our hypothesis. However, other interpretations are possible. One is that there may have been postmortem seepage of enzyme from the underlying normal media, which might be more prominent in thin than in thick lesions. This possibility is difficult either to prove or to disprove; it might be tested by obtaining a fresh aorta after a very short postmortem interval and taking sequential samples over a period of time to determine rate of seepage; but we have not as yet had the opportunity to do this.

Another possibility suggested by PEARSON et al. [1975], whose results are similar to ours, is that thick fibrous plaques do not arise from the

Table II. Distribution of atherosclerotic lesions in G-6-PD heterozygotes by thickness and frequency of 1 and 2 G-6-PD variants

Lesion thickness, μm	Black female 1[1]		Black female 2[1]	
	1 var.	2 var.	1 var.	2 var.
<200	0	15	1	4
200–299	0	12	0	8
300–399	1	5	3	2
400–499	7	5	3	1
>499	12	2	8	1
Total	20	39	15	61

[1] For normal aorta female 1 has 41 % A, 59 % B; female 2 has 53 % A, 47 % B.

Table III. Frequency of A vs. B type monotypism among atherosclerotic lesions of 5 women G-6-PD heterozygotes[1]

	Type	Case				
		1	2	3	4	5
Monotypic lesions	A	2	27	0	15	14
	B	18	1	8	0	2

[1] Ratios of A to B in the normal parts of the aorta determined by densitometry were respectively 41:59, 53:47, 41:59, 65:35 and 50:50.

thin fatty streaks. We do not think that this is likely but we made a point of including not only fatty streaks but also nonfatty streak foci of thickening of similar degree to that of fatty streaks. These too failed to show monotypism.

In the course of our studies of atherosclerotic lesions in G-6-PD mosaics we made another observation which is summarized in table III [THOMAS *et al.,* 1976c]. In this table are shown the distribution of A and B type monotypic lesions from the five individuals we have studied thus far who were found to have at least eight monotypic lesions. Looking at the overall data, one sees tthat both A and B type lesions are found, suggesting that the monotypism is not related to the A or B G-6-PD type.

However, when one looks at the ratio of number of A to B type lesions in a single individual, it is apparent that in this series the monotypic lesions tend to be predominantly of one type in a given individual. According to the hypothesis of LYON [1962], cellular mosaicism in females is a result of inactivation of one of the X chromosomes early in embryonic life. The inactivation occurs in a random fashion and is permanent. Thus if an individual is heterozygous for one of more genes on the X chromosome, some cells will have one genotype and some the other. A G-6-PD mosaic is obviously heterozygous for the G-6-PD gene but may also be heterozygous for other genes on the X chromosome, for which we did not assay in these studies. One or more of these genes for which the individual is heterozygous could be providing a selective advantage for survival and multiplication in the abnormal environment of the atherosclerotic lesion.

The data in table III suggest that the above mechanism is a factor in the development of monotypism in atherosclerotic lesions. However, it cannot be the only factor or else all monotypic lesions in a given individual would be of the same genotype as indicated by the G-6-PD marker enzyme. Instead there are some exceptions. This would suggest that more than one factor is involved in the development of montypism. We postulate that one other factor may be the heterogeneity of division potential suggested by our studies of SMC population dynamics in atherogenesis in swine.

In summary, we have shown that atherosclerotic lesions produced by HL diet in experiments with swine were multicellular in origin. The SMC involved in initiation of the lesions in the swine showed wide variability in cell cycle times, with the progeny of some going through as many as five generations in a 60-day period while others pass through only one.

We have carried out studies of atherosclerotic lesions in human G-6-PD mosaics which suggest that monotypism may appear during the course of development of an atherosclerotic lesion and thus does not necessarily indicate monoclonal origin of the lesion. The heterogeneous SMC division patterns observed in HL diet induced lesions in swine suggest one possible mechanism for eventual development of oligoclonal or even monoclonal foci. The tendency for monotonic lesions in a given individual to be mostly of one genotype suggests another. Monoclonal origin is still another possibility that has not as yet been eliminated. One can also envisage some combinations among the above possibilities and perhaps others as yet unknown. Atherosclerosis is a disease with a variety of temporal and spatial manifestations; and it should come as no surprise to find that lesions can develop in more than one fashion.

References

BENDITT, E.P. and BENDITT, J.M.: Evidence for a monoclonal origin of human atherosclerotic plaques. Proc. natn. Acad. Sci. USA 70: 1753–1756 (1973).

FLORENTIN, R.A.; NAM, S.C.; LEE, K.T.; LEE, K.J., and THOMAS, W.A.: Increased mitotic activity in aortas of swine after three days of cholesterol feeding. Archs. Path. 88: 463–469 (1969).

LYON, M.F.: Sex chromatin and gene action in the mammalian X-chromosome. Am. J. Hum. Genet. 14: 135–148 (1962).

McMILLAN, G.C. and DUFF, G.L.: Mitotic activity in the aortic lesions of experimental atherosclerosis in rabbits. Archs. Path. 46: 179 (1948).

McMILLAN, G.C. and STARY, H.C.: Preliminary experience with mitotic activity of cellular elements in the atherosclerotic plaques of cholesterol for rabbits studied by labelling with tritiated thymidine. Ann. N.Y. Acad. Sci. 149: 699 (1968).

PEARSON, T.A.; WANG, A.; SOLEZ, K., and HEPTINSTALL, R.H.: Clonal characteristics of fibrous plaques and fatty streaks from human aortas. Am. J. Path. 81: 379–387 (1975).

STARY, H.C. and McMILLAN, G.C.: Kinetics of cellular proliferation in the atherosclerotic lesion of cholesterol-fed rabbits. Archs Path. 89: 173 (1970).

THOMAS, W.A.; FLORENTIN, R.A.; NAM, S.C.; REINER, J.M., and LEE, K.T.: Alterations in population dynamics of arterial smooth muscle cells during atherogenesis. I. Activation of interphase cells in cholesterol-fed swine prior to gross atherosclerosis demonstrated by 'postpulse salvage labelling'. Expl molec. Path. 15: 245–267 (1971).

THOMAS, W.A.; FLORENTIN, R.A.; REINER, J.M.; LEE, W.M., and LEE, K.T.: Alterations in populations of arterial smooth muscle cells during atherogenesis. IV. Evidence for a polyclonal origin of hypercholesterolemic diet-inducing atherosclerotic lesions in young swine. Expl molec. Path. 24: 244–260 (1976a).

THOMAS, W.A.; REINER, J.M.; FLORENTIN, R.A.; LEE, K.T., and LEE, W.M.: Population dynamics of arterial smooth muscle cells. V. Cell proliferation and cell death during initial 3 months in atherosclerotic lesions induced in swine by hypercholesterolemic diet and intimal trauma. Expl molec. Path. 24: 360–374 (1976b).

THOMAS, W.A.; REINER, J.M.; FLORENTIN, R.A.; JANAKIDEVI, K., and LEE, K.J.: Arterial smooth muscle cells in atherogenesis. Births, deaths, and clonal phenomena. Proc. IVth Int. Symp. on Atherosclerosis, Tokyo (in press, 1976c).

Dr. W.A. THOMAS, Albany Medical College, *Albany, N.Y.* (USA)

Prog. biochem. Pharmacol., vol. 14, pp. 46–51 (Karger, Basel 1977)

Ultrastructural Changes in the Lipid Inclusions of Arterial Smooth Muscle Cells after Reduction of High Serum Cholesterol Levels[1]

H.C. STARY

Department of Pathology, Louisiana State University School of Medicine, New Orleans, La.

Introduction

The intimal atherosclerotic lesions of hypercholesterolemic human subjects and of experimental animals are characterized by cells containing intracytoplasmic lipid droplets. At least two morphological types of smooth muscle cells occur in lesions and accumulate lipid droplets [2, 4, 8]. In addition, intimal macrophages [1, 2, 4] and endothelial cells covering lesions also contain lipid inclusions. The extent to which accumulation occurs and the morphological structure of lipid droplets varies according to the cell type. The present report deals with the ultrastructure of accumulated lipid droplets of arterial smooth muscle cells, and in particular with the fate of the droplets after the elevated level of serum cholesterol has been reduced to normal.

Methods

The design of the experiments on which these observations were based has been described elsewhere in detail [6, 7]. Briefly, 53 mature, male rhesus monkeys, divided into 12 groups, were given a high-cholesterol diet (commercial diet supplemented with butter, beef tallow, casein, cholesterol, vitamins, and water) for 12 weeks. At the end of that

1 Supported by USPHS NIH, grant HL 08974

period, one group was killed to determine the extent and nature of the atherosclerotic lesions induced with the diet. The high-cholesterol diet was then changed to low-cholesterol food (unsupplemented commercial diet), and the remaining groups were killed after 2, 3, 4, 8, 12, 16, 24, 32, 40, 64, and 128 weeks. In addition, the experiments included 11 control monkeys divided into 4 groups that received only low-cholesterol food for varying periods. Tissue for electron microscopy was taken from the proximal left coronary artery, as described previously [5, 6], and from three standard sites in the thoracic and one standard site in the abdominal segment of the aorta. The tissues were fixed in buffered osmium tetroxide, and embedded in the epoxy resin Maraglas. Fine sections were stained with lead citrate and uranyl acetate.

Results

Control animals that had received only low-cholesterol food had mean serum cholesterol levels in the range of 110–165 mg/dl. Extensive segments of the coronary artery and aortic intima of every one of these monkeys contained smooth muscle cells. Intimal smooth muscle cells were of two main types. Myofilament-rich smooth muscle cells containing mainly myofilaments were the more frequent type whereas the less frequent type, rough endoplasmic reticulum (RER)-rich smooth muscle cells contained a variable but always smaller number of myofilaments. RER-rich smooth muscle cells were more frequent in intimal cushions near arterial bifurcations than in the more prevalent diffuse intimal thickening. Intimal smooth muscle cells of normocholesterolemic control monkeys infrequently contained lipid inclusions. When present, inclusions were small, homogeneous droplets that did not occupy a significant portion of the cell cytoplasm.

Animals given the high-cholesterol diet had mean serum cholesterol levels in the range of 230–640 mg/dl during the 12-week period on the diet. Lesions of the advanced fatty streak type occurred in predisposed segments of the coronary arteries and in the aorta. The two smooth muscle cell types found in the intima of control animals also occurred in lesions, although the number of RER-rich smooth muscle cells was increased. In lesions, both types of smooth muscle cells contained lipid droplets, and the cytoplasm of many was packed with droplets (fig. 1). Droplets were homogeneous although the periphery was granular and more osmiophilic than the less electron-dense inner aspects. Visible droplets were presumably created through aggregation of small lipid particles and enlarged in size by further accretion. The process of uptake across the plasma membrane, and the process of fusion to form visible droplets, could not be visualized with the electron microscope. The number of micropinocytic vesicles in smooth muscle cells was similar in hypercholesterolemic and in normocholesterolemic animals suggesting that uptake occurs by some mechanism other than micropinocytosis. The Golgi complex and the endoplasmic reticulum, particularly smooth-surfaced endoplasmic reticulum (SER), responded to lipid droplets by hyperplasia. Nevertheless, during the hypercholesterolemic phase, most lipid droplets remained morphologically unaltered; only a few showed evidence of conversion of the granular periphery to double-contoured membranes.

After change from high- to low-cholesterol food, elevated serum cholesterol declined to normal levels during a 4- to 8-week period in most animals. After serum cholesterol had returned to normal, there was no apparent further progression in the number and size of smooth muscle cell lipid droplets. Nor was there evidence of rapid regression of droplets in the weeks immediately after return to normal serum cholesterol levels, although increased activity and progressive morphological alterations developed at the granular droplet periphery. A decrease in the size of lipid droplets became apparent about 24 weeks after change to low-cholesterol food. Before a reduction became apparent, there was increasing prominence of the Golgi complex and of SER in both types of smooth muscle cells containing droplets. Small vesicles and tubules budded from the hyperplastic Golgi complex and from portions of the SER and accumulated at, and seemed to fuse with, the granular droplet periphery. As droplets decreased in size, membranes formed around the droplet periphery, apparently by alignment and fusion of smooth vesicles. Vesicles formed by the Golgi complex and by certain portions of the SER carry hydrolytic enzymes [3] and represent primary lysosomes. Fusion of vesicles with lipid inclusions represents the formation of secondary lysosomes. With time, peripheral membranes became multilayered, forming finely laminated stacks that usually were asymmetrically layered to one side of a droplet. Although droplets continued to acquire additional layers of peripheral membranes, the overall size of the inclusions decreased. After 64 weeks, inclusions were much smaller than the earlier lipid droplets and a smaller number of intimal smooth muscle cells

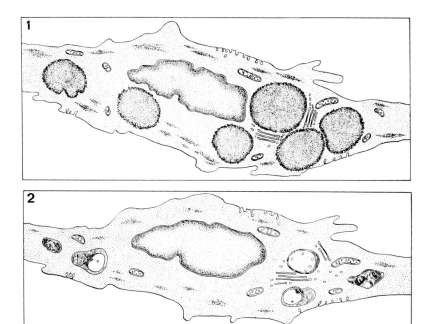

Fig. 1. Drawing of an intimal smooth muscle cell with cytoplasmic lipid droplets during the phase of lipid accumulation.

Fig. 2. Drawing of an intimal smooth muscle cell showing the residuals of cytoplasmic lipid droplets about 1 year after return of elevated serum cholesterol levels to normal.

contained inclusions, indicating that some smooth muscle cells might have metabolized inclusions completely. Residual inclusions were pleomorphic bulbous structures usually surrounded by a limiting membrane, containing a matrix made up partly of dense granules, finely laminated arrays of membranes, and occasional translucent vacuoles (fig. 2). Some cells also contained multivesicular bodies. Hyperplasia of the Golgi complex and of the SER had decreased. Residual inclusions were residual bodies or telolysosomes with probably very low enzyme activity. After 128 weeks, there was no further change in the morphology of residual bodies, and no appreciable decrease in their number. Animals with the highest serum cholesterol elevation during lesion progression had the largest number of intimal smooth muscle cells with residual inclusions.

Comment

The study of regressing lesions showed that intimal smooth muscle cells overloaded with lipid droplets can, when the serum cholesterol is reduced to a sufficiently low level over a sufficiently long period, reduce the size of droplets and that at least some can completely clear inclusions. After having temporarily assumed predominantly phagocytic, lipid storage, and digestive functions, smooth muscle cells can revert to their original morphology and presumably to their original functions of being contractile cells or producers of intercellular substances.

In normocholesterolemic animals, intracytoplasmic lipid droplets occurred infrequently in intimal smooth muscle cells, indicating that cellular digestive enzymes were adequate for the degradation of small amounts of lipid normally taken up into cells. Oversaturation of the cellular enviroment in hypercholesterolemic animals resulted in uncontrolled influx into cells, enzyme insufficiency, and accumulation of droplets. Smooth muscle cells became storage sites of undigested lipid. The present experiments showed that enzyme deficiency was only temporary and relative, since droplet degradation resumed as soon as normocholesterolemia returned and influx of lipid into cells ceased.

All residuals persisting after 1 year of regression were morphologically different from the original droplets. Residuals had great stability, because further degradation was increasingly sluggish. Although the larger portion of the original droplets had been solubilized, and either utilized by the cell or transferred out across the plasma membrane, alternate pathways for the eventual removal of undigestible residuals may exist.

We have also studied the morphology of lipid inclusions in intimal macrophages both in hypercholesterolemia and after serum cholesterol reduction. There are striking differences between macrophages and smooth muscle cells in the rate of droplet degradation and also in the ability to dispose of the altered inclusions. These differences between cell types will be the subject of a future report.

Summary

Intimal smooth muscle cells overloaded with lipid droplets can, when the serum cholesterol is reduced to a sufficiently low level over a sufficiently long period, reduce the size of droplets and at least some can completely clear inclusions.

References

1   ANITSCHKOW, N.: Über die Veränderungen der Kaninchenaorta bei experimenteller Cholesterinsteatose. Beitr. path. Anat. *56:* 379–404 (1913).
2   GEER, J.C. and HAUST, M.D.: Smooth muscle cells in atherosclerosis. Monogr. Atheroscler., vol. 2 (Karger, Basel 1972).
3   NOVIKOFF, A.B.: Lysosomes. A personal account; in HERS and VAN HOOF Lysosomes and storage diseases, pp. 1–41 (Academic Press, New York 1973).
4   STARY, H.C.: Coronary artery fine structure in rhesus monkeys. The early atherosclerotic lesion and its progression. Prim. Med., vol. 9, pp. 359–395 (Karger, Basel 1976).
5   STARY, H.C. and STRONG, J.P.: Coronary artery fine structure in rhesus monkeys. Nonatherosclerotic intimal thickening. Prim. Med., vol. 9, pp. 321–358 (Karger, Basel 1976).
6   STARY, H.C. and STRONG, J.P.: The fine structure of nonatherosclerotic intimal thickening, of developing, and of regressing atherosclerotic lesions at the bifurcation of the left coronary artery. Adv. expl Med. Biol., vol. 67, pp. 89–108 (Plenum Press, New York 1976).
7   STARY, H.C.; EGGEN, D.A., and STRONG, J.P.: The mechanism of atherosclerosis regression; in: Atherosclerosis IV. Proc. 4th Int. Symp. on Atherosclerosis, Tokyo 1976 (Springer, Berlin, in press).
8   THOMAS, W.A.; JONES, R.; SCOTT, R.F.; MORRISON, E.; GOODALE, F., and IMAI, H.: Production of early atherosclerotic lesions in rats characterized by proliferation of 'modified smooth muscle cells'. Expl molec. Path. *2:* suppl. 1, pp. 40–61 (1963).

HERBERT CHRISTIAN STARY, MD, Professor of Pathology, Louisiana State University School of Medicine, 1542 Tulane Avenue, *New Orleans, LA 70112* (USA)

Prog. biochem. Pharmacol., vol. 14, pp. 52–54 (Karger, Basel 1977)

Immunofluorescence in the Identification of Differentiating Arterial Smooth Muscle Cells in Culture

W. Hofmann and D. Goger[1]

Department of Pathology, University of Heidelberg, Heidelberg

In human and in the long line of animals one recognizes a continuous principle in the architecture of all vessels: the endothelium and the accessoria (fig. 1). The term endothelium was already defined by W. His sen. in 1865. The accessoria include the tunica adventitia and the tunica media which again consists of smooth muscle cells, collagen elastin, and glycosaminoglycans. If one wants to perform investigations on the metabolism in these cells in regard to the atherogenesis, it is necessary, to some extent, to grow pure fractions of smooth muscle cells. That will be sucessful if one strips the tunica adventitia and the endothelium with adjoining 'mesenchymal layer' of the tunica intima from the tunica media (fig. 2). At first fibroblasts grow out of the explants which are transported in a culture medium and some days later smooth muscle cells [Hofmann and Goger 1974, 1976; Groeschel-Stewart et al. 1974, 1975, 1976, 1977].

The morphologic differentiation of vascular smooth muscle cells and fibroblasts in tissue culture is difficult if not impossible. By direct immunofluorescence, it is possible to distinguish between vascular smooth muscle cells and fibroblasts after 6–10 days in tissue culture. Microfilaments appear from the 6th to the 10th day. After an incubation period of *30 min* with antibodies against smooth muscle actomyosin *at room tempe-*

[1] We are indebted to Prof. Dr. U. Groeschel-Stewart, Zoologisches Institut der Technischen Hochschule Darmstadt, for preparation and provision of FITC-labelled antiactomyosin.

Fig. 1. Architecture of the vascular wall. Notice 'Langhans cells' of the intima.
Fig. 2. Materials and methods. Stripping of the tunica intima and the tunica adventitia from the tunica media.

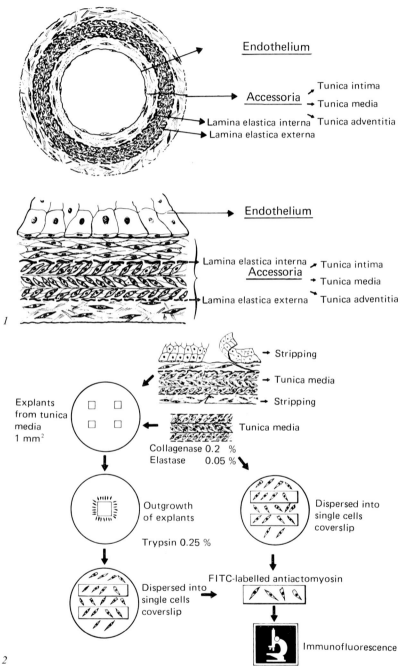

1

2

rature, microfilaments are demonstrable in smooth muscle cells. In contrast, fibroblasts, if incubated for the same period, show perinuclear, respectively nuclear fluorescence and a primary fluorescence of the cytoplasm, but filaments are not visible. If fibroblasts are incubated with antiactomyosin for *1 h at 37° C,* however, microfilaments are easily detectable.

With this method it is possible to differentiate in a simple manner vascular smooth muscle cells from fibroblasts in a heterogeneous culture.

References

HOFMANN, W. and GOGER, D.: Report on the differentiation of vascular wall smooth muscle cells with the aid of immunofluorescence. Virchows Arch. Abt. A Path. Anat. Histol. *363:* 225 (1974).

HOFMANN, W. and GOGER, D.: A simple method for differentiation of vascular smooth muscle cells and fibroblasts. Virchows Arch. Abt. A Path. Anat. Histol. *370:* 77 (1976).

GROESCHEL-STEWART, U. and GROESCHEL, D.: Immunological evidence for the presence of smooth muscle-type contractile fibres in mouse macrophages. Experientia *30:* 1152 (1974).

GROESCHEL-STEWART, U.; CHAMLEY, J.H.; McCONNELL, J.D., and BURNSTOCK, G.: Comparison of the reaction of cultured smooth and cardiac muscle cells and fibroblasts to specific antibodies to myosin. Histochemistry *43:* 215 (1975).

GROESCHEL-STEWART, U.; SCHREIBER, J.; MAHLMEISTER, C., and WEBER, K.: Production of specific antibodies to contractile proteins, and their use in immunofluorescence microscopy. I. Antibodies to smooth and striated chicken muscle myosins. Histochemistry *46:* 229 (1976).

GROESCHEL-STEWART, U.; CEURREMANS, S.; LEHR, I.; MAHLMEISTER, C., and PAAR, E.: Production of specific antibodies to contractile proteins, and their use in immunofluorescence microscopy. II. Species-specific and species-nonspecific antibodies to smooth and striated chicken muscle actin. Histochemistry *50:* 271 (1977).

Prof. Dr. W. HOFMANN, Department of Pathology, University of Heidelberg, *D-6900 Heidelberg* (FRG)

Prog. biochem. Pharmacol., vol. 14, pp. 55–58 (Karger, Basel 1977)

Smooth Muscle Cells of Intimal Cushions and the Localization of Atherosclerotic Lesions[1]

B.A. Kottke, M.T.R. Subbiah, G.E. Tesar and K.K. Unni

Mayo Clinic and Foundation, Rochester, Minn.

The possibility that intimal cushions of smooth muscle cells might represent predisposed locations for the development of atherosclerotic plaques was first suggested by Dock in 1946. In subsequent studies Neufeld et al. [1962] noted that the cushions were present near the branching areas of the major coronary arteries of the fetus at 34 weeks of gestation. They noted that in young children, prior to puberty, the cushions were more prominent in males than in females. The locations of the cushions, at branching points of the arteries, were similar to the locations in which atherosclerotic plaques were commonly seen in adult life. In a similar series of studies Wilens [1951] described similar areas of thickening in the aorta and femoral arteries which also corresponded reasonably well to the common locations of atherosclerotic plaques. Recently, Pesonen et al. [1975] of Finland have used morphometric methods to quantitate intimal thickening in 141 infants under 1 year of age who died of noninfectious causes. They determined the geographic birthplace of the parents and grandparents of these infants and compared the degree of thickening in infants whose parents and grandparents came from Eastern Finland with the thickening in those whose parents and grandparents came from Western Finland. The intimal thickening was much more marked in the infants whose parents, and particularly whose grandparents, came from Eastern Finland, an area which is known to have a higher incidence of coronary heart disease than Western Finland. This difference was particularly prominent in the case of the anterior descending coronary artery in the male infants. This evidence adds a

[1] Supported by a SCOR (Specialized Center of Research) grant, HL 14196 from the National Heart, Lung, and Blood Institute.

further indirect indication that intimal thickening may be related to the subsequent development of atherosclerotic plaques. Recently, STARY [1976] has described such intimal cushions in rhesus monkeys. The cushions are present at branching points in the general vicinity where coronary lesions develop after prolonged cholesterol feeding.

The White Carneau and Show Racer pigeons provide ideal animal models for the further evaluation of this phenomenon. The White Carneau develops grossly evident aortic atherosclerosis in an intimal cushion near the origin of the celiac arteries on a genetic basis with an incidence of nearly 100 % by age 3 years while on a cholesterol-free diet. In contrast, the Show Racer pigeon living in the same environment and eating an identical diet has a less than 5 % incidence of such lesions. Intimal cushions near the origin of the celiac artery are present at birth in both species.

In histologic and transmission electron microscopic studies of this intimal cushion area in both species, we have noted the presence of detectable lipid by 1–3 months of age. It is detectable by oil red O staining of cryostat sections and by transmission electron microscopy. It appears to be present in both the intracellular and extracellular locations. In many areas within the lesion this lipid appears to separate the smooth muscle cells from each other and is usually closely associated with what appears to be an accumulation of proteoglycans. During the early period of lesion development, up to 12 months of age, we have noter a striking accumulation of basement membrane-like material in the White Carneau breed. This has not been a prominent feature in the Show Racer breed. These findings are preliminary and will need confirmation by studies in larger groups of birds. In some of the intimal cushions massive amounts of this basement membrane material are present between the smooth muscle cells. After 12 months of age histologic and transmission electron microscopic evidence of lipid accumulation indicates that the accumulation becomes stable or possibly a bit reduced in the Show Racer breed. In contrast, in the White Carneau breed, there is a dramatic increase in lipid accumulation with the development of large pools of confluent lipid material. This is associated with a striking accumulation of acid mucopolysaccharides detected by Hale's colloidal iron stain.

Biochemical studies in this model have demonstrated a dramatic two-fold increase in aortic steryl ester accumulation between 9 and 12 months of age in the White Carneau breed. This change is not seen in the Show Racer breed. Serum lipid levels and serum lipoprotein profiles on electrophoresis are similar between the two breeds. Recently, utilizing a rabbit antipigeon apo LDL antiserum for immunofluorescent microscopy, we have noted that the localization of apo LDL in early lesions is limited to the intimal cushion area of both breeds and that the localization closely matches the localization of oil red O stained lipid in adjacent cryostat sections. My associate, Dr. M.T. RAVI SUBBIAH, has compared the levels of arterial microsomal cholesteryl ester synthetase and the levels of microsomal and supernatant cholesteryl ester hydrolase in both species. At 9 months of age, just prior to the period of biochemically detectable lipid accumulation, the microsomal cholesteryl ester synthetase increases and the microsomal cholesteryl ester hydrolase decreases in the White Carneau breed. This change is not seen in the control Show Racer breed.

As reviewed in the Workshop on Arterial Cell Injury, Doctors FUSTER and LEWIS of our group have identified differences in platelet factor 4-like activity as well as differences in the characteristics of thrombocyte adhesion to glass between these two breeds of pigeons. In the past 6 months Doctor LEWIS has demonstrated the spontaneous occurrence of localized endothelial damage and thrombocyte adherence on the surface overlying the intimal cushion area in the White Carneau breed. Such a change was not seen in the Show Racer breed.

Because of the predictable and constant location of aortic lesions in this model it is possible to study sequential changes during the pathogenesis of atherosclerosis. Our current working hypothesis is that atherosclerosis results from a precise sequence of critical events including: endothelial interaction with platelets or thrombocytes and mononuclear cells; the uptake of specific lipoproteins; cholesteryl ester removal; and production of collagen, elastin and proteoglycans by activated smooth muscle cells. Thus, both the filtration hypothesis and the thrombogenic hypothesis for the pathogenesis of atherosclerosis appear to be correct. They can be integrated into a combined hypothesis based on the sequence of critical events. We feel different specific factors in this sequence may be altered by specific risk factors. In future studies we hope to further delineate the precise sequence of these events and determine whether or not a number of risk factors can alter this sequence or modify its individual factors.

Summary

Atherosclerosis results from a precise sequence of endothelial interaction with platelets or thrombocytes and mononuclear cells, uptake of specific lipoproteins, cholesteryl ester removal, production of collagen, elastin and proteoglycans by activated smooth muscle cells. Thus, both the filtration hypothesis and the thrombogenic hypothesis for the pathogenesis of atherosclerosis appear to be correct.

References

DOCK, W.: The predilection of atherosclerosis for the coronary arteries. J. Am. med. Ass. *131:* 875–878 (1946).

NEUFELD, H.N.; WAGENVOORT, C.A., and EDWARDS, J.E.: Coronary arteries in fetuses, infants, juveniles, and young adults. Lab. Invest. *11:* 837–844 (1962).

PESONEN, E.; NORIO, R., and SARNA, S.: Thickenings in the coronary arteries in infancy as an indication of genetic factors in coronary heart disease. Circulation *51:* 218–225 (1975).

STARY, H.C.: Coronary artery fine structure in rhesus monkeys: the early atherosclerotic lesion and its progression; in STRONG Primates in medicine, vol. 9, pp. 359–395 (Karger, Basel 1976).

WILENS, S.L.: The nature of diffuse intimal thickening of arteries. Am. J. Path. *26:* 825–839 (1951).

B.A. KOTTKE, MD, PhD, Mayo Clinic and Foundation, 200 First Street, SW, *Rochester, MN 55901* (USA)

Prog. biochem. Pharmacol., vol. 14, pp. 59–68 (Karger, Basel 1977)

Some Aspects of Aortic Medial Explant Morphology and Lipid Metabolism

Ross G. Gerrity, John B. Somer, Dianne J. Bernas and Colin J. Schwartz

Department of Atherosclerosis and Thrombosis Research,
The Cleveland Clinic Foundation, Cleveland, Ohio

Introduction

Smooth muscle cells are an important cellular component of atheroma [1], and in recent years it has become increasingly important to define the metabolism of these cells. This is appropriately undertaken in the controlled environment of tissue culture, in which studies may be performed in two ways, using either passaged cells or primary explant cultures. In this preliminary study we report some observations on lipid biosynthesis and cellular ultrastructure in primary cultures derived from the inner media of the young pig aorta, and compare these with similar findings obtained from intact intima-media preparations.

Material and Methods

The culture methods employed are essentially those described and developed by Fischer-Dzoga *et al.* [2]. Medial explant cultures were grown in Eagles minimum essential media with Hanks' salts for periods of 4–7 weeks. Isotopic precursors employed were 1-^{14}C-acetate (1.87 μCi/ml); U-^{14}C-D-glucose (1.56 μCi/ml); 1-^{14}C-oleic acid (0.31 μCi/ml); and ^{32}P-phosphoric acid (6.25 μCi/ml). All incubations were for 5 h. ^{14}C-acetate incorporation was initially studied in cultures 4, 5, and 7 weeks of age. Subsequent incorporation studies for the four precursors were undertaken in 4-week cultures, in which the influence of differing concentrations of calf, normo- and hyperlipemic human serum were compared. Lipid classes were separated by TLC using the solvent system hexane:diethyl ether:glacial acetic acid (146:50:4). Representative cultures were prepared for both scanning and transmission electron microscopy.

Results

Figure 1 indicates that acetate incorporation into lipids was greatest in 4-week, relative to 5- or 7-week-old cultures. In table I, the percentage distribution of ^{14}C-acetate, ^{14}C-glucose, and ^{14}C-oleic acid among the major lipid classes in aortic medial explant cultures is presented, and is compared with the percentage distribution obtained in aortic intima-media preparations. In explant cultures, the major incorporation of acetate ocurred in phospholipid, sterol + diglycerides, and triglycerides. With both glucose and oleic acid, incorporation was, as expected, greatest in both phospholipids and triglycerides. Table II presents similar data for the distribution of ^{32}P into the individual phospholipids. It is readily apparent that the percentage distribution of glucose and oleic acid is similar in both culture and aortic intima-media incubations (table I), but that significant differences exist with respect to both ^{14}C-acetate (table I) and ^{32}P-phosphoric acid (table II).

The influence of both hyperlipemic and normolipemic human serum

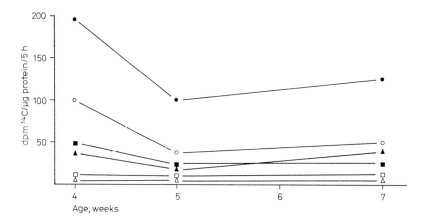

Fig. 1. Incorporation of 1-^{14}C-acetate into lipids at various culture ages: no vitamin supplement. ● = TL, ○ = PL, ■ = S+DG, ▲ = FFA, □ = Tri, △ = CE.

Table 1. Percentage distribution of lipid precursors among lipid classes; comparison of 4-week primary SMC cultures and *in vitro* aorta incubation

Lipid class	1-14C-acetate		U-14C-D-glucose		1-14C-oleic acid	
	SMC culture[1]	aortic incubation[2]	SMC culture[1]	aortic incubation[2]	SMC culture[1]	aortic incubation[3]
Total lipid	100	100	100	100	100	100
PL	61.5±2.6	34.0	45.8±1.8	45.0	76.0±1.1	75.1
S+DG	21.8±2.1	9.3±2.6	7.8±1.7	4.0	1.6±0.1	–
FFA	2.0±0.3	9.8±2.6	1.2±0.6	trace	–	–
TG	13.5±1.0	42.0±2.9	44.1±1.5	49.0	22.4±1.1	18.2
CE	1.2±0.1	4.9±1.0	0.9±0.2	trace	0.5±0.1	0.7
n	12	8	15	8	23	

[1] 4-week cultures, 5 h incubation.
[2] Whole aorta, 3 h incubation.
[3] Whole aorta, 4 h incubation.

Table II. Percentage distribution of ^{32}P-phosphoric acid into phospholipids; comparison of 4-week primary cultures and *in vitro* aorta incubation

Phospholipids	Primary SMC cultures	Aortic incubation
Total	100	100
Lysophosphatidyl choline	5.4 ± 1.5	–
Sphingomyelin	1.9 ± 0.2	1.1
Phosphatidyl choline	65.1 ± 1.5	30.0
Phosphatidyl inositol + phosphatidyl serine	23.9 ± 0.9	65.5
Phosphatidyl ethanolamine	5.1 ± 0.5	3.7
n	21	–

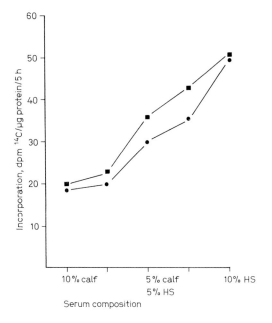

Fig. 2. Effect of HLHS and NLHS on incorporation of 1-^{14}C-acetate into triglycerides. ■ = NLHS, ● = HLHS.

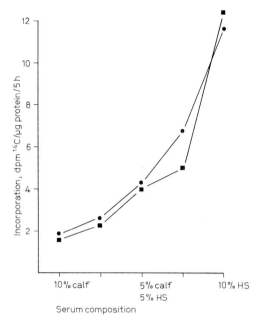

Fig. 3. Effect of HLHS and NLHS on incorporation of 1-¹⁴C-acetate into cholesterol esters. ● = NLHS, ■ = HLHS.

in concentrations of 2, 5, 7.5 and 10 % on the incorporation of 1-¹⁴C-acetate into triglycerides is presented in figure 2. It can be seen that both human sera significantly and similarly enhance the incorporation of acetate into triglycerides relative to the basal level obtained with 10 % fetal calf serum. Human serum exhibits a similar effect on the incorporation of 1-¹⁴C-acetate into cholesteryl esters (fig. 3). Again no significant difference between hyperlipemic and normolipemic serum was observed.

Ultrastructurally, the cells grown from medial explants were typically kite-shaped, with many surface projections prior to confluence, as seen in the scanning electron microscope (fig. 4). From 4 weeks onward, in the stationary phase, the cells became elongated in shape, with less surface detail, and the cultures were frequently multi-layered (fig. 5). In section, these cells exhibited well-developed and numerous organelles in the perinuclear areas, while the peripheral cytoplasm was filled with myofilaments (fig. 6), which often ran in tracts (fig. 7). Short profiles of rough endoplasmic reticulum were common, the Golgi was well-devel-

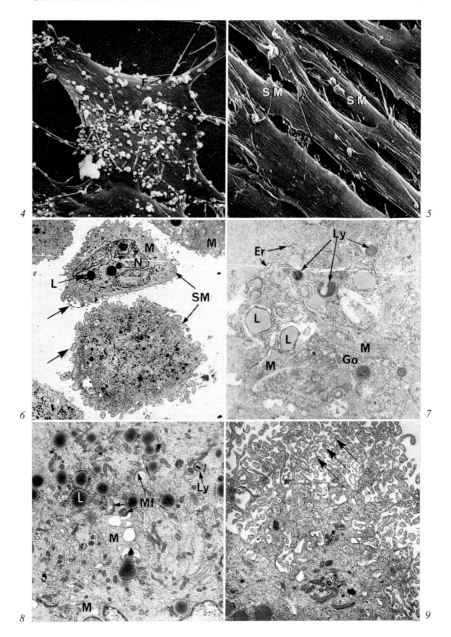

Fig. 4–9.

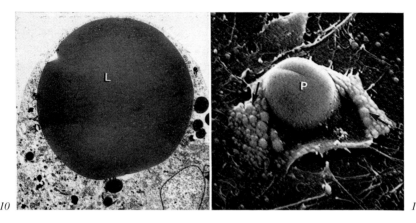

10   *11*

Fig. 10. Transmission electron micrograph of a cultured smooth muscle cell incubated in hyperlipemic human serum. A large lipid droplet (L) is prominent in the peripheral cytoplasm. ×3,000.

Fig. 11. Scanning electron micrograph of a cultured smooth muscle cell incubated in hyperlipemic human serum. A large bulbous protrusion (P), probably representing a lipid droplet as in figure 10, and numerous small protrusions (arrows) in the peripheral cytoplasm, are visible. ×1,750.

Fig. 4. Scanning electron micrograph of a smooth muscle cell from a 3-week-old explant culture. Cell is kite-shaped, with numerous globular (G) and filamentous (F) surface projections. ×2,200.

Fig. 5. Scanning electron micrograph of a 7-week-old culture. Smooth muscle cells (SM) are elongate and polarized, with few surface projections. Cells are overlapped and frequently multilayered. ×4,300.

Fig. 6. Transmission electron micrograph of smooth muscle cells (SM) from a 4-week culture. Nuclei (N) are multilobular, and organelles are mainly perinuclear. Lipid droplets (L) are visible in the cytoplasm. Peripheral cytoplasm is filled with myofilaments (M), and surfaces show many projections (arrows). ×2,100.

Fig. 7. Transmission electron micrograph of perinuclear cytoplasm from a 4-week-old cultured smooth muscle cell. Membrane-bound lipid inclusions (L) can be seen, as well as lysosomes (Ly), rough endoplasmic reticulum (Er) and Golgi (Go). Myofilaments (M) run in tracts through the cytoplasm. ×13,000.

Fig. 8. Transmission electron micrograph of perinuclear cytoplasm from 7-week-old cultured smooth muscle cell. Membrane-bound lipid inclusions (L), myelin forms (Mf) and lysosomes (Ly) are visible. Myofilaments (M) are randomly distributed in the cytoplasm. ×6,300.

Fig. 9. Transmission electron micrograph of peripheral cytoplasm of a 4-week-old cultured smooth muscle cell incubated in normal human serum. Cell surface is thrown into numerous complex projections (arrows), which are cut in section. ×6,300.

oped, and lipid inclusions and lysosomes were seen in all cells at 4 weeks
(fig. 7). With increasing age, degenerative changes were frequently observed. Lipid inclusions increased in number and in osmophilia. Lysosomes and myelin forms were more frequently seen, and myofilaments
became less orientated and more dispersed (fig. 8). Mitochondria were
more numerous, and were thinner and more elongate than previously
(fig. 8).

The addition of human serum to the medium induced an increase in
the number and extent of surface projections from the cell (fig. 9), while
cells grown in hyperlipemic human serum additionally contained large,
nonmembrane-bound lipid inclusions in their cytoplasm (fig. 10). In the
scanning electron microscope, these inclusions were seen as bulbous protrusions under the plasma membrane (fig. 11).

Discussion

Tissue culture systems provide a unique means of studying the metabolism and biology of cells in the absence of uncontrollable physiological
or pathological stimuli present in the intact animal. In this study we have
employed the primary medial explant techniques, and have compared
lipogenesis in medial smooth muscle cells in culture with that of incubated whole intima-media preparations. This study has clearly established in primary medial explant cultures that lipogenesis from 1-^{14}C-
acetate is dependent upon the age of the culture, and that incorporation is
greatest in 4-week-old cultures, relative to those at 5 and 7 weeks. This
set of observations has important implications in the design and interpretation of metabolic studies in tissue culture, and indicates that culture
age is an important determinant of metabolic activity. It should be com-
mented that at 4 weeks the cultures were in the stationary phase; the
influence, if any, of growth phase has not been independently assessed
in these studies. The diminished incorporation of acetate in cultures at
5 and 7 weeks may reflect decreasing cellular viability. This possibility is
consistent with the ultrastructural observations that older cultures exhibit
increasing numbers of lipid inclusions, myelin forms, lysosomes, and
autophagocytic vacuoles, together with an increased disorientation of
myofilaments.

With the precursors, 1-^{14}C-acetate, U-^{14}C-D-glucose, 1-^{14}C-oleic acid,
and ^{32}P-phosphoric acid, two important observations have emerged with

respect to lipogenesis in both 4-week primary medial explant cultures, and whole intima-media incubations. The percentage distribution of labeled glucose among the major lipid classes was essentially similar in the two systems as was that of oleic acid. However, the percentage distribution of labeled acetate into the major lipid classes, and that of ^{32}P-phosphoric acid into the individual phospholipids differed markedly between the explant cultures and intima-media preparations. These findings indicate that there are both qualitative and quantitative differences in *in vitro* lipogenesis between cells in explant culture and cells in the intact intima-media. These differences serve to point out the need for caution in extrapolating data derived from either system to the other. At least one explanation for the differences may reside in the absence of an endothelial layer in the explants, which has been suggested to exert some regularity control over medial metabolism.

It is significant that the addition of both normo- and hyperlipemic human serum to the explant cultures significantly increases the incorporation of 1-^{14}C-acetate into triglycerides and cholesteryl esters relative to the basal incorporations with fetal calf serum. No difference between the two human sera was observed. These observations have a number of implications, one of which relates to the metabolic changes which may result from manipulating the serum composition of the culture or incubation media. Additionally, significant structural changes can be observed after the addition of hyperlipemic human serum not only with respect to surface morphology, but also in organelle content and structure, and the extent of lipid inclusion in the cytoplasm.

Summary

This study has examined some aspects of lipogenesis in both primary aortic medial explant cultures and intact aortic intima-media preparations. It has been shown that both lipogenesis and cellular ultrastructure vary with the age of the culture. Additionally, data has been presented indicating marked qualitative and quantitative differences in lipogenesis between explant cultures and intima-media incubations. Finally, it has been shown that the addition of either normo- or hyperlipemic human serum to explant cultures can significantly modify acetate incorporation into both triglycerides and cholesteryl esters and induce significant changes in ultrastructural morphology. It is concluded that one should interpret cell culture data with caution, particularly with respect to culture age, serum composition, and ultrastructural cellular viability.

References

1   HAUST, M.D.; MORE, R.H., and MOVAT, H.Z.: The role of smooth muscle cells in the fibrogenesis of arteriosclerosis. Am. J. Path. *37:* 377–389 (1960).
2   FISCHER-DZOGA, K.; FRASER, R., and WISSLER, R.W.: Stimulation of proliferation in stationary primary cultures of monkey and rabbit aortic smooth muscle cells. I. Effects of lipoprotein fractions of hyperlipemic serum and lymph. Expl molec. Path. *24:* 346–359 (1976).

Dr. R.G. GERRITY, Department of Atherosclerosis and Thrombosis Research, The Cleveland Clinic Foundation, *Cleveland, OH 44106* (USA)

Prog. biochem. Pharmacol., vol. 14, pp. 69–72 (Karger, Basel 1977)

Derivation of Intimal Smooth Muscle Cells in Normal Arteries and Atherosclerotic Plaques. An Overview

ROBERT M. O'NEAL

Department of Pathology, University of Oklahoma, Oklahoma City, Okla.

For the past 20 years, there has been gradually increasing acceptance of a central role for a type of smooth muscle cell in the formation of atherosclerotic lesions [2]. These cells, variously referred to as 'myo-intimal cells', 'intimacytes', 'modified smooth muscle cells', or often now simply 'SMC', lie between the endothelium and the media. There is such great variability in their appearance, depending primarily on the extent of vacuolization of the cytoplasm by lipid, that most investigators have now concluded that essentially all intimal foam cells are modified SMC [4]. Other major characteristics of these intimal SMC that distinguish them from medial SMC have been enumerated by BENDITT [1]: They appear smaller, produce more collagen than elastin, have fewer cell junctions, and lack orderly arrangement.

Although much has been learned about the conditions required for their proliferation, very little information is available that would indicate their origin. Knowledge of their derivation will be important to our understanding of atherogenesis, regardless of the particular theory of the pathogenesis of the lesions that we favor.

At least four possibilities exist. They could be derived from medial SMC, from endothelial cells, from undifferentiated cells in the subendothelial space, or from immigrant cells from the circulating blood.

The first of these presently has the widest acceptance, although direct supporting evidence is not available and will be difficult to get. In favor of this origin is the proximity of the media. We have all been impressed with the placement of medial SMC at fenestrae in the internal elastic lamella, with cell processes reaching upward toward the intima as if ready to leap; perhaps only waiting for the signal from a platelet! Ross and

GLOMSET [9], who have given us such a much better insight concerning stimuli causing proliferation, has stated that 'five to seven days after balloon-catheter injury, SMC can be observed within fenestrae of the internal elastic lamina apparently in the process of migrating into the intima'. His illustrations also indicate a diffuse invasion of the SMC from the media immediately below the intima. However, experimental evidence for such a migration has not been obtained; with our usual methods, detection of cell movement is obviously impossible. The studies of THOMAS et al. [12] have not established that cell division is more likely in this first medial layer than in other cells of the aortic wall–including the endothelium–even when mitotic activity has been enhanced by choles- terol feeding. Perhaps, under conditions of increased mitotic activity, there is less concomitant cell death in the inner than in deeper medial layers, providing excess cells to allow for migration to the intima.

The second possibility–that endothelial cells proliferate and extend downward, become 'buried' in the intima, and thereafter transform into SMC–presently has little support. However, recognizable endothelial cells can be fairly frequently found, by transmission electron microscopy (TEM), extending deep into the intima with only an elongated tail at- tached to the surface endothelial lining. Also, there has been increasing recognition of the ability of endothelium, under certain conditions such as hypertension, to develop increased numbers of supposedly contractile filaments, as described by STILL and DENNISON [10], suggesting a transi- tion to SMC. The interpretations of IMPARATO et al. [5] also suggest that the identities of these two cell lines are not distinct: they describe, by TEM, replacement of endothelium by a continuous layer of modified SMC near the site of an arteriovenous anastomosis in dogs.

The third possibility, that a sparse population of undifferentiated primitive cells inhabits the normal subendothelial space, has had frequent support [11]. Such cells, properly stimulated, could well be the pre- cursors of intimal SMC, and a cell consistent with this possibility was de- scribed as early as 1866 by LANGHANS [6]. Similar undifferentiated mono- nuclear cells are often found by TEM, probably in all species, lying directly beneath the endothelium in supposedly normal vessels [7]. The blood that are being seen in an early stage of transit through the vessel damage remains obscure [3]. They may be only cells from the circulating blood that are being seen in an early stage of transit through the vessel wall.

The fourth possibility, that the precursor cells are derived from cells

of the circulating blood, has little general support and would seem somewhat remote, in view of the other, more similar, potential precursor cells
lying nearby. But there is considerable evidence that penetration of the
endothelium by mononuclear cells is frequent, and that this frequency is
markedly increased by hypertension. STILL and DENNISON [10], in particular, have systematically and continuously added to the evidence that
this process of invasion of the intima by circulating mononuclear cells is
of significant frequency; use of the scanning electron microscope has
made the results of study of this phenomenon much more easily demonstrable and dramatic.

Another bit of support for the presence of circulating cells that are
capable of acting as precursors of SMC comes from the collaborative
studies that were performed in Houston, Texas, at Baylor College of
Medicine several years ago, by members of the Departments of Pathology
and Surgery [8]. It had been noted that, occasionally, small isolated
endothelialized plaques formed on dacron aortic prostheses in man, and
well-formed plaques of smooth muscle cells rapidly covered large dacron
patches placed over septal defects in children. To determine whether or
not formation of these neointimas depended upon the underlying connective tissue or adjacent vessel wall, small squares of dacron were suspended by polyethylene sutures in the center of aortic dacron prostheses,
and these were placed in the thoracic aortas of young pigs and dogs. In
several weeks a neointima covered isolated, suspended dacron squares.
The presence of the neointima, covered by endothelium and containing
collagen and spindle cells which appeared to be smooth muscle in type,
did not appear to depend upon the presence of a 'bridge' of ttissue from
the wall of the prosthesis. Although these bridges between the wall and the
centrally suspended dacron square occasionally formed, the composition
of the neointima covering the square was the same in those with and
without demonstrable connecting bridges, and in all instances was indistinguishable from the inner lining of the wall of the prosthesis.

Summary

We have no evidence of the precise derivation of myointimal cells,
either in 'normal' intima or in atherosclerotic lesions. Neither has any
derivation been eliminated. Efforts to establish the origin of the cells
might be as helpful to our understanding of the lesions as have been the

studies of proliferation of SMC, regardless of which one of the various theories of the pathogenesis of atherosclerosis we happen to support.

References

1   BENDITT, E.P.: Implications of the monoclonal character of human athero-sclerotic plaques. Beitr. path. Anat. *158:* 405–416 (1976).
2   GEER, J.C. and HAUST, M.D.: Smooth muscle cells in atherosclerosis. Monogr. Atheroscler., vol. 2 (Karger, Basel 1972).
3   HOFF, H.F. and GOTTLOB, R.: Ultrastructural changes of large rabbit blood vessels following mild mechanical trauma. Virchows Arch. path. Anat., Abt. A *345:* 93–106 (1968).
4   IMAI, H.; LEE, K.T.; PASTORI, S.; PANLILIO, E.; FLORENTIN, R., and THOMAS, W.A.: Atherosclerosis in rabbits. Architectural and subcellular alterations of smooth muscle cells in aortas in response to hyperlipemia. Expl molec. Path. *5:* 273–310 (1966).
5   IMPARATO, A.M.; BAUMANN, F.G.; PEARSON, J.; KIM, G.E.; DAVIDSON, T.; IBRAHIM, I., and NATHAN, I.: Electron microscopic studies of experimentally produced fibromuscular arterial lesions. Surgery Gynec. Obstet. *139:* 497–504 (1974).
6   LANGHANS, T.: Beitrag zur normalen und pathologischen Anatomie der Arterien. Virchows Arch. path. Anat. *36:* 187–226 (1866).
7   LEE, K.T.; LEE, K.J.; LEE, S.K.; IMAI, H., and O'NEAL, R.M.: Poorly differ-entiated subendothelial cells in swine aorta. Expl molec. Path. *13:* 118–129 (1970).
8   O'NEAL, R.M.; JORDAN, G.L., jr.; RABIN, E.R.; DEBAKEY, M.E., and HALPERT, B.: Cells grown on isolated intravascular dacron hub. An electron microscopic study. Expl molec. Path. *3:* 403–412 (1964).
9   ROSS, R. and GLOMSET, J.A.: The pathogenesis of atherosclerosis. New Engl. J. Med. *295:* 369–377, 420–425 (1976).
10 STILL, W.J.S. and DENNISON, S.: The arterial endothelium of the hypertensive rat. Archs Path. *97:* 337–342 (1974).
11 STILL, W.J.S. and O'NEAL, R.M.: Electron microscopic study of experimental atherosclerosis in the rat. Am. J. Path. *40:* 21–35 (1962).
12 THOMAS, W.A.; FLORENTIN, R.A.; NAM, S.C.; REINER, J.M., and LEE, K.T.: Alterations of population dynamics of arterial smooth muscle cells during atherogenesis. 1. Activation of interphase cells in cholesterol-fed swine prior to gross atherosclerosis demonstrated by 'post-pulse salvage labelling'. Expl molec. Path. *15:* 245–267 (1971).

Dr. R.M. O'NEAL, Department of Pathology, University of Oklahoma, *Oklahoma City, OK 73190* (USA)

Prog. biochem. Pharmacol., vol. 14, pp. 73–77 (Karger, Basel 1977)

Modulations of the Vascular Smooth Muscle Cells During Spontaneous or Diet-Induced Arterial Changes in Pigs

G. HOLLE, J. MASSMANN and H. WEIDENBACH

Institute of Pathology, Karl Marx University, Leipzig

Introduction

The aim of this study was to examine the relations between spontaneous and induced changes of the intima and to determine the range of modulations of the arterial smooth muscle cells.

Material and Methods

The investigations were carried out in castrated male pigs of a modern breed (initial weight 25–30 kg). The animals were given a standard diet containing 15 % butter and 1.5 % cholesterol (group A, n = 4), or 0.8 % cholesterol (group B, n = 5), or no cholesterol (group C, n = 2). 8 animals received the standard feed containing 1.25 % raw fat (group D). The animals were killed after the following test periods: group A after 2, 5, and 7 months; group B after 4 months; group C after 5 and 7 months; group D after 2, 4, 5, and 7 months. Light-microscopical examinations included at least 11 standard sites of the arterial system while 5–8 sites were analysed electron-microscopically. Total serum cholesterol and triglyceride values were checked.

Results and Discussion

Under normo- and hypercholesterolaemic conditions, quantitatively and qualitatively different intimal changes are developed in pigs in

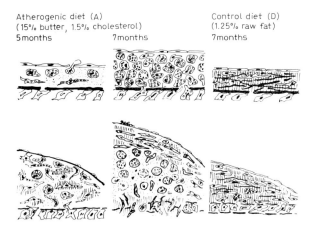

Atherogenic diet (A)
(15% butter, 1.5% cholesterol)
5 months   7 months

Control diet (D)
(1.25% raw fat)
7 months

Fig. 1. Scheme of different arterial reactions under normal and atherogenic diet. Intimal changes in the elastic thoracic aorta and elastic carotid arteries (a), and in the muscular abdominal aorta, extramural coronary arteries and iliac arteries (b).

dependence upon calibre and structural type of the arteries. Figure 1 shows in a schematic representation the different responses of the arterial wall. After 7 months of diet A, complicated atheromas developed at sites which under normal conditions develop fibromuscular plaques (abdominal aorta, the intima of the thoracic aorta showed, after 5 and 7 months of diet A, lipoproliferative changes were found at these sites. On the other hand, the intima of the thoracid aorta showed, after 5 and 7 months of diet A, relatively thin foam cell infiltrates and under normal conditions (group D) diffuse fibroelastic intimal thickenings. Similarly different reactions of the arteries were also observed in chickens [8], rabbits [6], and primates [3]; these may be due to local haemodynamic influences and metabolic differences in the arterial walls. Distribution, degree of affection and histogenesis of the spontaneous and induced lipoproliferative changes in pigs show a marked similarity to atherogenesis in humans. Similar to the findings in other animals, the degree of the intimal changes was dependent upon the serum cholesterol level. After 2 months of diet in group A, for example, the changes corresponded to those found in group B after 4 months and in group C after 7 months of diet with mean serum cholesterol values of 400, 250, and 175 mg/100ml. They consisted in an increase in the extra and intracellular lipid contents, in fibromuscular plaques, and

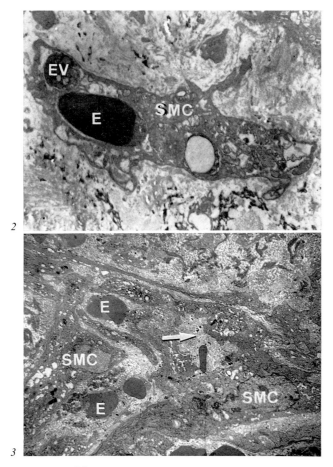

Fig. 2. Modified smooth muscle cell (SMC) with erythrophagocytosis in different stages of digestion. E = Engulfed erythrocyte, EV = erythrophatocytic vacuole. × 6,900.

Fig. 3. Modified smooth muscle cells (SMC) forming primitive capillary-like structures in the atherosclerotic plaque. E = Erythrocytes, arrow = capillary-like lumen. × 1,950.

in an increase in poorly differentiated subendothelial cells [5]. From these findings one may conclude that spontaneous thickenings of the intima with low-degree hypercholesterolaemia mainly accumulate lipids.

The main cell of the spontaneous and induced changes is the smooth muscle cell and its respective modulation: in spontaneous changes in the form of activated and fibroblast-like muscle cells, in induced changes in addition lipid-storing and poorly differentiated muscle cells. Some new observations could be made with regard to stenosing atheromas, complicated by ulceration, microthrombi, vascularization and haemorrhages. Precursors of myogenic capillary formations were solid cell cords which were formed by activated muscle cells. After the formation of a lumen (fig. 2), these are modulated into endothelial and pericyte-like cells. Thus, the atheroma capillaries may not only be formed from endothelial sprouts [8], but also from stimulated muscle cells. The stimuli causing these modulations of myointimal cells have been found to be blood components getting into the arterial wall by capillary haemorrhages. Temporary endothelial functions of the smooth muscle cells have been described by other authors [9, 10] after experimental endothelial destruction. Besides, in atheroma haemorrhages an erythrophagocytosis caused by activated muscle cells could be found in the intima and media. While in the early stages of phagocytosis and endocytosis there still were signs of the smooth muscle cells, the contractile system was largely reduced in the stage of intracellular digestion with the occurrence of primary and secondary lysosomes (fig. 3). Thus, the ability of the smooth muscle cells to develop phagocytosis [1, 2] which had already be found in the tissue culture could also be observed *in vivo*. The demonstrated changes in the structure of the arterial muscle cells corroborates and extends WISSLER's [11] hypothesis according to which under the influence of special stimuli the muscle cells can take over functions of a mesenchymal cell [4].

References

1   COLTOFF-SCHILLER, B.; GOLDFISCHER, S.; ADAMANY, A.M., and WOLINSKY, H.: Endocytosis by vascular smooth muscle cells *in vivo* and *in vitro*. Am. J. Path. *83:* 45–53 (1976).

2   GARFIELD, R.E.; CHACKO, S., and BLOSE, S.: Phagocytosis by muscle cells. Lab. Invest. *33:* 418–427 (1975).

3   GRESHAM, G.A. and HOWARD, A.N.: Experimental atherosclerosis in baboons. Ann. N.Y. Acad. Sci. *162:* 99–102 (1969).

4   KATENKAMP, P. und STILLER, D.: Der Myofibroblast – eine kontraktile Bindegewebszelle? Übersicht zur Orthologie und Pathologie. Dt. GesundhWes. *32:* 865–871 (1977).

5   LEE, K.T. LEE, K.J.; LEE, S.K.; IMAI, H., and O'NEAL, R.M.: Poorly differentiated subendothelial cells in swine aortas. Expl molec. Path. *13:* 118–129 (1970).

6   MASSMANN, J. und HELBIG, W.: Morphologische und biochemische Untersu-
    chungen zur unterschiedlichen Ausbildung der cholesterolinduzierten Athero-
    sklerose von Aorta und Koronararterien. Expl Path. *7:* 60–70 (1972).

7   MOSS, N.S. and BENDITT, E.P.: The ultrastructure of spontaneous and experi-
    mentally induced arterial lesions. III. The cholesterol-induced lesions and the
    effect of a cholesterol and oil diet on the preexisting spontaneous plaque in the
    chicken aorta. Lab. Invest. *23:* 521–535 (1970).

8   SCHOEFL, G.I.: Studies on inflammation. III. Growing capillaries: their
    structure and permeability. Virchows Arch. path. Anat. Physiol. *337:* 97–141
    (1963).

9   SCHWARTZ, S.M.; STEMERMAN, M.B., and BENDITT, E.P.: The aortic intima. II.
    Repair of the aortic lining after mechanical denudation. Am. J. Path. *81:*
    15–42 (1975).

10 TSAO, C.: Myointimal cells as a possible source of replacement for endothelial
    cells in rabbit. Circulation Res. *23:* 671–682 (1968).

11 WISSLER, R.W.: The arterial medial cell – smooth muscle or multifunctional
    mesenchym? J. Atheroscler. Res. *8:* 201–213 (1968).

Prof. Dr. sc. med. G. HOLLE, Institute of Pathology, Karl Marx University,
Liebigstrasse 26, *DDR-701 Leipzig* (DDR)

Prog. biochem. Pharmacol., vol. 14, pp. 78–83 (Karger, Basel 1977)

A Method to Measure the Pinocytic Uptake of [125] I-Labelled Polyvinylpyrrolidone by Pig Aortic Smooth Muscle and Endothelial Cells in Culture[1]

D.S. LEAKE and D.E. BOWYER

Department of Pathology, University of Cambridge, Cambridge

Lipids, particularly cholesteryl oleate, accumulate in engorged secondary lysosomes of arterial smooth muscle cells (SMC) in athero-sclerotic lesions, probably because lipoproteins in the arterial tissue fluid are taken up by pinocytosis into the lysosomes, and when present in high concentrations overload their sterol-ester hydrolase activity [5, 8]. Plasma lipoproteins probably enter the tissue fluid, at least partly, because of diacytosis by endothelial cells (EC), i.e. pinocytosis, translocation of the resulting pinosome and exocytosis at the opposite surface of the cell. Thus, pinocytosis by both arterial SMC [7] and EC is of significance in atherogenesis.

The technique of WILLIAMS et al. [9], to measure the rate of pinocytic uptake of ^{125}I-labelled polyvinylpyrrolidone (PVP), has been adapted for aortic SMC and EC in culture. ^{125}I-labelled PVP is a useful marker for pinocytosis, because it cannot be degraded in lysosomes and its mean molecular weight of 30,000–40,000 prevents it from permeating cellular membranes. Its rate of uptake was expressed by WILLIAMS et al. [9] as the volume of culture medium whose ^{125}I-labelled PVP content was taken up per unit time per unit mass of cellular protein, and was defined to be the endocytic index for this compound. This method of expressing uptake aids comparison between the rates of uptake of the same or different substances at different concentrations [10].

[1] We thank Nattermann GmbH & Cie, Köln, West Germany for support and D.S.L. thanks the Medical Research Council (London) for a research studentship.

Isolation and Culture of Cells

SMC were obtained by outgrowth from cultured explants of media from pig thoracic aortas by the method of Ross [6]. EC were isolated by a modification of the technique of JAFFE *et al.* [3], as follows. After cannulation of the aorta and ligation of the branches, the lumen was washed with Hanks' balanced salt solution and filled with collagenase (type I; Sigma) 500 μg/ml, in this buffer. After incubation at 37° C for 30 min, the contents were drained and about half of it was returned to the aorta, which was then inverted about 50 times to provide the necessary shear to remove the vast majority of the isolated cells, which were then washed and cultured. The culture medium consisted of 4 vol of medium 199 with Earle's balanced salts mixed with 1 vol of fetal bovine serum and contained L-glutamine (2 mM), penicillin G (200 iu/ml), streptomycin sulphate (200 μg/ml) and kanamycin sulphate (200μg/ml). Cultured were incubated at 37° C in humidified air/CO_2 (95:5). SMC were grown in 35 mm diameter dishes (Falcon) and experiments performed with 3rd to 6th subcultures. EC were grown in 25 cm² flasks (Falcon), because they consistently detached from the dishes before reaching confluency, and 7th to 8th subcultures were used for experiments.

Accumulation of ^{125}I-Labelled PVP

After incubation of SMC in dishes (or EC in flasks) with 2 ml (or 5 or 6 ml for EC) of medium containing ^{125}I-labelled PVP (Radiochemical Centre, Amersham, Bucks.) the culture vessels were washed six times with ice-cold buffer (Hanks' balanced salt solution) and the cells detached by trypsinisation. After centrifugation at 4° C for 10 min at 250 g, they were washed in buffer, recentrifuged, sonicated in water and assayed for radioactivity by gamma-spectroscopy and for protein.

During incubation with ^{125}I-labelled PVP (30 μg/ml), cellular accumulation was directly proportional to the time of incubation over 48.5 h for both SMC and EC (fig. 1a). The rate of accumulation, as measured by the gradient of the linear regression line, was 2.45 (95 % confidence limits 2.12, 2.78) and 1.03 ng/h/mg cellular protein (0.87, 1.18) for SMC and EC, respectively. Although the rates of accumulation by the two cell types were different in these experiments, this was not always the case. This variability *between* experiments may possibly be due to differing cell densities or batches of serum.

Figure 1b shows that for both cell types accumulation of ^{125}I-labelled PVP over 48 h was directly proportional to its concentration in the medium and indicates that within the range of 5–100 μg/ml it neither stimulated nor inhibited pinocytosis.

Release of ^{125}I-Labelled PVP

20 dishes of SMC (or flasks of EC) were incubated with 2 ml (or 5 ml for EC) of medium containing ^{125}I-labelled PVP (100 μg/ml). After 48 h the medium was removed and the culture vessels washed six times with non-radioactive medium and then reincubated with it. After various times the media from the vessels were removed, centrifuged at 4°C as described above, to remove any detached cells, and assayed for radio-activity. The cells in the vessels were detached, washed and assayed for radioactivity as described above.

There was a progressive release of radioactivity into the cell-free reincubation medium of both SMC and EC (fig. 2). As discussed previously [4], there are several potential sources of this released material, as follows: (a) leakage from extracellular spaces inaccessible to the washing procedure; (b) desorption from the vessel surface; (c) cell lysis; (d) desorption from the cell surface and (e) exocytosis of previously pinocytosed material. Because of the unknown contributions of sources (a) to (d), the rate of release of ^{125}I-labelled PVP exocytosis cannot be determined from the rate of appearance of radioactivity in the medium.

A linear regression analysis of the ^{125}I-labelled PVP associated with the *total* cells isolated from each vessel revealed no significant decrease ($0.10 > p > 0.05$ for SMC; $p > 0.10$ for EC) over the 48-hour reincubation period (fig. 2). The 95% confidence interval for the percentage change in the cell-associated label, over this period, extended from a decrease of about 50 and 20%, for the SMC and EC respectively, to an increase of a few per cent for both cell types. The cells therefore probably retained the majority (if not all) of their previously pinocytosed ^{125}I-labelled PVP over this period.

It might have been anticipated that EC, which are normally trans-ferring substances between the plasma and the tissue fluid by diacytosis, would have shown a greater percentage release of label. It is possible, however, that diacytosis by EC was inhibited by contact with the plastic surface of the culture vessel.

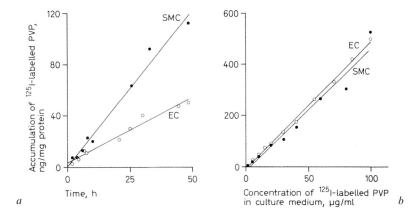

Fig. 1. Accumulation of ^{125}I-labelled PVP by SMC and EC in culture. Each point corresponds to the SMC (●) or EC (○) isolated from a single culture vessel after incubation with culture medium containing (a) ^{125}I-labelled PVP (30 *μ*g/ml) for various times or (b) various concentrations of ^{125}I-labelled PVP for 48 h.

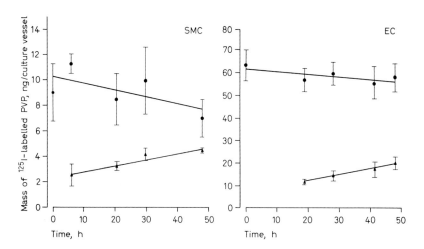

Fig. 2. Release of ^{125}I-labelled PVP during reincubation of SMC and EC with non-radioactive medium. Dishes containing SMC and flasks containing EC were incubated with ^{125}I-labelled PVP (100 *μ*g/ml) for 48 h, washed six times and reincubated with non-radioactive medium. The mass of ^{125}I-labelled PVP associated at various times with the cells (●) and cell-free medium (▲) are shown. A point and error bar corresponds to the mean value ± SD from four culture vessels.

Uptake of ^{125}I-Labelled PVP

The rate of cellular of ^{125}I-labelled PVP would have been equal to its combined rates of accumulation and release. The 95 % confidence limits of the release experiment thus indicate that the rate of uptake would probably have been somewhere between 1 and about 1.5 times, and between 1 and about 1.2 times the rate of accumulation by SMC and EC, respectively. Therefore, the rate of uptake during the time course experiment, in which cells were incubated with 30 °g of this substance/ml, was estimated to have been somewhere between about 2.4 and 3.7, and between about 1.03 and 1.23 ng/h/mg protein for the SMC and EC, respectively. When expressed as the endocytic indices for ^{125}I-labelled PVP (see above), the estimates for this experiment would lie somewhere between about 82 and 123, and between about 34 and 41 nl/h/mg protein for the SMC and EC, respectively. However, the rates of accumulation varied between individual experiments (see above) and so the indices would also have varied in this way.

Applications of the Method

There are few published quantitative studies of pinocytosis by non-macrophage mammalian cells in culture. The adaptation reported here of the method of WILLIAMS *et al.* [9] provides a simple and accurate way of measuring the rate of accumulation by cultured arterial cells of a non-degradable marker molecule for pinocytosis.

The system may be used to investigate factors of relevance to atherogenesis that may modify the pinocytic process in arterial SMC and EC. For example, one of these factors may be the fluidity of the plasma membrane, which may be modified by its cholesterol to phospholipid ratio [2] and also by polyunsaturated phospholipids, such as the thera-peutic agent, essential phospholipids [1]. The method may also be used to investigate the possibility of feedback inhibition of pinocytosis due to lipid-engorged secondary lysosomes. A comparison of the endocytic index of a substance of interest (such as a lipoprotein) with that of ^{125}I-labelled PVP may demonstrate whether the pinocytic uptake of that substance involves either high affinity binding or only low affinity, or no, binding to the plasma membrane before internalisation [10].

References

1 HEGNER, D.: Effect of essential phospholipids on the ATPases and on the fluidity of liver plasma membranes; in PEETERS Phosphatidylcholine. Biochemical and clinical aspects of essential phospholipids, pp. 87–96 (Springer, Berlin 1976).

2 HEINIGER, H.J.; KANDUTSCH, A.A., and CHEN, H.W.: Depletion of L-cell sterol depressed endocytosis. Nature, Lond. 263: 515–517 (1976).

3 JAFFE, E.A.; NACHMAN, R.L.; BECKER, C.G., and MINICK, C.R.: Culture of human endothelial cells derived from umbilical veins. J. clin. Invest. 52: 2745–2756 (1973).

4 LEAKE, D.S. and BOWYER, D.E.: Quantitative studies of pinocytic uptake of ^{125}I-labelled polyvinylpyrrolidone by pig aortic smooth-muscle cells in culture. Biochem. Soc. Trans. 5: 130–133 (1977).

5 PETERS, T.J.: Lysosomes of the arterial wall; in DINGLE and DEAN Lysosomes in biology and pathology, vol. 4, pp. 47–73 (North Holland, Amsterdam 1975).

6 ROSS, R.: The smooth muscle cell. II. Growth of smooth muscle in culture and formation of elastic fibres. J. Cell Biol. 50: 172–186 (1971).

7 SCHILLER, B.; GOLDFISCHER, S.; ADAMANY, A.M., and WOLINSKY, H.: Endocytosis by vascular smooth muscle cells in vivo and in vitro. Am. J. Path. 83: 45–60 (1976).

8 SCHILLER, B.; GOLDFISCHER, S.; WOLINSKY, H., and FACTOR, S.M.: Lipid accumulation in human aortic smooth muscle cell lysosomes. Am. J. Path. 83: 39–44 (1976).

9 WILLIAMS, K.E.; KIDSTON, E.M.; BECK, F., and LLOYD, J.B.: Quantitative studies of pinocytosis. I. Kinetics of uptake of [^{125}I]polyvinylpyrrolidone by rat yolk sac cultured in vitro. J. Cell Biol. 64: 113–122 (1975).

10 WILLIAMS, K.E.; KIDSTON, E.M.; BECK, F., and LLOYD, J.B.: Quantitative studies of pinocytosis. II. Kinetics of protein uptake and digestion by rat yolk sac cultured in vitro. J. Cell Biol. 64: 123–134 (1975).

Dr. D.S. LEAKE, Department of Medicine, Royal Postgraduate Medical School, Hammersmith Hospital, Du Cane Road, London W12 OHS (England)

Prog. biochem. Pharmacol., vol. 14, pp. 84–87 (Karger, Basel 1977)

Ultrastructural and Functional Aspects of Vascular Smooth Muscle Cells

Anna Kádár, Éva Csonka, B. Veress, G. Chaldakov and Magdolna Bihari-Varga

2nd Department of Pathology, Central Electron Microscope Laboratory, Semmelweis Medical University, Budapest, and Department of Anatomy and Histology, Medical Faculty, Varna

Introduction

Various functions are attributed to the vascular smooth muscle cells (SMC), i.e. they have to maintain the contractility of vessels [5] and produce the precursors of connective tissue elements, i.e. elastin protein, glycosaminoglycans, glycoproteins and collagen [7, 10].

Ultrastructural characteristics and cell surface properties may be indicative of the actual functional state of SMC. Aging or pathological conditions as well as a particular physiological requirement may induce the predominance of one of these original functions over the other.

Material and Methods

Aortas from normal embryonic and adult rats, experimental intima proliferation, aortas from copper-deficient and BAPN-treated chicken, untreated as well as cholesterol, lipoprotein or colchicine-treated cultured SMC from mini pig aortas or atherosclerotic human aortas, incorporation of human arterial prosthesis were studied by transmission (TEM) and by scanning (SEM) electron microscope. In addition to conventional TEM and SEM methods ruthenium red and concanavalin A reactions were performed. The experimental methods were described elsewhere [7, 8].

Results

In cultured SMC myofilament bundles and dense bodies are seen along the plasmalemma. In the hyaloplasm the endoplasmic reticulum is filled with a granular substance. Microtubules, microfilaments and plasma membrane-associated transport vesicles can be observed. In the extracellular space, a basement membrane-like material is accompanied by a granular-filamentous structure corresponding to precollagen and/or preelastin.

The smooth-surfaced and elongated cultured SMC possess bundles of contractile filament. The number of myofilaments is inversely proportional to the amount of extracellular substance. The roundish cells contain intracellular microtubules and concanavalin A positive proteoglycans. The surface of the cultured SMC becomes irregular after administration of colchicine (concentration 10^{-4} M) and microtubules and microfilaments are reduced in their number.

In the *atherosclerotic lesions* of humans two types of cells can be distinguished. (1) Cells with dilated endoplasmic reticulum and a few myofilaments, surrounded by large amounts of extracellular substance. (2) Cells resembling to matured 'resting' SMC surrounded by mature elastic and collagen fibers.

Two cell types can be distinguished in the neomedia of *vascular prostheses* of humans: cells characterized by intensive extracellular matrix production or others which remind the resting SMC. Cells which are not active participants of protein synthesis are smooth-surfaced and elongated. The surface characteristics of the resting SMC revealed by SEM are in accordance with the TEM findings.

SMC actively contributing in extracellular matrix production visualized by TEM contain less contractile filaments and their surface is uneven. These phenomena are reflected under the SEM. The cells surface is irregular, the protrusions may represent proteins attached to the surface. This represents a transitory state between the 'resting' SMC and those primarily involved in protein synthesis.

In the protein synthetizing state the surface of the cell is uneven by SEM while dilated endoplasmic reticulum and a Golgi system can be noted by TEM.

Discussion

We suppose that SMC are capable of altering their shape, surface properties, arrangement of subcellular organelles including changes in their number and shape, according to their actual functional state. The 'resting' SMC can be found in the mature and fully developed arterial media.

Surface and ultrastructural properties of SMC involved in active protein or glycoprotein synthesis are different. These cells resemble the dedifferentiated SMC [2], and/or 'myofibroblast' in granulation tissue [5, 9]. In our opinion in these cells the contractile activity is depressed in favor of their connective tissue protein synthesis. The colchicine-caused microtubulous deficiency, depletion of the Golgi system and lack of transport vesicles suggests that not only the Golgy system and the transport vesicles but the microtubules too may play a role in the extracellular matrix production.

There is only few evidence in the literature concerning the SEM of cultured SMC [3, 6]. We found evidence by SEM that the *'resting'* mature SMC are elongated and smooth-surfaced except some areas where the vesicles open to the surface. The bundles of myofilaments can be noted running parallel to the long axis.

The actively protein synthetizing 'modified' SMC are roundish by SEM, displaying numerous surface protrusions. Actively protein synthetizing (modified) SMC can be found in embryos, in early phases of intima proliferation and of incorporation of vascular prostheses as well as in the early stage of atherosclerosis or under some experimentally induced pathological condition like copper deficiency, or β-aminoproprionitrile, colchicine treatment, and in SMC cultures engaged actively with protein synthesis.

The resting, mature SMC can be found in adult aorta, in the late phase of atherosclerosis in the properly incorporated vascular prosthesis and are those cells of the SMC cultures which are maintaining the function and are directing the proliferation and synthesis.

References

1 BLOSE, S.H.; LAZARIDES, E., and CHAKO, S.K.: Loss of differentiated phenotype in the progeny of aortic smooth muscle cells. J. Cell Biol. *67:* 34 (1975).

2   CHAMLEY, J.H. and CAMPBELL, G.R.: Mitosis of contractile smooth muscle cells in tissue culture. Expl Cell. Res. *84:* 105–110 (1974).

3   CHOCK, E. and SHAIN, W.: Dissociation and continuous cell culture of human smooth muscle cells. J. Cell Biol. *67:* 68 (1975).

4   GABBIANI, G.; HIRSCHEL, B.J.; RYAN, G.B.; STATKOV, P.R., and MAJNO, G.: Granulation tissue as a contractile organ. A study of structure and function. J. exp. Med. *135:* 719–734 (1972).

5   GABBIANI, G.; LELOUS, M.; BAILEY, A.J.; BAZIN, S., and DELUNAY, A.: Collagen and myofibroblasts of granulation tissue. A chemical, ultrastructural and immunologic study. Virchows Arch. Abt. B Cell Path. *21:* 133–145 (1976).

6   JONES, R.M.; FISCHER-DZOGA, K., and WISSLER, R.W.: Scanning and transmission electron microscopic studies of the effects of hyperlipemic serum on cultured rhesus monkey aortic medial cells. Am. J. Path. *91:* 82 (1976).

7   KÁDÁR, A.: The ultrastructure of elastic tissue. Pathol. Eur. *9:* 133–146 (1974).

8   KÁDÁR, A.; CSONKA, É., and JELLINEK, H.: Cultured smooth muscle cells of blood vessel. Front. Matrix Biol., vol. 3, pp. 100–112 (Karger, Basel 1976).

9   ROSS, R.; EVERETT, N.B., and TYLER, R.: Wound healing and collagen formation. VI. The origin of the wound fibroblasts studied in parabiosis. J. Cell Biol. *44:* 645–654 (1970).

10   ROSS, R. and KLEBANOFF, S.J.: The smooth muscle cell. I. *In vivo* synthesis of connective tissue protein. J. Cell Biol. *50:* 159–171 (1971).

Dr. A. KÁDÁR, 2nd Department of Pathology, Central Electron Microscope Laboratory, Semmelweis Medicine University, *Budapest* (Hungary)

Prog. biochem. Pharmacol., vol. 14, pp. 88–93 (Karger, Basel 1977)

Proliferation of Arterial Smooth Muscle: Glucocorticoid Effect

C. CAVALLERO, P. SARTI and L.G. SPAGNOLI

IInd Institute of Pathological Anatomy, University of Rome, Rome

Introduction

It is generally accepted that proliferation of arterial smooth muscle cells occurs in several physiological and pathological conditions [1, 2]. Smooth muscle proliferation is a key event in the initiation and progress of the atherosclerotic lesion; actually, smooth muscle cells are the main components of the atherosclerotic plaque.

Recently, particular attention has been paid to the mechanisms triggering or supporting cell proliferation; platelet factor(s) [3, 4], insulin [5], low molecular weight lipoproteins [6] have been implicated. In order to give further insight on this problem we have investigated the effect on cell proliferation of several hormones known to influence the atherosclerotic process. This paper is a short account of the results so far obtained.

Studies on Cholesterol Atherosclerosis

Preliminary colchicine and ^{3}H-thymidine studies carried out on cholesterol-fed rabbits have confirmed that the initiation and the evolution of the atherosclerotic plaque are associated to a proliferative reaction of the arterial wall involving both the medial smooth muscle cells and the cellular constituents of the intimal lesions. Colchicine-blocked mitoses and tritium-labelled nuclei were particularly numerous in early plaques [7, 8]. Subsequent observations have shown that proliferation of arterial smooth muscle in hyperlipemic cholesterol-fed rabbits is under the influ-

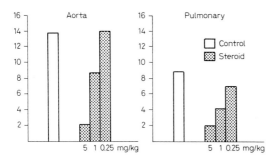

Fig. 1. Inhibition of ³H-thymidine uptake in aortic and pulmonary plaques of cholesterol-fed rabbits 24 h after a single administration of cortisol; dose-response effect. On the ordinate the mean number of labelled nuclei per 1,000 cell population is reported.

ence of several hormones, including glucocorticoids, mineralocorticoids, adrenaline and insulin [9–11]. In these experiments a clear-cut inhibitory effect on cell proliferation by cortisol was ascertained; actually this steroid, even after 1 day of treatment and at a relatively low dose, decreases sharply the deoxyribonucleic synthesis in the intimal plaques (fig. 1).

The inhibitory effect on DNA synthesis was duplicated by other synthetic steroids endowed with antiinflammatory activity. The hormonal influence on (³H)-thymidine uptake was found to be dose-dependent. Moreover a close correlation between the inhibitory effect on (³H)-thymidine uptake by glucocorticoids and their relative antiinflammatory potency was noticed.

In contrast, hypertensive and sodium-retaining active mineralocorticoids, such as aldosterone and DOC, increased the number of labelled nuclei in the plaques. In this connection it is worth mentioning that a stimulation of DNA synthesis in the arterial wall of normal and cholesterol-fed animals has been already noticed after angiotensin injection, renal ischemia [12], adrenal enucleation [13] and epinephrine administration [14].

From the results obtained it was concluded that the antiatherogenic effect of glucocorticoids on cholesterol-fed rabbits may be due, at least partly, to the inhibitory effect of these steroids on the DNA synthesis of the cellular constituents of the intimal plaques, namely of the myo-intimal cells.

Studies on Disendothelized Arteries

Further studies have been performed with the aim to ascertain whether the inhibitory effect of glucocorticoids on cell proliferation occurs also in normolipemic animals. In these experiments we have employed the new technique developed by FISHMAN *et al.* [15] to study the endothelial regeneration in the rat.

In the rabbit, like in the rat, disendothelization of the common carotid artery by air drying is followed by a rapid endothelial ingrowth from the ends of the injured segment of the vessel; the endothelial sheet of the injured area appears to be restored after 7–10 days. In addition, the loss of endothelium stimulates the smooth muscle cells of the underlying media to migrate and proliferate so that a myofibroelastic thickening between endothelium and internal elastic lamina develops. Electron microscopy and radioautographic observations show that the intimal thickening is composed by modified smooth muscle cells and is closely related to migration and proliferation of medial muscle cells.

The effect on intimal thickening and on cell proliferation of a potent synthetic glucocorticoid, triamcinolone (1 mg/day/kg body weight), was tested. As shown in figure 2, in steroid-treated animals the intimal thickening was evidently less marked at each stage after surgery. The results of radioautographic studies with ^{3}H-thymidine are reported in figure 3. There it appears that steroid treatment decreases sharply the labelling of smooth muscle cells of the media.

Inhibition of DNA synthesis was practically complete in the animals sacrificed 15 days after surgery. In addition it is worth noting that the steroid did not modify the uptake of the label by the regenerating endothelium and that labelling of the modified smooth muscle cells of the intimal thickening was only moderately inhibited.

From the results reported it appears that *in vivo* the inhibitory effect of glucocorticoids on DNA synthesis and mitotic rate of arterial smooth muscle is not related to hyperlipemia and that the endothelial barrier does not play any important role in such inhibition. The steroid effect seems to be cell specific; actually in steroid-treated animals no inhibition on the growth of regenerating endothelium was observed. It is very likely that adrenal steroids act directly at a cellular level as suggested for other tissues, namely for the skeletal muscle [16–19]. Our findings, therefore, should indicate that arterial smooth muscle is equipped by specific receptor sites for steroid action, membrane linked or more likely intracellularly

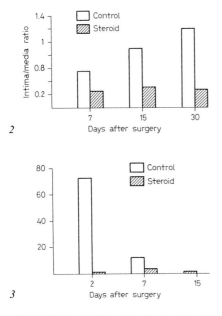

2

3

Fig. 2. Intimal thickening in the denuded carotid artery of control and steroid-treated rabbits.

Fig. 3. ^{3}H-thymidine labelling in the tunica media of the denuded carotid artery of control and steroid-treated rabbits. On the ordinate the mean number of labelled nuclei per 1,000. No label in steroid group 15 days after surgery.

located. As to the exact mechanism of the inhibitory effect, DNA polymerase activity, histones, and lysosomes may be implicated, but at present these are only speculations and the problem remains still open to future investigation. Besides, the possibility that steroids may interfere also with some plasmatic factor stimulating smooth muscle growth cannot be discarded.

Summary

Tritiated thymidine radioautography was employed to study the effect of glucocorticoids on smooth muscle proliferation in rabbit arteries. In the aorta and pulmonary artery of rabbits with cholesterol atherosclerosis, labelled cell counts showed that these steroids decrease the deoxyribonucleic acid synthesis in the intimal plaques. The inhibitory effect on thymidine uptake was found to be dose dependent and closely related to the antiinflammatory potency of the steroid tested. In another set of experiments the smooth muscle proliferation occurring in the rabbit carotid artery after disendothelization was studied. In these normolipemic animals the inhibition of DNA synthesis was particularly evident in the medial smooth muscle cell; concomitantly, in steroid-treated animals the myointimal thickening in the denuded area was less prominent. It is concluded that very likely the glucocorticoid effect on the artery is due to a direct interaction of the steroid with smooth muscle cells.

References

1   CAVALLERO, C.; LELLIS, C. DE; TONDO, U. DI; MINGAZZINI, P.; NATOLI, S.; PERICOLI, N.; PESANDO, P.; SPAGNOLI, L.G., and VILLASCHI, S.: Reactive and proliferative changes of the arterial smooth muscle in experimental athero-sclerosis: hormonal control; in CAVALLERO The arterial wall in atherogenesis, pp. 25–42 (Piccin, Padua 1975).

2   ROSS, R. and GLOMSET, J.A.: The pathogenesis of atherosclerosis. New Engl. J. Med. *295:* 369–377, 420–425 (1976).

3   ROSS, R.; GLOMSET, J.; KARIYA, B., and HARKER, L.: A platelet-dependent serum factor that stimulates the proliferation of arterial smooth muscle cells *in vitro.* Proc. natn. Acad. Sci. USA *71:* 1207–1210 (1974).

4   RUTHERFORD, B.R. and ROSS, R.: Platelet factors stimulate fibroblasts and smooth muscle cells quiescent in plasma-serum to proliferate. J. Cell Biol. *69:* 196–204 (1976).

5   STOUT, R.W.; BIERMAN, E.L., and ROSS, R.: Effect to insulin on the prolifera-tion of cultured primate arterial smooth muscle cells. Circulation Res. *36:* 319–327 (1975).

6   BIERMAN, E.L. and ALBERS, J.J.: Lipoprotein uptake by cultured human arterial smooth muscle cells. Biochim. biophys. Acta *388:* 198–202 (1975).

7   CAVALLERO C.: Le rôle de la paroi artérielle dans l'athérogénèse; dans Collo-ques int. Cent. natn. rech. scient., pp. 893–916 (Centre national de la recherche scientifique, Paris 1967).

8   CAVALLERO, C.; TUROLLA, E., and RICEVUTI, G.: Cell proliferation in the athero-sclerotic plaques of cholesterol-fed rabbits. I. Colchicine and (^{3}H) thymidine studies. Atherosclerosis *13:* 9–20 (1971).

9   CAVALLERO, C.: in WOLF The artery and the process of arteriosclerosis. Advances in experimental medicine and biology, vol. 16A, p. 179 (Plenum Press, New York 1971).

10 CAVALLERO, C.; TONDO, U. DI; MINGAZZINI, P.L.; PESANDO, P.C., and SPAGNOLI, L.G.: Cell proliferation in the atherosclerotic lesions of cholesterol-fed rabbits. II. Histological, ultrastructural and radioautographic observations on epineph-rine-treated rabbits. Atherosclerosis *17:* 49–62 (1973).

11 CAVALLERO, C.; TONDO, U. DI; MINGAZZINI, P.L.; NICOSIA, R.; PERICOLI, M.N.; SARTI, P.; SPAGNOLI, L.G.; and VILLASCHI, S.: Cell proliferation in the athero-sclerotic plaques of cholesterol-fed rabbits. III. Histological and radioauto-graphic observations on glucocorticoid-treated rabbits. Atherosclerosis 25: 145–152 (1976).

12 SCHMITT, G.; KNOCHE, K.; JUNGE-HÜLSING, G.; POCH, R., und HAUSS, W.H.: Über die Reduplikation von Aortenwandzellen bei arterieller Hypertonie. Z. Kreislaufforsch. 58: 461–487 (1970).

13 CRANE, W.A.J. and DUTTA, L.P.: The utilisation of tritiated thymidine for deoxyribonucleic acid synthesis by the lesions of experimental hypertension in rats. J. Path. Bact. 86: 83 (1963).

14 CAVALLERO, C.; TONDO, U. DI; MINGAZZINI, P.L.; SPAGNOLI, L.G., and CAVAL-LERO, M.: Cellular proliferation in the arterial walls of epinephrine-treated rabbits. Experientia 28: 265–266 (1972).

15 FISHMAN, J.A.; GRAEME, B.R., and KARNOWSKY, M.J.: Endothelial regeneration in the rat carotid artery and the significance of endothelial denudation in the pathogenesis of myointimal thickening. Lab. Invest. 32: 339–351 (1975).

16 THOMPSON, E.B. and LIPPMAN, M.E.: Mechanism of action of glucocorticoids. Metabolism 23: 159 (1974).

17 MAYER, M.; KAISER, M.; MILHOLLAND, R.J., and ROSEN, F.: The binding of dexamethasone and triamcinolone acetonide to glucocorticoid receptors in rat skeletal muscle. J. biol. Chem. 249: 5236 (1974).

18 MAYER, M.; KAISER, N.; MILHOLLAND, R.J., and ROSEN, F.: Cortisol binding in rat skeletal muscle. J. biol. Chem. 250: 1207 (1975).

19 MAYER, M. and ROSEN, F.: Glucocorticoid receptors in skeletal muscle; in SHAFRIR Contemporary topics in the study of diabetes and metabolic endo-crinology, pp. 173–181 (Academic Press, New York 1975).

Dr. C. CAVALLERO, IInd Institute of Pathological Anatomy, University of Rome, Viale Regina Elena 324, I-00161 Rome (Italy)

Prog. biochem. Pharmacol., vol. 14, pp. 94–98 (Karger, Basel 1977)

Smooth Muscle Cell Response to Endothelial Injury

L. G. Spagnoli, R. Nicosia, S. Villaschi and C. Cavallero

IInd Institute of Pathological Anatomy, University of Rome, Rome

Introduction

In recent years, a good deal of data has been accumulated on the arterial wall responses to injury. It is now ascertained that every mechanical damage to the arterial wall stimulate smooth muscle cell (SMC) proliferation in the intima with production of a thickening. Myointimal cells seem to derive by migration and proliferation of medial SMC in the intima [6].

SMC proliferation, in the media of elastic arteries, has been reported in autoradiographic studies on early lesions of hypercholesterolemic animals [7, 9] and during the response of the arterial wall to mechanical injuries, always including lesions of the tunica media [5, 10]. Moreover, a proliferative response of the tunica intima has been induced by a selective injury of the endothelium [4, 8].

The aim of our study has been to investigate with autoradiographic and electron microscopic methods, the response of the tunica media to a selective endothelial injury and to collect data on the dynamic of the relationships between medial SMC intima proliferation.

Material and Methods

30 New Zealand rabbits of either sexes, weighing 1–1.5 kg, have been used. Endothelium of the left common carotid arteries was air-dried following the technique previously used in rats by Fishman et al. [4], with minor modifications. Groups of animals were then sacrificed at 1, 2, 3, 7, 15, 30, 90 and 300 days after surgery.

Left carotid arteries as well as the right ones, used as controls, were fixed by perfusion with Karnovsky's fluid (1:2). Thin rings, obtained by slicing each carotid perpendicularly to the main axis, were processed in part for electron microscopy and the most for light microscopy. For the autoradiographic studies 2–3 animals per group were injected intravenously, 1 h before sacrifice, with 1 mCi of ^{3}H-thymidine (Radiochemical Center, Amersham; specific activity 16.2–20.2 Ci/mmol) per kilogram body weight. Sections of 2 μm were exposed for 15 days, after coating with KODAK NTB 2, and developed in KODAK D 19. Labeled nuclei among the endothelial cells of the edges of the lesion, the SMC in the inner half of the tunica media and the cells present in the intima, were counted and expressed as ratio to 1,000 unlabeled nuclei.

The maximal width of the intimal thickening was measured and expressed as ratio to the width of the media, measured at the same point. Finally, each carotid ring, in the groups of 1, 2, 3, 7 and 15 days, was searched for the presence of SMC in the gaps of the IEL. The number of these 'migrating cells' was expressed as a mean for each group.

Results

Table I summarizes the main results of our investigation. Integrity of the medial SMC was ascertained electron microscopically in the carotid arteries 1 day after surgery and in one case by the dye exclusion test following the method of Björkerud and Bondjers [1]. However electron microscopic studies showed an edematous swelling of the amorphous ground substance mainly in the innermost interlamellar spaces together with an apparent decrease in number of SMC. All the animals, displaying more than 2–3 leukocytes per carotid ring, were discarded.

Migrating SMC were observed in light and electron microscopy by 24 h up to 15 days after injury, but exceptionally low values were registered in all carotids at 2 days. Obviously, no 'migrating cells' were found in the controls. Starting from day 3, also labeled 'migrating cells' could be seen.

It is of interest that the labeling index of the media reached its maximum 2 days after injury, while in the intima the highest number of labeled cells was observed at 3 days. No labeled cells were observed in the media of the control carotid over 15,000 cells counted, whilst in the endothelium $0.96 \pm 0.6 \, ^0/_{00}$ labeled cells were found.

Table I. Summary of the experimental data

Days	³H-thymidine labeled cells, ‰			Semiquantitative morphological observations	
	endothelium	Intima	media	IT:M	'migrating cells'
1	none		none		1.72
2	207 ± 34.25		72.8 ± 13.25		0.14
3	69.09 ± 9.78	49.72 ± 4.22	26.32 ± 2.40	0.15 ± 0.09	3.25
7	18.52 ± 2.62	46.28 ± 5.32	12.76 ± 2.37	0.55 ± 0.00	3.55
15	none	3.57 ± 2.61	1.54 ± 0.80		2.20
30	1.64 ± 0.82	7.45 ± 3.02	2.26 ± 0.86	1.08 ± 0.08	
90	none	none	none		
300	none	none	none	0.59 ± 0.07	

Thickening of the intima was observed starting from day 3 after surgery and reached its maximum at day 15; at this stage its width was practically the same as that of underlying media. Our observations on the late stages of the intimal thickening will be presented elsewhere.

Discussion

The SMC proliferation in the media of arteries, subjected to various injuries, has been a matter of different interpretations [5, 7, 9, 10]. In this concern, the main results of our research may be summarized as follow: (1) the early reaction of the arterial wall to the disendothelialization is represented by proliferation of medial SMC whilst the intimal thickening occurs later; (2) migration of medial SMC may be ascertained soon before the start of the proliferative response of the tunica media; (3) it seems likely that migration in its earliest stages leads to some hypocellularity of the media.

These findings support the view that, after endothelial injury, migration rather than proliferation, probably due to some chemotactic factor, is the key event for the intimal thickening. In this connection it is noteworthy that in other experimental models, such as in epinephrine-treated animals, thickening of the intima does not occur, in spite of a marked proliferation of the media [2, 3].

Summary

Electron microscopy and autoradiography with ^{3}H-thymidine have been employed to study the cellular dynamic of intimal thickening occurring in the rabbit carotid artery after selective endothelial injury. The results obtained suggest that migration of SMC of the tunica media rather than proliferation is the key event in the development of the intimal thickening.

References

1   BJÖRKERUD, S. and BONDJERS, G.: Endothelial integrity and viability in the aorta of the normal rabbits and rats as evaluated with dye exclusion tests and interference contrast microscopy. Atherosclerosis 15: 285–300 (1972).

2   CAVALLERO, C.; DI TONDO, U.; MINGAZZINI, P.; SPAGNOLI, L.G., and CAVALLERO, M.: Cellular proliferation in the arterial walls of epinephrine-treated rabbits. Experientia 28: 263–265 (1972).

3   CONSTANTINIDES, P.; GUTMANN-AERSPERG, N., and HOSPES, D.: Accelerattion of intima atherogenesis through prior medial injury. Archs Path. 66: 247–254 (1958).

4   FISHMAN, J.A.; RYAN, G.B., and KARNOVSKY, M.J.: Endothelial regeneration in the rat carotid artery and the significance of endothelial denudation in the pathogenesis of myointimal thickening. Lab. Invest. 32: 339–351 (1975).

5   HASSLER, O.: The origin of the cells constituting arterial intima thickening: an experimental autoradiographic study with the use of ^{3}H-thymidine. Lab. Invest. 22: 286–293 (1970).

6   ROSS, R. and GLOMSET, J.A.: Atherosclerosis and the arterial smooth muscle cell: proliferation of smooth muscle is a key event in the genesis of the lesions of atherosclerosis. Science 180: 1332–1339 (1973).

7   STARY, H.C. and MCMILLAN, G.C.: Kinetics of cellular proliferation in experimental atherosclerosis: radioautography with grain counts in cholesterol-fed rabbits. Archs Path. 89: 173–183 (1970).

8   STEMERMAN, M.B. and ROSS, R.: Experimental arteriosclerosis. I. Fibrous plaque formation in primates, an electron microscope study. J. exp. Med. 136: 769–789 (1972).

9   THOMAS, W.A.; FLORENTIN, R.A.; NAM, S.C.; KIM, D.N.; JONES, R.M., and LEE, K.T.: Preproliferative phase of atherosclerosis in swine fed cholesterol. Archs Path. 86: 621–643 (1968).

10 WEBSTER, W.S.; BISHOP, S.P., and GEER, J.C.: Experimental aortic intimal thickening. I. Morphology and source of intimal cells. Am. J. Path. 76: 245–259 (1974).

Dr. L.G. SPAGNOLI, IInd Institute of Pathological Anatomy, University of Rome, Viale Regina Elena, 324, I-00161 Rome (Italy)

Prog. biochem. Pharmacol., vol. 14, pp. 99–102 (Karger, Basel 1977)

Abnormal Maturation of Elastic Fibres in the Atherosclerotic Intima

IAN RANNIE

Department of Pathology, Dental School, University of Newcastle upon Tyne, Newcastle upon Tyne

While not departing from the DUGUID [1976] proposition that incorporation of mural thrombi is responsible for much of the intimal lesion in atherosclerosis, it has to be admitted that a good deal of the tissue is the product of vascular smooth muscle cells which migrate from the media when the vessel is injured [KÁDÁR, 1976]. These cells are known to produce collagen, elastic fibres and ground substance. That this process is not always carried out in the normal way can be seen in medio-necrosis, where there is an imbalance between ground substance and fibre production which may lead to dissecting aneurysm and also experimentally in copper-deficient developing embryos and in lathyrism. Discussing this recently, LEVENE and MURRAY [1977] postulated that lysyl oxidase, the enzyme responsible for the cross-linking of both the collagen and the elastic fibres, was both copper dependent and vitamin B_6 dependent. They suggested that a failure in cross-linking could lead to the fraying and splitting lesions of the elastic laminae found in the coronary arteries of infants dying in the perinatal period and this could be produced by B_6 deficiency in the pregnant woman.

There is considerable evidence now [COTTA-PEREIRA et al., 1976] that three types of elastic fibre can be identified and they have characterised the EM appearances of these as follows. The mature elastic fibre shows an amorphous appearance with peripheral microfibrils and these authors go on to describe another fibre which they call elaunin which has only a small amount of the structureless material which they equate with elastin and the majority of the fibre is made up of microfibrillar material. The third type of fibre they identify as oxytalan fibre – first described by

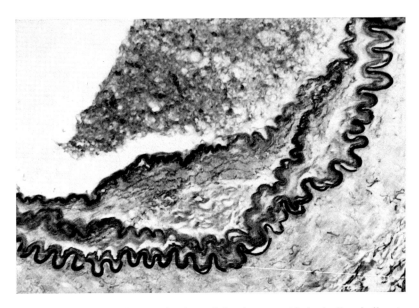

Fig. 1. Oxidised orcein. Newly formed laminae morphologically similar to elastica but differing in intensity of staining reaction with orcein. ×190.

FULLMER and LILLIE in 1958. This fibre they say is made up entirely of microfibrils and has no amorphous element.

Oxytalan fibres are well seen in the human periodontal membrane and can be stained with many dyes following oxidation of the tissue with oxone [RANNIE, 1963]. These fibres have a considerable affinity for orcein after oxidation and are then indistinguishable from elastica. Indeed we reserve the term oxytalan for those fibres such as are found in the periodontal membrane or in the tympanic membrane [CAMERON *et al.,* 1970] where one ordinarily does not find elastic fibres.

When we apply oxone to developing embryonal tissues or to healing tissues, orcein-positive fibres are shown in situations where eventually elastic fibres will be found. These fibres we term pre-elastic. It is possible that it is only after maturation that the microfibrillar element will show strong affinity for the elastic tissue stains and there is some evidence that it is the microfibrillar element and not the amorphous element of the mature fibre which stains with some of these dyes such as aldehyde thionine.

When the tissue of atherosclerotic lesions is stained with orcein after oxidation with oxone we find that there is positive staining and this suggests that microfibrillar material is being laid down, but when we come to look at the more severe lesions such as those seen in Buerger's disease, we see that the newly formed elastic tissue does not have the same tinctorial qualities as the original laminae and this suggests that its make-up may be different (fig. 1).

So far we have not disagreed with the suggestion that this new tissue may be produced in certain circumstances by smooth muscle cells, but one has to be reminded that it is also accepted that following certain injuries to the vessel the active cells are not myocytes but are cells invading from the blood stream [HAUSS, 1973]. It is entirely possible that these cells are not programmed to produce mature elastic fibrils such as are found in blood vessels. We do not know which cells produce the oxytalan fibres in the periodontal membrane but it would seem likely that these are fibroblasts.

In conclusion we would suggest that the electron microscopists should accept that there is a recognisable pre-elastic stage in the developing elastic fibre where the appearances may be more like that of the oxytalan fibre, and that they should be on the look-out for these appearances.

Summary

It is probable that the conditions obtaining during cellular proliferation occurring as a result of damage to the vessel wall will not be at optimum level. The amino oxidase, lysyl oxidase, is copper-dependent and is required for proper cross-linkage in the maturing fibre. Elastic tissue in blood vessels is normally produced by smooth muscle cells and in circumstances where other cells derived from the blood are involved the production of fibres and ground substance may be altered. Orcein staining alone, or after oxidation with oxone, shows different tinctorial affinities for the fibres in the thickened intima and may indicate some departure from normality in their make-up.

References

CAMERON, D.S.; JENNINGS, E.H., and RANNIE, I.: Oxytalan fibres in the human tympanic membrane. J. Lar. Otol. 84: 1235–1239 (1970).

Cotta-Pereira, G.; Guerra, R.F., and David-Pereira, J.F.: The use of tannic acid-glutaraldehyde in the study of elastic and elastic-related fibres. Stain Technol. *51:* 7–11 (1976).

Duguid, J.B.: The dynamics of atherosclerosis, p. 19 (Aberdeen University Press, Aberdeen 1976).

Fullmer, H.M. and Lillie, R.D.: A previously undescribed connective tissue fibre. J. Histochem. Cytochem. *6:* 425–430 (1958).

Hauss, W.H.: Tissue alterations due to experimental arteriosclerosis; in Vogel Connective tissue and ageing. Workshop Conference Hoechst, vol. 1, pp. 23–33 (Excerpta Medica, Amsterdam 1973).

Kádár, A.: Smooth muscle cells and elastic fibres in connection with the development of the morphological lesions of arteriosclerosis. Atherogenese *1:* 61–75 (1976).

Levene, C.I. and Murray, J.C.: The etiological role of maternal vitamin-B_6 deficiency in the development of atherosclerosis. Lancet *i:* 628–629 (1977).

Rannie, I.: Observations on the oxytalan fibre of the periodontal membrane. Trans. Eur. orthod. Soc. *39:* 127–136 (1963).

Dr. I. Rannie, Department of Pathology, Dental School, University of Newcastle upon Tyne, *Newcastle upon Tyne NE1 8TA* (England)

Prog. biochem. Pharmacol., vol. 14, pp. 103–110 (Karger, Basel 1977)

Proliferation of Primary Cultures from Rat Aortic Media

Effects of Hyperlipemic Serum[1]

M.C. BOURDILLON, J.P. BOISSEL and B. CROUZET

INSERM, Vascular Physiopathology, Lyon-Bron

In the development of the atherosclerotic (AS) plaque, cell proliferation is commonly held to be a constant factor. The smooth muscle cell (SMC) of the media and/or intima is viewed by several investigators as the main reactive cell in the atherogenic process [13, 14, 19, 20, 24]. An increased and localized mitotic activity could be seen as a primary cytological alteration before histological lesions [1, 21]. In relation to arterial biopathology, it seems particularly interesting to study arterial SMC cytodynamics: an *in vitro* study may provide some indications on SMC growth. For this purpose we have used a culture pattern from rat aortic explants.

First, we shall describe the cell growth in our 'normal' conditions of culture and afterwards we shall study the effects of hypercholesterolemic serum (HCS) added to the medium.

Growth Pattern of Aortic Medial Cells

The thoracic aorta was removed from 7-week-old rats. The adventitia was stripped off. Each explant (aortic ring 0.5 mm in length) was placed in the central area of a Falcon flask. It was overlaid with MEM medium Earle's salts supplemented with 10 % calf serum. Renewal of medium was made twice a week (pH 7.4). Histological and ultrastructural controls showed endothelium disappearing during this procedure. Thus it could be reasonably asserted that the culture cells are issued from the media [2, 3].

Three *parameters* related to time were measured weekly: the surface

---

[1] Supported by a grant from the DGRST No. 75.7.0938.

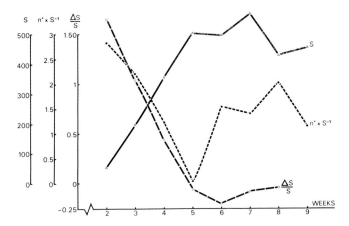

Fig. 1. Kinetics of cell proliferation of primary aortic cultures represented by three parameters related to time: S = surface area of cultures; ΔS/S = relative increase of surface; n* $\times$ S^{-1} = number of ^{3}H-thymidine labelled cells per unit surface.

of the culture (S), the relative increase of surface area (ΔS/S) and the number of labelled cells per unit surface following ^{3}H-thymidine incorporation (n* $\times$ S^{-1}). The curve of primary culture surface showed a continuous growth until the fifth week and reaches a plateau beyond that time (fig. 1). The two other parameters decreased regularly during the first phase to attain a minimum at the beginning of the plateau period.

These *results* showed two distinctive phases in the primary cultures [4]. The graph of the first phase corresponds to the surface extension of the neo-tissue; but ΔS/S is not constant, as shown in figure 2, and many hypotheses could explain this phenomenon. The second plateau period does not correspond to an absence of DNA synthesis since the cells incorporate thymidine during this period. But there is a lack of correlation between the surface evolution and the number of cells in S phase per unit surface. This phenomenon may result from a block of cells in S phase, or a cellular mortality rate which compensates the number of divisions, or a stratified outgrowth of the culture.

Some *characteristics* of primary cultures of rat aorta may be noted: (a) some cells are still capable of mitosis, since subcultures are possible; (b) the neo-tissue is multilayered as shown in histological preparations in vertical sections; (c) the plateau phase seems to correspond to a particular ultrastructural state of the neo-tissue [2, 5], and (d) the growth stop

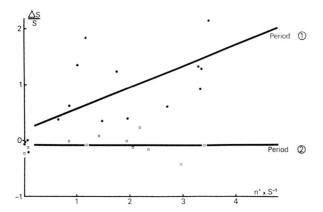

Fig. 2. Relation between relative increase of surface and S phase cell number per unit surface, during the growth phase (period 1) and the plateau phase (period 2). ● = Period 1: $\Delta S/S = 0.368(n^* \times S^{-1}) + 0.187$, $p < 0.01$; □ = period 2: $\Delta S/S = 0.007(n^* \times S^{-1}) - 0.063$, n.s.

phenomenon is different from contact inhibition, since the disposable surface is not completely covered [4].

In vitro outgrowth of cells yielded a possible pattern of the proliferation of mediacytes involved in the atherogenesis process. This event may be not entirely illusory, since during the plateau phase some cells appear with ultrastructural aspects showing some resemblances to foam cells of the AS plaque.

Effects of Hypercholesterolemic Serum

The growth of medial cells may be altered by different factors, particularly by hyperlipemic serum. We studied the effect of homologous HCS on proliferation of SMC *in vitro* using this culture pattern [6].

The *object* of this work was essentially to: (1) Determine whether the growth effect of HCS was also observed with cells of rat aortic media. This animal is known to be particularly 'resistant' to experimental AS produced by dietary fat [22]. (2) Determine whether there exists a relationship between the growth effect and the cholesterol level of HCS. (3) Determine whether the stage of the culture at which the serum is incubated has any marked effect on the cell proliferation.

Table I. Combination of tested factors

Final cholesterol concentration in culture medium g/l	NCRS	0.040	0.030	0.035	0.050
	HCRS	0.128	0.400	0.230	0.415
Age of the cultures at start of experiments			0	0	growth phase	plateau phase
Incubation time, weeks			3	3	5	4

Methods. Four experiments were performed using culture media supplemented with one of the following concentrations of pooled serum: 5 % calf serum +5 % hypercholesterolemic rat serum (HCRS); 5 % calf serum +5 % normocholesterolemic rat serum (NCRS).

The final concentrations of cholesterol in the culture medium are presented on table I. Serum was added to cultures of different ages, namely, the initial time, the growth phase or the plateau period. The time of serum incubation varied from 3 to 5 weeks. The surface area of the proliferative sheet of primary cells surrounding the aortic explant was measured weekly.

Results. They were analyzed by a global test using analysis of variance with three controlled factors (media, rats and time). They are presented on figures 3 and 4.

(1) When sera are tested at the beginning of the culture, with HCRS 3-fold the NCRS cholesterol level, no difference occurred between the two homologous sera within 3 weeks of culture.

(2) In the same culture conditions but with higher cholesterol level (HCRS 13-fold the NCRS), the mean surface of cultures incubated with HCRS was doubled and the difference with NCRS was very significant within 3 weeks ($p < 0.01$).

(3) When the sera were incubated during the growth period before the stabilization of the culture, HCRS induced a higher proliferation than did NCRS; in this experiment HCRS was nearly 7-fold NCRS cholesterol level. A marked difference was observed between the two homologous sera ($p < 0.001$).

(4) During the plateau phase, with serum incubated during 4 weeks, no difference occurred between the two homologous sera in spite of HCRS cholesterol being 8-fold the corresponding concentration of NCRS.

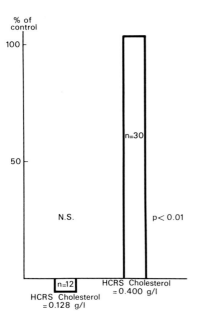

Fig. 3. Increase or decrease of surface cultures with two HCRS different in cholesterol level, expressed as % of control NCRS, within 3 weeks.

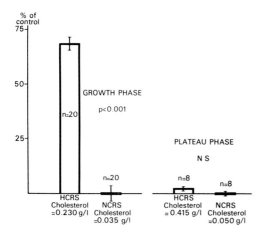

Fig. 4. Increase of surface cultures incubated with HCRS, expressed as % of control NCRS, during the growth phase and the plateau phase.

Some *comments* can be pointed out from the above results:

(1) The homologous HCS has an *in vitro enhancing effect* on growth of cells from *rat* aortic media.

(2) This effect depends on the cholesterol level in the culture medium: no effect with low concentration (0.128 g/l) and it was present with higher cholesterol levels (0.400 g/l).

(3) This effect is related to the *chronology of incubation* with HCRS: marked effect at the beginning of the culture; still appreciable during the growth phase; absent at the beginning of the plateau phase. This last result is apparently different from those reported by FISCHER-DZOGA [9] who observed an enhancing effect of hyperlipemic serum incubated at this time on monkey cells.

(4) The final concentrations of cholesterol used in culture media are low compared to *in vivo* blood levels. Thus, *human or experimental hyper-lipemic* sera might have a marked effect on cell growth. But it is not the only serum factor involved in cell proliferation, as suggested by the variability of growth curves obtained with calf serum [6].

(5) Cells derived from rat aortic media showed an appreciable response to hypercholesterolemic stimulus *in vitro,* as in the case of cells from other species. The effect of homologous HCS was reported on primary cultures of aortic media from monkey and rabbit and a second growth phase was observed by adding HCS [9, 10]. The surface of cultures of SMC from monkey aorta was increased 4-fold with 5 % HCS as compared to NCS [15]. At initial stages of rabbit aorta cultures, 20 % homologous HCS stimulated both cell migration and proliferation and the rate of outgrowth from AS aortae exceeded that of the intact aortae [18]. But with respect to growth behavior in long-term culture, the replicative life-span of human AS plaque cells was equal to or less than that of the corresponding normal medial cells [17]. Increased mitotic index was also observed in cultures and explants of swine aorta exposed to HCS [8, 11].

Cells in primary cultures closely resemble cells in the *in vivo* artery where similar observations have been reported. Therefore, initial proliferation and migration of SMC occurring in intima of AS arteries *in vivo* might be influenced by hypercholesterolemia. Many investigators noted an increased arterial cell proliferation ocurring in *in vivo* hypercholestero-lemia [7, 12, 16, 21, 23].

In conclusion, this study provides some information concerning the kinetics of rat aorta primary cultures and effects of HCS. Some appreciable response to hypercholesterolemic stimulus was obtained in cells from rats, who are known to be rather resistant to such treatment *in vivo*. It is a possible pattern of the proliferation of mediacytes involved in atherogenesis process.

Summary

Tissue cultures have been made from explants of thoracic aortas to study the growth pattern of rat aortic mediacytes. Three parameters were measured weekly: the surface of the culture, the relative increase of this surface and the number of ^{3}H-thymidine labelled cells per unit surface. The primary cultures showed two distinctive phases: a first phase with continuous growth followed by a plateau phase. We studied the growth effect of homologous hypercholesterolemic serum added to the cultures. The cell proliferation was affected by the cholesterol level in the medium and the stage of the culture at which serum incubation was initiated. An enhancing effect occurred in the rat resistant to such treatment *in vivo*.

References

1 BENDITT, E.P. and BENDITT, J.M.: Evidence for a monoclonal origin of human atherosclerotic plaques. Proc. natn. Acad. Sci. USA 70: 1753–1756 (1973).

2 BOISSEL, J.P.; BOURDILLON, M.C.; CROUZET, B.; SUPPLISSON, A.; PETIOT, M. et PERRIN, A.: Evolution ultrastructurale de cultures primaires de media aortique de rats. Arterial Wall 2: 105–121 (1974).

3 BOISSEL, J.P.; BOURDILLON, M.C.; LOIRE, R., and CROUZET, B.: Histological arguments for collagen and elastin synthesis by primary cultures of rat aortic media cells. Atherosclerosis 25: 107–110 (1976).

4 BOURDILLON, M.C.; BOISSEL, J.P.; CROUZET, B., and PERRIN, A.: Primary cultures of rat aortic media: a growth stop phenomenon different from contact inhibition. Biomedicine 25: 263–267 (1976).

5 BOURDILLON, M.C.; BOISSEL, J.P. et CROUZET, B.: Formation de cellules xanthomateuses *in vitro* à partir de media aortique de rat. Arterial Wall 3: 101–104 (1976).

6 BOURDILLON, M.C.; BOISSEL, J.P., and CROUZET, B.: Effects of hyperlipemic serum on the growth of primary cultures of rat aortic media. Artery 2: 438–450 (1976).

7 CAVALLERO, C.; TUROLLA, E., and RICEVUTI, G.: Cell proliferation in the atherosclerotic plaques of cholesterol-fed rabbits. I. Colchicine and ^{3}H-thymidine studies. Atherosclerosis 13: 9–20 (1971).

8 DAOUD, A.S.; FRITZ, K.E.; JARMOLYCH, J., and AUGUSTYN, J.M.: Use of aortic medial explants in the study of atherosclerosis. Expl. molec. Path. 18: 177–189 (1973).

9 FISCHER-DZOGA, K.: Response of aortic medial cells to hyperlipemic serum *in vitro;* in SCHETTLER and WEIZEL Atherosclerosis III, pp. 172–174 (Springer, Berlin 1974).

10 FISCHER-DZOGA, K. and WISSLER, W.: Stimulation of proliferation in stationary primary cultures of monkey aortic smooth muscle cells. II. Effect of varying concentrations of hyperlipemic serum and low density lipoproteins of varying dietary fat origins. Atherosclerosis *24:* 515–525 (1976).

11 FLORENTIN, R.A.; CHOI, B.H.; LEE, K.T., and THOMAS, W.A.: Stimulation of DNA synthesis and cell division *in vitro* by serum from cholesterol-fed swine. J. Cell Biol. *41:* 641–645 (1969).

12 FLORENTIN, R.A.; NAM, S.C.; LEE, K.T.; LEE, K.J., and THOMAS, W.A.: Increased mitotic activity in aortas of swine after three days of cholesterol feeding. Archs Path. *88:* 463–469 (1969).

13 GEER, J.C. and HAUST, M.D.: Smooth muscle cells in atherosclerosis, pp. 27–38 (Karger, Basel 1972).

14 HAUST, M.D.; MORE, R.H., and MOVAT, H.Z.: The role of smooth muscle cells in the fibrogenesis of arteriosclerosis. Am. J. Path. *37:* 377–389 (1960).

15 KAO, V.C.Y.; WISSLER, R.W., and DZOGA, K.: The influence of hyperlipemic serum on the growth of medial smooth muscle cells of rhesus monkey aorta *in vitro.* Circulation *38:* VI–12 (1968).

16 MCMILLAN, G.C. and STARY, H.C.: Preliminary experience with mitotic activity of cellular elements in the atherosclerotic plaques of cholesterol-fed rabbits studied by labeling with tritiated thymidine. Ann. N.Y. Acad. Sci. *149:* 699–709 (1968).

17 MOSS, N.S. and BENDITT, E.P.: Human atherosclerotic plaque cells and leiomyoma cells. Am. J. Path. *78:* 175–190 (1975).

18 MYASNIKOV, A.L. and BLOCK, Y.E.: Influence of some factors on lipoidosis and cell proliferation in aorta tissue cultures of adult rabbits. J. Atheroscler. Res. *5:* 33–42 (1965).

19 ROSS, R. and GLOMSET, J.A.: Atherosclerosis and the arterial smooth muscle cell. Science *180:* 1332–1339 (1973).

20 ROSS, R. and GLOMSET, J.A.: The pathogenesis of atherosclerosis. New Engl. J. Med. *295:* 369–377 (1976).

21 STARY, H.C. and MCMILLAN, G.C.: Kinetics of cellular proliferation in experimental atherosclerosis. Radioautography with grain counts in cholesterol-fed rabbits. Archs Path. *89:* 173–183 (1970).

22 THOMAS, W.A.; SCOTT, R.F.; LEE, K.T.; DAOUD, A.S., and JONES, R.M.: Experimental atherosclerosis in the rat; in ROBERTS and STRAUS comparative atherosclerosis, pp. 93–108 (Harper & Row, New York 1965).

23 THOMAS, W.A.; FLORENTIN, R.A.; NAM, S.C.; KIM, D.N.; JONES, R.M., and LEE, K.T.: Preproliferative phase of atherosclerosis in swine fed cholesterol. Archs Path. *86:* 621–643 (1968).

24 WISSLER, R.W.: The arterial medial cell, smooth muscle or multifunctional mesenchyme? J. Atheroscler. Res. *8:* 201–213 (1968).

Dr. M.C. BOURDILLON, INSERM, Unité 63, 22, avenue Doyen Lépine, *F-69500 Lyon-Bron* (France)

Prog. biochem. Pharmacol., vol. 14, pp. 111–114 (Karger, Basel 1977)

Twin Tracer Technique to Follow Up the Increased Permeability

Harry Jellinek[1]

2nd Department of Pathology, Semmelweis Medical University, Budapest

In our previous studies colloidal iron was used to study the changes of vessel permeability in experimental hypertension, hypoxia and excess cholesterol feeding.

The sequence of changes of permeability was studied in a 'time lapse' experiment. Hypoxia was maintained for 1 min and recirculation lasted for 1, 2, 5, 15 or 20 min. The appearance of colloidal iron was detectable already after 1 min hypoxia and 1 min recirculation. The amount of iron in the vessel wall increased parallel to the duration of hypoxia and recirculation.

Colloidal iron was present in the intima in the intercellular space and in the damaged smooth muscle cells as well as in the connective tissue cells of the adventitia. During its transmural transport the tracer was considerably diluted. This fact rendered its demonstration in the lymph vessels quite difficult. Therefore we developed a new method for the study of transmural material transport, i.e. we administered together with the colloidal iron an equal amount of Lipofundin S (B. Brown, Med. Pharm. Werke, Melsungen). Following hypoxia of 1 h duration the Lipofundin-iron mixture was injected directly into the aortic sac between the two ligatures. The presence of Lipofundin chylomicrons in the intima was demonstrated light microscopically in preparations stained with Sudan and Prussian blue. Sudan positivity was observed in the media already after 48 h.

In semi-thin sections Lipofundin droplets were seen in both the

[1] Technical coworker: Andrea Vicenty; operations: Iringo Németh, Teréz Zombori; EM engineer: Z. Saródy; photo assistants: Emöke Kádár, Katalin Kovács.

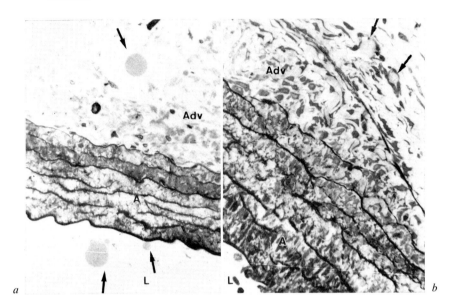

Fig. 1. a Toluidine blue stained semi-thin section. At the luminal surface and in the adventitia (Adv) the grayish Lipofundin droplets of various sizes (→) can be seen. *b* Semi-thin section from an acid-painted vessel. In the adventitia there is a dilatated lymph vessel containing the grayish droplets of Lipofundin (→). L = Lumen; A = aortic wall.

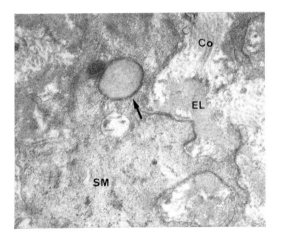

Fig. 2. In the medial smooth muscle cells (SM) a iron-coated Lipofundin droplet (→) is seen. Co = Collagen; EL = elastic lamina.

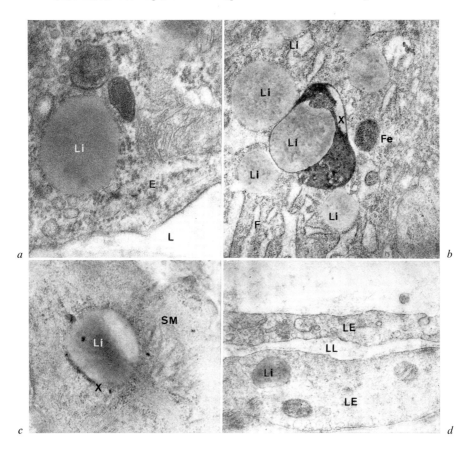

Fig. 3. a Endothelium (E) of an acid-painted aorta. The cell contains iron-coated Lipofundin (Li). L = Lumen. *b* Medial smooth muscle cell (SM) from an acid-painted aorta containing iron-coated (X) Lipofundin (Li) chylomicron. *a and b* Uranyl acetate contrasted preparations. *c* In the adventitial connective tissue cell (F) Lipofundin (Li) chylomicrons are seen; some of them carry attached iron (X). Free iron (Fe) granules are also present. Uranyl-lead contrasted preparation. *d* Part of an adventitial lymph vessel is shown. Nn its endothelium (LE) there is an iron-coated Lipofundin droplet (Li). LL = Lumen.

lumen and the adventitia (fig. 1a). The presence of Lipofundin in the endothelial cells was demonstrable by transmission electron microscopy. The colloidal iron was usually attached to the surface of the Lipofundin granules giving a sharp contour to the latter. Lipofundin contoured by

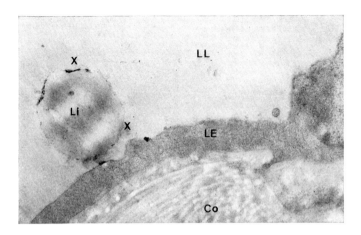

Fig. 4. Part of a lymph vessel exhibiting in its lumen (LL) over an endothelial
cell (LE) a Lipofundin droplet (Li) with occasional bound iron granules (X).
Co = Adventitial collagen. Contrasted only with uranyl.

iron was demonstrable also in the media of aortas damaged by hypoxia
(fig. 2).

In the second series of experiments we studied the changes in
permeability after acid-painting of the aorta. The presence of Lipofundin
and iron was demonstrable in the endothelial cells and the media by
light microscopy. In semi-thin sections the presence of Lipofundin
droplets was observed in the dilatated lymph vessels of the adventitia
(fig. 1b). In transmission electron micrographs the iron-coated Lipofundin
droplets were clearly visible in the aortic endothelial cells as well as in
the media (fig. 3). In the adventitial connective tissue cells and lymph
vessels (fig. 3) as well as in the latters lumen (fig. 4) there were also the
iron-coated droplets of Lipofundin detected.

The twin tracer technique appeared to be useful in the study not only
of the increased intimal permeability but also of that of the transmural
transport and drainage of material.

Dr. H. JELLINEK, Professor of Pathology, 2nd Department of Pathology,
Semmelweis Medical University, *Budapest* (Hungary)

Prog. biochem. Pharmacol., vol. 14, pp. 115–122 (Karger, Basel 1977)

Further Studies on the Effect of Regenerated Endothelium on Intimal Lipid Accumulation[1]

C.R. Minick, M.M. Litrenta, D.R. Alonso, M.F. Silane and M.B. Stemerman

Department of Pathology, Cornell University Medical College, New York, N.Y.

Introduction

Atherosclerosis is characterized by lipid accumulation in the thickened intima. Notwithstanding many years of research, the pathogenesis of the intimal thickening and lipid accumulation remains poorly understood. Experimental and clinicopathologic evidence indicates that injury to the arterial wall favors deposition of blood lipids at the site of injury and leads to atherosclerosis [1, 2, 4, 5, 8–15, 17–20]. Endothelial damage appears to be an early feature common to many types of arterial injury. This finding, together with other experimental evidence, has led to the hypothesis that endothelial damage will result in changes in the endothelial barrier thus exposing underlying smooth muscle cells to increased blood elements, in particular low density lipoprotein and platelets, which leads to smooth muscle proliferation and intimal thickening [6, 15, 16]. In addition, it is suggested that the continued absence of the endothelium will lead to increased transport of lipoprotein into the thickened intima where it accumulates and results in atherosclerosis.

Results of previous experiments reported from this laboratory are at variance with the above hypothesis and suggested that intimal thickening covered by regenerated endothelium was more prone to lipid accumulation than intimal thickening without endothelium or normal arterial wall [14]. In experiments reported here we further tested the hypothesis that rege-

[1] Supported by grants from The Cross Foundation, and research grants HL-01803, HL-18828, and HL-19109 from the National Heart, Lung and Blood Institute of the National Institutes of Health.

nerated endothelium favors lipid accumulation in the underlying intima and predisposes to atherosclerosis.

Materials and Methods

22 New Zealand white male rabbits weighing 2,000–3,500 g were divided into two groups. Group I was fed commercial rabbit chow low in total lipid and group II a diet supplemented with 0.5 % cholesterol by weight [12]. 30 days later, aortas were de-endothelialized as described previously [20]. Briefly, a 4-F embolectomy catheter with its balloon inflated at a pressure of approximately 500 mm Hg was drawn through the aorta of anesthetized rabbits. Following de-endothelialization all rabbits were continued on their assigned diets and sacrificed at 4 days and 1, 2, 4, 8 and 9 weeks following injury.

In order to distinguish endothelialized from de-endothelialized areas by gross examination, all rabbits were injected intravenously with 4 ml of 0.45 % Evans blue 40 min prior to sacrifice. Following fixation by perfusion full-thickness specimens of aorta, including de-endothelialized and re-endothelialized areas, were taken at four standard sites for light microscopy, scanning, and transmission electron microscopy as described previously [14]. Tissue sections for light microscopy were stained with hematoxylin and eosin, Weigert-van Gieson for elastic tissue, oil red O for fat, and alcian blue for proteoglycans. The amount of lipid in the intima and media of de-endothelialized areas, stained blue, and re-endothelialized areas, unstained and appearing nonblue, was graded as slight, moderate, and marked, as described previously [14]. The thickness of the intima in the blue and nonblue areas was measured at its thickest point using an ocular micrometer. Cellularity of the intima and underlying media in blue and nonblue areas was assessed using a point counting technique and counting the number of intersects that overlay nuclei or extracellular material. Observations made by light microscopy were confirmed by scanning and transmission electron microscopy on blocks taken from blue and nonblue areas.

Results

Prior to feeding the cholesterol-supplemented diet, the total serum cholesterol concentrations for rabbits of groups I and II were normal,

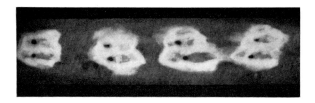

Fig. 1. Luminal surface of the thoracic portion of the aorta of rabbit de-endothelialized 14 days prior to sacrifice. Rabbit fed cholesterol-supplementted diet (group II) and injected with Ewans blue 40 min prior to sacrifice. De-endothelialized aorta, stained blue, surrounds unstained islands of regenerated endothelium appearing white. × 3.

40–80 mg/100 ml. Serum cholesterol concentration for rabbits of group I remained within normal range for the experimental period. During feeding of the cholesterol-supplemented diet, the average total serum cholesterol concentration for these rabbits increased to between 327 and 1,009 mg/100 ml with an overall mean of 723 mg/100 ml.

Grossly, the luminal surface of previously de-endothelialized segments of aorta revealed readily distinguishable regions that were stained or unstained by Evans blue dye. These regions were present in the same distribution in the two experimental groups and were characterized by a continuous blue-stained area surrounding approximately 35 unstained islands. In group I animals, each nonblue island consisted of a central gray zone surrounded by a thin intensely white, often incomplete, ring-like zone bordering on the blue area. With regard to number, distribution and size of blue and nonblue areas the luminal surface of aortas of cholesterol-fed animals (group II) were similar to group I. However, in contrast to group I animals, in group II the intensely white zone was usually much broader and often involved nearly the entire endothelial island (fig. 1).

Microscopically, three distinct types of change were regularly observed in animals of group I that corresponded to the grossly visible blue areas and gray and intensely white zones of unstained islands. The aortic wall in blue areas of rabbits of group I was characterized by fibromuscular intimal thickening containing 5–10 layers of smooth muscle cells. The luminal surface lacked an endothelial lining and was covered by smooth muscle cells. The aortic wall in the intensely white zone in the outer portion of nonblue islands was characterized by similar fibromuscular intimal thickening but, in contrast to blue areas, the thickened intima was covered by endothelial cells. The intima of intensely white zones of

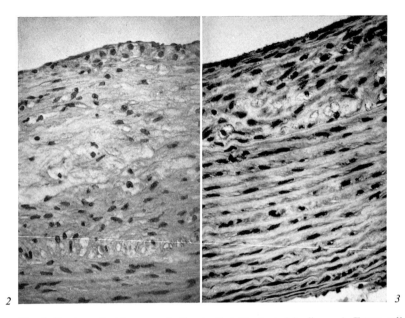

Fig. 2. Section of white area similar to that illustrated in figure 1. Foam cells and extracellular lipid accumulation are prominent. HE. × 200.

Fig. 3. Section of blue-stained area similar to that illustrated in figure 1. Intima is not as thick as in the adjacent white area (fig. 2) and lacks an endothelial covering. Only occasional foam cells are present deep in the intima. HE. × 200.

nonble areas was significantly thicker than the intima of adyacent blue areas (Wilcoxon Signed Ranks test, p <0.01). The intima of intensely white zones was less cellular than adjacent blue areas. In addition, preliminary observations indicate increased alcianophilia in white zones of nonblue areas as compared to blue areas. The aortic wall in gray zones was characterized by comparatively slight fibromuscular intimal thickening covered by endothelium. Slight to moderate fatty change was observed in the white zone of nonblue areas of some animals in group I; adjacent blue areas showed no fatty change. However, in the majority of animals of group I, no fatty change was seen in the aortic wall of any of the regions.

Histologic changes, consisting of the presence or absence of intimal thickening and presence or absence of endothelium, were similar in blue areas and intensely white zones of nonblue areas in animals of group I and II. As was the case in animals of group I, the intima was thicker in the intensely white zone of nonblue areas than in the adjacent blue areas and the intensely white zones were not as cellular as blue areas. However, in contrast to animals of group I, aortas of animals of group II revealed marked microscopic fatty change in cells and extracellular tissue of intima and subjacent media of blue and nonblue areas. The amount of fatty change was significantly greater in the intensely white zones of nonblue areas than in the adjacent blue areas (fig. 2, 3). Thus, 92 % of blue areas showed either no change or only slight fatty change; 80 % of nonblue areas showed moderate or marked fatty change ($\chi_1^2 = 42.90$, p <0.001). In contrast to animals of group I, intimal thickening often extended from the edge of the endothelial island to the ostium of the artery; hence there was either no gray zone or only a small gray zone.

Discussion

The purpose of experiments reported here was to further test the hypothesis that in hypercholesterolemic rabbits the absence of endothelium would lead to increased transport of lipid into the arterial wall and lipid accumulation in the intima and thereby predispose to atherosclerosis. Results of these experiments indicate that the quantity of lipid was much greater in areas of intimal thickening within endothelial islands covered by regenerated endothelium than in areas of intimal thickening not covered by endothelium. Thus, these results support those of our previous experiments [14] but do not support the hypothesis that the absence of endothelium favors lipid deposition and atherosclerosis.

The pathogenesis of the increased lipid accumulation in re-endothelialized areas of intimal thickening is not clear. Conceivably, re-endothelialization might favor accumulation of lipid by enhancing the uptake of lipid by endothelium and its transport to underlying tissue, by inhibiting release of lipid back into the blood, or by leading to changes in the structure of the intimal plaque or alteration of metabolism of smooth muscle cells within the plaque.

An increased number of smooth muscle cells in intima of nonblue areas could lead to increased avidity for lipid. However, results of experiments reported here indicate that increased cellularity in re-endothelialized area of intimal thickening does not account for the increased lipid accumulation since our results demonstrate that areas of intimal thickening lacking an endothelial covering are more cellular than intimal thickening covered by regenerated endothelium. Alternatively, an increased amount of extracellular material in nonblue areas could lead to increased avidity for lipid since elastin and glycosaminoglycans have been shown to bind to lipids both *in vitro* and *in vivo* [3, 7, 21]. Preliminary results support the latter possibility since there appears to be increased alcianophilic material in intensely white zones of nonblue areas of animals in group I, suggesting the presence of increased proteoglycans.

Results of experiments reported here indicate that the thickness of intima covered by regenerated endothelium was significantly greater than intimal thickening in adjacent blue areas devoid of endothelium, especially in animals of group II. The pathogenesis of the increased intimal thickness in areas covered by regenerated endothelium is also unknown. However, results of these experiments suggest that as a result of increased lipid accumulation or other mechanisms regenerated endothelium stimulates and sustains intimal thickening.

The design of these experiments differs from that of our previous experiments [14] in that hypercholesterolemia was induced prior to balloon injury. Thus animals were hypercholesterolemic at the time of injury, and during initiation of intimal thickening and endothelial regeneration. The results of the experiments were also different. In previous experiments, the intensely white zone formed a narrow rim around the endothelial island. In these experiments, the intensely white zone was much broader and in many instances extended from the ostium to the edge of the island. We believe these findings are in keeping with the interpretation that recently regenerated endothelium is associated with increased lipid accumulation and thereby enhances intimal thickening. Results could also be interpreted to indicate that increased serum lipids enhance intimal thickening around the ostium; and this intima is then re-endothelialized. After re-endothelialization, the thickened intima in the area of the ostium is then more likely to accumulate lipid.

In conclusion, results of our experiments are consistent with the hypothesis that endothelial damage or loss leads to smooth muscle proliferation and intimal thickening. However, these results do not support the hypothesis that the absence of endothelium favors lipid accumulation. Our findings indicate that thickened intima covered by regenerated endothelium is particularly prone to accumulate lipid. Although the pathogenesis of the increased lipid accumulation and increased intimal thickness in re-endothelialized areas remains unknown, the finding is intriguing and may be fundamental to our understanding of the pathogenesis of lipid accumulation in blood vessels and the development of atherosclerosis in man.

References

1 ALONSO, D.R.; STAREK, P.K., and MINICK, C.R.: Studies on the pathogenesis of atheroarteriosclerosis induced in rabbit cardiac allografts by the synergy of graft rejection and hypercholesterolemia. Am. J. Path. (in press, 1977).

2 ANITSCHKOW, N.N.: Experimental arteriosclerosis in animals; in COWDRY Arteriosclerosis, a survey of the problem, pp. 271–322 (MacMillan, New York 1933).

3 BERENSON, C.S.; SRINIVASAN, S.; DOLAN, P., and RADHAKRISHNAMURTHY, B.: Lipoprotein-acid mucopolysaccharide complexes from fatty streaks of human aorta. Circulation 44: 11–6 (1971).

4 CONSTANTINIDES, P.: Experimental atherosclerosis, pp. 1–88 (Elsevier, Amsterdam 1965).

5 DUFF, G.L.: Experimental cholesterol arteriosclerosis and its relationship to human arteriosclerosis. Archs Path. 20: 80–123, 259–304 (1935).

6 FISHER-DZOGA, K.; CHEN, R., and WISSLER, R.W.: Effects of serum lipoproteins on the morphology, growth and metabolism of arterial smooth muscle cells; in WAGNER and CLARKSON Advances in experimental biology and medicine, vol. 43; pp. 229–311 (Plenum Press, New York 1974).

7 GERÖ, S.; GERGELY, J.; DEVENYI, T.; JAKAG, L.; SZEKELY, J., and VIRAG, S.: Role of intimal mucoid substance in the pathogenesis of atherosclerosis. I. Complex formation in vitro between mucopolysaccharides from atherosclerotic intimas and plasma B-lipoproteins and fibrinogen. J. Atheroscler. Res. 1: 67 (1961).

8 HARDIN, N.J.; MINICK, C.R., and MURPHY, G.E.: Experimental induction of atherosclerosis by the synergy of allergic injury to arteries and lipid-rich diet. III. The role of earlier acquired fibromuscular intimal thickening in the pathogenesis of later developing atherosclerosis. Am. J. Path. 73: 301–326 (1973).

9 HARKER, L.A.; SLICHTER, S.J.; SCOTT, C.R., and ROSS, R.: Homocystinemia: vascular injury and arterial thrombosis. New Engl. J. Med. 291: 537–543 (1974).

10 HASS, G.L.: Observations on vascular structure in relation to human and experimental arteriosclerosis; in Symposium on Atherosclerosis, pp. 24–32 (National Academy of Sciences, Washington 1955).

11 HAUST, M.D.: Arteriosclerosis; in BRUNSON and GALL Concepts of disease: a textbook of pathology, pp. 451–487 (MacMillan, New York 1971).

12 MINICK, C.R.; MURPHY, G.E., and CAMPBELL, W.G., jr.: Experimental induction of athero-arteriosclerosis by the synergy of allergic injury to arteries and lipid-rich diet. I. Effect of repeated injections of horse serum in rabbits fed a dietary cholesterol supplement. J. exp. Med. 124: 635–652 (1966).

13 MINICK, C.R. and MURPHY, G.E.: Experimental induction of athero-arteriosclerosis by the synergy of allergic injury to arteries and lipid-rich diet. II. Effect of repeatedly injected foreign protein in rabbits fed a lipid-rich, cholesterol-poor diet. Am. J. Path. 73: 265–300 (1973).

14 MINICK, C.R.; STEMERMAN, M.B., and INSULL, W., jr.: Effect of regenerated

endothelium on lipid accumulation in arterial wall. Proc. natn. Acad Sci. USA (in press, 1977).

15 Ross, R. and Glomset, J.A.: Atherosclerosis and the arterial smooth muscle cell. Science *180:* 1332–1339 (1973).

16 Ross, R.; Glomset, J.A.; Kariya, B., and Harker, L.: A platelet-dependent serum factor that stimulates the proliferation of arterial smooth muscle cells *in vitro*. Proc. natn. Acad. Sci. USA *71:* 1207–1210 (1974).

17 Ross, R. and Glomset, J.A.: The pathogenesis of atherosclerosis. New Engl. J. Med. *295:* 369–376, 420–425 (1976).

18 Ross, R. and Harker, L.: Hyperlipidemia and atherosclerosis, chronic hyperlipidemia initiates and maintains lesions by endothelial cell desquamation and lipid accumulation. Science *193:* 1094–1100 (1976).

19 Stemerman, M.B. and Ross, R.: Experimental arteriosclerosis. I. Fibrous plaque formation in primates, an electron microscopic study. J. exp. Med. *136:* 769–789 (1972).

20 Stemerman, M.B.: Thrombogenesis of the rabbit arterial plaque, an electron microscopic study. Am. J. Path. *73:* 7–26 (1973).

21 Woodard, J.F.; Srinivasan, S.R.; Zimny, M.L.; Radhakrishmamurthy, B., and Berenson, C.S.: Electron microscopic features of lipoprotein-glycosaminoglycan complexes from human atherosclerotic plaques. Lab. Invest. *34:* 516–521 (1976).

Dr. C.R. Minick, Department of Pathology, Cornell University Medical College, *New York, N.Y.* (USA)

Prog. biochem. Pharmacol., vol. 14, pp. 123–133 (Karger, Basel 1977)

Arterial Uptake and Synthesis of Low Density Lipoproteins[1]

WILLIAM HOLLANDER, JOHN PADDOCK and MARILYN A. COLOMBO

Boston University Medical Center, Boston, Mass.

Introduction

One of the characteristic findings in atherosclerosis is the accumulation of low density lipoproteins (LDL) and very low density lipoproteins (VLDL) in the arterial intima [1]. The manner in which these lipoproteins are deposited in the arterial wall has not been established. However it appears likely that a number of mechanisms operate in lipoprotein deposition and these include the uptake, transport and degradation of plasma lipoprotein by the arteries as well as the biosynthesis of lipoproteins in the arteries. Recent studies of human vessels [2] suggest that the intracellular and extracellular transport of LDL and VLDL in atherosclerotic lesions may be impaired as a result of the interaction of these lipoproteins with acid mucopolysaccharides (AMPS) and the binding of these complexes to the connective tissue proteins of the plaque. The present study in subhuman primates is an extension of these studies and was undertaken to further clarify the mechanism involved in the accumulation of LDL and cholesterol in the atherosclerotic plaque.

Methods

Three groups of adult male cynomolgus monkeys *(Macaca fascicularis)* were studied on controlled diet. The control group of 10 animals was fed a low cholesterol diet containing monkey Purina chow while the

[1] Supported by USPHS Grant HL-13262.

atherosclerotic group of 10 animals was fed an atherogenic diet containing 2 % cholesterol and 10 % butter. The diets were fed for 6 months. A third group of 7 animals (regression group) was fed the atherogenic diet for 6 months following which the group received the low cholesterol diet for 12 months.

The composition and concentration of plasma lipoproteins were determined chemically following their separation by differential density ultracentrifugation [3]. Plasma LDL (d 1.019–1.063) isolated from each group of animals was iodinated with ^{125}I by the method of Mac Farlane as modified by BILHEIMER et al. [4]. Analyses of the ^{125}I-LDL preparation revealed that the percent of soluble counts in 10 % trichloroacetic acid (TCA) was less than 3 % and the percent of counts extractable by chloroform:methanol (2:1) was less than 4 %. The ^{125}I-LEL showed β-mobility on electrophoresis and gave immunoprecipitation lines of complete identity to unlabeled LDL. The preparation was shown to be free of contamination with other plasma proteins or lipoproteins by immunoelectrophoresis and immunodiffusion. For complexing radioactive cholesterol to serum lipoproteins, serum from each group was incubated with [4-^{14}C]-cholesterol (specific radioactivity 58 mCi/mM; New England Nuclear, Boston, Mass.) according to the method of GOODMAN and NOBLE [5].

Under phencyclidine sedation, ^{125}I-LDL prepared from a given experimental group was injected into the same group through an indwelling venous catheter in a dose of 5 μCi/kg. The ^{14}C-cholesterol preparations were similarly administered in a dose of 6 μCi/kg. Blood samples were collected in glass tubes containing EDTA at 10 and 30 min and at 1, 2, 3 and 4 h. Aliquots of plasma were assayed for ^{125}I radioactivity and for free and ester cholesterol content and radioactivity [6].

The lipoproteins in the final plasma sample (4-hour sample) were separated in the preparative ultracentrifuge and analyzed as described above. Over 95 % of the plasma ^{125}I radioactivity was recoverable in d 1.063–1.019 and more than 98 % of ^{125}I radioactivity in the isolated LDL and plasma samples were precipitable in 10 % TCA. Less than 3 % of the radioactivity in these samples was extractable by chloroform:methanol (2:1).

4 h after the injection of the radioactive preparations, the animals were sacrificed with intravenous pentabarbital. The thoracic aortae were removed immediately and maintained at 4° C while they were trimmed of surrounding connective tissue and fat and opened longitudinally. After washing the aorta in saline for 2 min, the inner portion of the aorta (in-

tima-media) was stripped from the adventitia and rinsed in saline again to assure the removal of contaminating plasma radioactivity from the surface of the vessel. The intima-media was transferred to counting tubes for direct counting of ^{125}I radioactivity. A portion of the tissue was finely minced and extracted with 1.65 M NaCl containing 0.1 % EDTA, pH 7.4, for 18 h at 4° C. Aliquots of the saline extract were assayed for ^{125}I radioactivity before and after dialysis against 0.15 M NaCl and following precipitation in 10 % TCA after the addition of carrier protein. The TCA soluble supernatant and the saline dialyzate were analyzed respectively for free-iodide radioactivity [7] and for heparin and manganese precipitable ^{125}I-LDL [8]. The saline-extracted tissue fragments were digested sequentially with collagenase and elastase or with a mixture of chondroitinase A, B, C and collagenase as previously described [2, 9, 10]. The digests were analyzed for ^{125}I radioactivity and for AMPS content [11].

For cholesterol and ^{14}C-cholesterol analyses a separate portion of minced intima-media was extracted with chloroform:methanol (2:1) and analyzed for free and total cholesterol content and radioactivity [6].

The subclavian carotid, iliac and femoral arteries were used to determine the distribution of ^{125}I-LDL by the technique of subcellular fractionation [6]. Representative sections of arterial tissue were taken for histological examination [2].

Lipoprotein Biosynthesis by Arterial Smooth Muscle Cells

Segments of thoracic aorta were obtained from normal cynomolgus monkeys and stripped of adventitia and outer portion of the media under sterile conditions and smooth muscle cells were grown from these explants according to the method of Ross [12].

One or more radioactive substrates were added to the incubation medium containing 10 % fetal calf serum in a final concentration of 1 μCi/ml. These were supplied by the New England Nuclear Corporation and included sodium acetate-1-[14]C (specific activity 59.2 mCi/mM), L-leucine [4,5,[3]H(N)] (specific activity 33.6 Ci/mM) and ^{35}S-sodium sulfate (specific activity 558 mC/mM). Following incubation for 24 h, the incubation media was decanted and the cell layer was removed by trypsinization, spun and homogenized in 0.15 M NaCl. The lipoproteins contained in the trypsin supernatant, incubation media and saline extract from homogenized cells were analyzed separately by differential ultracentrifugation with deuterium oxide being used to adjust the solvent density to 1.063g/ml [13]. Radiosulfate activity was assayed after isolation in the lipoprotein fractions as ^{35}S-AMPS [11].

The ultracentrifugally isolated lipoprotein fractions also were assayed for radioactivity by the technique of radioimmunodiffusion and radio-immunoelectrophoresis [14] after the addition of carrier lipoprotein to the samples.

Results

During the feeding of the high cholesterol diet the serum cholesterol rose to 582 mg/100 ml without a change in serum triglycerides (table I). The hypercholesterolemia was due largely to increase in plasma LDL and to a small extent to elevation of VLDL. These changes, as described previously [15], were accompanied by marked reductions of plasma HDL. When the diet was changed to a low cholesterol one (regression diet) the plasma lipid and lipoprotein concentrations returned to control values.

Morphological and Chemical Changes in Aortae

On gross and histological examination, the aorta of the control animals appeared normal except for an occasional fatty streak whereas the aorta of the group fed the atherogenic diet showed extensive involvement with fibrofatty lesions. The animals fed the regression diet also had numerous atherosclerotic plaques which were markedly fibrotic. These lesions were less cellular and fatty than those observed during the feeding of the atherogenic diet. The distribution of oil red O stainable lipid in diseased arteries was similar to that of the AMPS.

Table I. Plasma lipids and lipoproteins in cynomolgus monkeys in mg/100 ml (mean ± SD)

	Control diet	Atherogenic diet	Regression diet
Cholesterol	125 ± 17	582 ± 87	129 ± 15
Triglyceride	34 ± 10	36 ± 12	32 ± 9
VLDL	15 ± 7	144 ± 17	13 ± 6
LDL	123 ± 16	862 ± 98	128 ± 18
HDL	287 ± 32	105 ± 14	282 ± 30

The changes in the cholesterol content of the aorta (table II) were consistent with the pathological findings. The aortic cholesterol content of the animals fed an atherogenic diet was about five times higher than that of the control group. About 56 % of the cholesterol was esterified as compared to about 11 % for the control group. During the regression diet the cholesterol content of the aorta remained above control values but was significantly reduced by about 60 % as compared to the values in the atherosclerotic group. The decrease in aortic cholesterol was largely due to a decrease in cholesteryl ester which made up only 21 % of the aortic cholesterol in regressed animals.

Influx of Plasma Cholesterol and LDL Into the Aorta

The influx of LDL into the artery was calculated from the ^{125}I radio-activity contained in the artery per gram of intima-media divided by the mean specific activity of LDL in the plasma. The influx of cholesterol into the aorta was similarly calculated.

The influx of plasma cholesterol into the aorta of control animals averaged 6.4 μg/g tissue over a 4-hour period (table II). During the feeding of the atherogenic diet, cholesterol influx increased more than 6-fold above the control values. During the regression diet, the influx decreased to or below control values. The changes in the influx of plasma LDL were similar to those for cholesterol. During a 4-hour period the uptake of LDL protein by the aorta averaged 0.52 μg/g tissue in the control group, 7.8 μg in the atherosclerotic group and 0.42 μg in the regression group.

Table II. Influx of plasma cholesterol and LDL into the aorta of the cyno-molgus monkey

	Aortic cholesterol		Aortic influx, μg/g/4 h	
	total cholesterol mg/gdt	% ester	cholesterol	LDL protein
Control	11.2 ± 1.5	10.7 ± 3.6	6.4 ± 1.5	0.52 ± 0.28
Atherogenic	56.6 ± 10.2	55.8 ± 8.4	42.3 ± 4.4	7.80 ± 1.23
Regression	22.9 ± 7.0	21.4 ± 5.3	5.1 ± 1.2	0.42 ± 0.24

Table III. Saline-extractable [125]-I-LDL from aorta of cynomolgus monkey

	[125]I radioactivity, %			
	saline-extractable	dialyzable	TCA soluble[1]	Heparin Mn^{2+} precipitable ^{125}I-LDL
Normal aorta	56.3 ± 5.7	56.3 ± 5.3	55.3 ± 3.7	37.3 ± 3.4
Atherosclerotic aorta	54.7 ± 5.1	55.7 ± 5.2	54.5 ± 5.6	38.3 ± 2.9

[1] Trichloracetic acid-soluble, iodide-free radioactivity.

Distribution and Degradation of ^{125}I-LDL in Aorta

Although the atherosclerotic aortae of the animals fed the atherogenic diet contained significantly more ^{125}I radioactivity than did the normal aorta of the control group, the percent distribution of the radioactivity was not significantly different in the groups. Of the total ^{125}I radioactivity in the aorta, about 55 % was extractable into 1.65 M NaCl (table III). Of the saline-extractable radioactivity about 55 % was dialyzable or soluble in 10 % TCA. This radioactivity which contained less than 3 % free iodide, was presumed to represent degradation products of ^{125}I-LDL. Of the nondialyzable ^{125}I radioactivity about 82 % was precipitable with heparin-mangenese. This precipitable radioactivity comprised about 38 % of the total saline-extractable ^{125}I radioactivity and was assumed to represent intact ^{125}I-LDL.

Most of the 125I radioactivity remaining in the tissue was released by sequential treatment with collagenase and elastase or sequential treatment with a mixture of chondroitinase A, B, C and collagenase (table IV). The release of [125]-I radioactivity from the tissues was accompanied by the release of AMPS suggesting a close relationship between ^{125}I-LDL with the AMPS as well as the connective proteins of the artery.

Subcellular fractionation of the peripheral arteries of animals fed a control or atherogenic diet (carotid, subclavian, femoral and iliac) also revealed that the ^{125}I radioactivity in these tissues existed in a soluble and tissue-bound form with 60.4 ± 6.4 % of the radioactivity being in the supernatant fraction and 30.0 ± 5.6 % in the tissue debris fraction. Only small amounts of ^{125}I radioactivity (less than 10 %) were detectable in the mitochondrial and microsomal fractions. About 64 % of the supernatant

Table IV. Distribution of [125I]-LDL in atherosclerotic aorta of cynomolgus monkey

	[125I] radioactivity %/0	Acid muco-polysaccharides %/0
Experiment I		
Saline	55.7 ± 4.8	42.2 ± 5.7
Collagenase	22.8 ± 5.5	41.8 ± 5.3
Elastase	18.4 ± 4.6	14.1 ± 3.8
Experiment II		
Saline	54.8 ± 4.3	40.8 ± 4.5
Chondroitinase	30.6 ± 4.7	46.1 ± 5.9
(A, B, C)		
Collagenase	9.1 ± 2.6	10.5 ± 2.7

Table V. Incorporation of [14C]-acetate, [3H]-leucine and [35S]-sulfate into lipoprotein fractions by monkey aortic smooth muscle cells in tissue culture

	cpm/1×10⁶ cells		
	µg protein protein	lipid	AMPS-³⁵SO₄
Cells			
Trypsin-releasable			
VLDL	– 200	200	100
LDL	– 1,200	7,200	1,000
HDL	– 2,500	8,200	1,300
Saline-extractable			
VLDL	59 300	500	200
LDL	30 3,200	16,000	1,200
HDL	50 6,500	20,500	1,500
Incubation media			
VLDL	37 500	300	500
LDL	94 5,900	36,000	5,500
HDL	224 10,400	45,000	1,300

[125I] counts were dialyzable. Of the nondialyzable counts, 84.7 ± 5.1 %/0 was precipitable with heparin and manganese.

Biosynthesis of Lipoproteins by Smooth Muscle Cells

Following incubation of arterial smooth muscle cells in a medium containing fetal calf serum and [14C]-acetate and [3H]-leucine, the lipid and

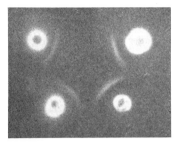

Fig. 1. Radioautograph of immunoprecipitin bands of LDL formed by the interaction of LDL antisera with LDL ultracentrifugally isolated from the culture media (right) and from the smooth muscle cells (left).

protein components of the ultracentrifugally isolated VLDL, LDL and HDL were radioactively labeled (table V). Only small amounts of radioactivity were detectable in the VLDL fraction. The incorporation of radioactively labeled substrates into LDL also was demonstrated by radioimmunodiffusion (fig. 1). When $^{35}SO_4$ was additionally incubated with the smooth muscle cells, ^{35}S-labeled AMPS were detectable in the lipoprotein fractions suggesting the formation of lipoprotein-AMPS complexes from newly synthesized lipoproteins and sulfated AMPS.

The labeled lipoproteins were detected not only in the incubation medium but also in the smooth muscle cells in close association with labeled AMPS. Significant amounts of lipoprotein and AMPS radioactivity also appeared to be bound to the surface of the cells as indicated by the trypsin-releasable radioactivity from the intact cells.

Discussion

The present study confirms earlier findings [15] that elevation of serum cholesterol induced by an atherogenic diet in the cynomolgus monkey is associated with an increase in the concentration of plasma LDL and VLDL and a decrease in the level of serum HDL. Similar changes in serum lipoproteins have been reported in man with coronary atherosclerotic heart disease [16]. The accumulation of cholesterol in the atherosclerotic aorta of the cholesterol-fed cynomolgus monkey was associated with an increased influx of plasma LDL and cholesterol into the arterial wall. Although these findings could result from an increase in vascular permeability caused by structural damage to the endothelial cells, they also could be due to an increased transendothelial transport of plasma LDL caused by high concentrations of serum LDL and low concentrations of HDL. That changes in the plasma levels of LDL and HDL may influence the binding and uptake of LDL by the endothelial cells is suggested by *in vitro* studies [17].

During the regression of atherosclerosis, the uptake of serum LDL and cholesterol returned to or below normal, suggesting that the retention of cholesterol in regressed lesions is due to a defect in the removal of cholesterol from the arterial wall rather than to an abnormality in vascular permeability. It is noteworthy that most of the cholesterol retained in the regressed lesion after feeding a low cholesterol diet for 1 year was in a nonesterified form and appeared to be closely associated with the AMPS. Some of the factors that might operate to reduce the entry of plasma LDL into the arterial wall during regression include repair of damaged endothelial cells, return of serum lipoproteins to normal and decrease in intimal permeability caused by fibrotic scar tissue in the regressed lesion.

Although atherosclerotic vessels contained significantly more ^{125}I-LDL than did the normal artery, the percent distribution of the labeled LDL, as revealed by subcellular fractionation and saline and enzyme treatment of the vessels, appeared similar. The results of these studies are consistent with earlier findings on the distribution of lipoproteins in human vessels and indicate that plasma LDL is present in the arterial wall in a saline-extractable form and in a tissue-bound form in close association with collagen, elastin and AMPS.

The percent degradation of ^{125}I-LDL in normal and atherosclerotic vessels did not appear significantly different. The degradation rate of labeled LDL by these arteries appeared constant over a 24-hour period since the percent of acid-soluble and dialyzable ^{125}I radioactivity contained in the arteries was comparable at 4 and 24 h after the intravenous administration of ^{125}I-LDL. Although the fractional degradation rate of ^{125}I-LDL was similar in normal and diseased vessels, the total amount of labeled LDL degraded by the diseased vessel was significantly increased. These findings suggest that arterial lipoproteins which equilibrate with plasma lipoproteins within 24 h are rapidly degraded in atherosclerotic vessels. However, the results do not exclude a possible defect in the degradation of the more slowly equilibrating pools of arterial lipoproteins in diseased vessels.

The present studies with cultured smooth muscle cells support earlier observations that the arterial wall is capable of synthesizing lipoproteins [1, 2, 12]. The detection of ^{35}S-labeled AMPS in the lipoprotein fractions also suggest that the newly synthesized AMPS may interact with the lipoproteins to form lipoprotein-AMPS complexes. These complexes appeared to be located extracellularly, intracellularly and on the plasma membrane of the smooth muscle cell as indicated by the release of labeled lipoproteins and AMPS following trypsin treatment of the intact cell. It is unlikely that the radioactivity in the lipoprotein fractions represented contamination by the radioactive precursors. In control studies, in which the radioactive substrates (^{14}C-acetate, ^{3}H-leucine and ^{35}S-sodium sulfate) were incubated with fetal calf serum but without smooth muscle cells, the isolated lipoprotein fractions contained no significant radioactivity. That the labeled lipoprotein fractions represented newly synthesized lipoproteins is supported by radioimmunodiffusion studies in which incorporation of radioactivity was demonstrated in the immunoprecipitin bands of LDL.

Summary

The accumulation of cholesterol in atherosclerotic lesions is associated with an icreased uptake of plasma cholesterol and LDL by the arterial wall. During the regression of atherosclerosis, the uptake of these macromolecules returns to or below normal, suggesting that the retention of cholesterol in regressed lesions is due to a defect in the removal of cholesterol from the arterial wall rather than to an abnormality in vascular permeability. Although increased amounts of ^{125}I-LDL were detected in atherosclerotic vessels, the percent distribution and fractional degradation rate of ^{125}I-LDL appeared similar in normal and diseased vessels. The present studies in support of earlier findings in human vessels indicate that LDL in the artery is contained in a number of different cellular and extracellular pools in close association with the AMPS. These lipoproteins appeared to be derived not only from the lipoproteins contained in the plasma but also from lipoproteins synthesized by the arterial wall.

References

1   HOLLANDER, W.: Influx, synthesis and transport of arterial lipoproteins in atherosclerosis. Expl molec. Path. *7:* 248–258 (1967).

2 HOLLANDER, W.: Unified concept on the role of acid mucopolysaccharides and connective tissue proteins in the accumulation of lipids, lipoproteins and calcium in the atherosclerotic plaque. Expl molec. Path. *25:* 106–120 (1976).

3 HAVEL, R.J.; EDER, H.A., and BRAGDEN, J.H.: Distribution and chemical composition of ultracentrifugally separated lipoproteins and chylomicrons. J. clin. Invest. *34:* 1345–1353 (1955).

4 BILHEIMER, D.W.; EISENBERG, S., and LEVY, R.I.: The metabolism of very low density lipoprotein proteins. I. Preliminary *in vitro* and *in vivo* observations. Biochim. biophys. Acta *260:* 212, 221 (1972).

5 GOODMAN, DE W.S. and NOBLE, R.P.: Turnover of plasma cholesterol in man. J. clin. Invest. *47:* 231–241 (1968).

6 HOLLANDER, W. and KRAMSCH, D.M.: The distribution of intravenously administered [³H] cholesterol in the arteries and other tissues. I. Tissue fractionation findings. J. Atheroscler. Res. *7:* 491–500 (1967).

7 GOLDSTEIN, J.L. and BROWN, M.S.: Binding and degradation of low density lipoproteins by cultured human fibroblasts. J. biol. Chem. *249:* 5153–5162 (1974).

8 BURSTEIN, M. et SAMAILLE, J.: Sur un dosage rapide du cholestérol lié aux α- et aux β-lipoprotéines du sérum. Clinica chim. Acta *5:* 609 (1960).

9 ROSENBERG, L.; JOHNSON, B., and SCHUBERT, M.: The protein-polysaccharides of human costal cartilage. J. clin. Invest. *48:* 543–552 (1969).

10 SAITO, M.; YAMAGATA, T., and SUZUKI, S.: Enzymatic methods for the determination of small quantities of isomeric chondroitin sulfates. J. biol. Chem. *213:* 1536–1542 (1968).

11 HOLLANDER, W.; KRAMSCH, D.M.; FARMELANT, M., and MADOFF, I.M.: Arterial wall metabolism in experimental hypertension of coarctation of the aorta of short duration. J. clin. Invest. *47:* 1221–1229 (1968).

12 ROSS, R.: The smooth muscle cell. II. Growth of smooth muscle cell in tissue culture formation of elastic fibers. J. Cell. Biol. *50:* 172–186 (1971).

13 SRINIVASAN, S.R.; DOLAN, P.; RADHAKRISHNAMURTHY, B., and BERENSON, G.S.: Isolation of lipoprotein-acid mucopolysaccharide complexes from fatty streaks of human aorta. Atherosclerosis *16:* 95–104 (1972).

14 HOCHWALD, G.M.; THORBECKE, G.J., and ASOFSKY, R.: Sites of formation of immune globulins and a component of C3. A new technique for the demonstration of the synthesis of individual serum proteins by tissues *in vitro.* J. exp. Med. *114:* 459–470 (1961).

15 HOLLANDER, W.; MADOFF, I.; PADDOCK, J., and KIRKPATRICK, B.: Aggravation of atherosclerosis by hypertension in a subhuman primate model with coarctation of the aorta. Circulation Res. *38:* suppl. II, pp. 63–72 (1976).

16 RHOADS, G.G.; GULBRANDSEN, C.L., and KAGAN, A.: Serum lipoproteins and coronary heart disease in a population study of Hawaii Japanese men. New Engl. J. Med. *294:* 293–298 (1976).

17 RECKLESS, J.P.D.; WEINSTEIN, D.B., and STEINBERG, D.: Lipoprotein metabolism by rabbit arterial endothelial cells. Circulation *54:* II-56 (1976).

W. HOLLANDER, MD, Boston University Medical Center, *Boston, Mass.* (USA)

Prog. biochem. Pharmacol., vol. 14, pp. 134–137 (Karger, Basel 1977)

Structural Correlates of Arterial Endothelial Permeability in the Evans Blue Model

Ross G. Gerrity and Colin J. Schwartz

Department of Atherosclerosis and Thrombosis Research,
The Cleveland Clinic Foundation, Cleveland, Ohio

Material and Methods

6 male Yorkshire-Landrace pigs, 6 weeks of age, were injected intravenously with Evans blue and 3 h subsequently with ferritin (10 mg/kg), and killed at intervals of 1, 5 and 15 min after ferritin injection. Samples of aortic arch from areas of dye uptake (blue areas) and devoid of dye uptake (white areas) were processed and sectioned for transmission electron microscopy. Some samples were block-stained with ruthenium red. Ten micrographs of endothelium were photographed at a magnification of 20,000 from each of five blocks taken from three blue and three white areas from each animal. The number of vesicles per μm^2 cross-sectional area of endothelium, the number of vesicles labelled with ferritin, the number of ferritin particles per vesicle, the number of large inclusions per cell, both labelled and unlabelled, and the number of ferritin particles per large inclusion were quantitated from these micrographs. Statistical comparisons were made between blue and white areas for each circulation time.

Results

Figure 1 depicts the ultrastructural appearance of ferritin granules in the endothelium and subendothelial space in a blue area 5 min after injection. Ferritin grains may be seen in vesicles, larger inclusions, and in the subendothelial space. The results of the quantitation of ferritin uptake are summarized in table I. No statistically significant differences were found with respect to the number of vesicles per μm^2 endothelium,

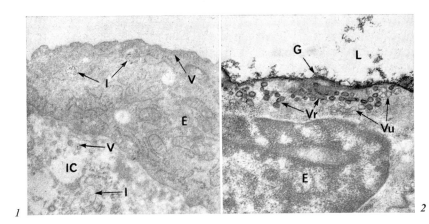

Fig. 1. Endothelium (E) and intimal cell (IC) in a blue area 5 min after intra-venous ferritin injection. Ferritin grains can be seen in vesicles (V) and large inclusions (I) in both the endothelial cell and the intimal cell. ×21,000.

Fig. 2. Endothelial cell (E) from a blue area stained with ruthenium red. Glycocalyx (G) is visible on luminal surface. Some vesicles (Vr) exhibit ruthenium red staining, while others (Vu), at a similar distance from the lumen (L), are un-stained. ×28,000.

Table I. Uptake of ferritin by aortic endothelium in the Evans blue model

Time post-injection	Perme-ability area	Vesicles/ endothelium, μm^2	% vesicles with FE	FE grains/ vesicle	% inclusion with FE	FE grains/ inclusion
1 min	white	39.7	10.3	1.0	34.9	3.2
	blue	25.7	22.1*	1.1	58.3	4.1
5 min	white	18.7	4.6	2.2	44.6	15.7
	blue	17.9	12.5*	2.9	37.2	4.0*
15 min	white	24.9	12.0	0.9	76.2	40.8
	blue	36.1	21.1*	1.3	51.3	20.0
Average	white	27.8	9.0	1.4	51.9	19.8
	blue	26.6	18.6*	1.8	48.9	9.4*

* $p < 0.05$.

the number of ferritin grains per vesicle, or the percentage of large inclu-sions containing ferritin. However, at all circulation times, blue areas had a significantly higher percentage of vesicles containing ferritin than did white areas. In addition, white areas showed a significantly greater number of ferritin grains in large inclusions as compared to blue areas at

5 and 15 minutes, but not at 1 min after injection. In samples which were block-stained with ruthenium red to demonstrate the glycocalyx, some cytoplasmic vesicles took up this stain. Other vesicles, at a similar distance from the lumen, did not show ruthenium red staining (fig. 2).

Discussion

There is now considerable evidence that areas of spontaneously occurring enhanced permeability to proteins, including ^{131}I-albumin and ^{131}I-fibrinogen [1], are readily and consistently demarcated *in vivo* in pigs and dogs by their uptake of the protein-binding azo dye, Evans blue [1]. These areas of dye uptake and enhanced permeability exhibit differences in cholesterol uptake and accumulation [2] and in endothelial ultrastructural morphology [3] compared to areas devoid of dye uptake. The present study presents preliminary data which suggest that the enhanced permeability of blue areas relates, not to the number of pinocytic vesicles, or the carrying capacity of each vesicle, but to the number of vesicles actively involved in the transport process. This concept indicates that there exists more than one functional type of vesicle, or that activation of vesicular transport is subject to controlling factors exerted on or by endothelial cells. In this respect it is of interest that blue areas have been shown to be sites of increased hemodynamic stress and early lipid accumulation [4], and that increased permeability has been associated with induced atherosclerosis [5]. The mechanism by which vesicles are activated is unclear, but it is tempting to suggest a possible role of the glycocalyx. This surface coat is significantly thinner in blue areas as opposed to white areas [3], and thinning of the glycocalyx has been described in hypercholesterolemia [6]. The present study, as well as previous studies [3] by us have shown that vesicles exhibit variable staining with ruthenium red, which stains glycocalyx material. The presence of ruthenium-stained vesicles is independent of their proximity to the luminal surface.

In summary, the results show that endothelial permeability is not homogeneous along the length of the aorta, and that areas of enhanced permeability may be explained, at least in part, by increased activation of vesicular transport which is subject to controlling factors. The glycocalyx, which is thinner in areas of enhanced permeability and in hypercholesterolemia, may serve to control access of macromolecules to the endothelial plasma membrane, the formation of caveolae, or the activation of vesicular uptake, thus serving as one factor which may modulate the influx of blood-borne macromolecules.

Summary

Normal young pigs were injected intravenously with the azo dye Evans blue, which is preferentially and consistently taken up by focal areas in the aorta known to be areas of enhanced permeability. Ferritin was intravenously injected into these animals, and its uptake was quantitated at the electron microscope level at 1, 5 and 15 min after administration. The number of vesicles, large inclusions or vacuoles, and junctions, both labelled and unlabelled, were counted in areas of normal and enhanced permeability. The results have revealed that the number of vesicles per μm^2 cross-section of endothelium, and the average number of ferritin grains per vesicle is the same in both areas. However, the percentage of vesicles containing ferritin is significantly higher in areas of enhanced permeability.

References

1   BELL, F.P.; ADAMSON, I.L.; GALLUS, A.S., and SCHWARTZ, C.J.: Endothelial permeability. Focal and regional patterns of ^{131}I-albumin and ^{131}I-fibrinogen uptake and transmural distribution in the pig aorta; in SCHETTLER and WEIZEL Atherosclerosis III. Proc. 3rd Int. Symp. (Springer, Berlin 1973).

2   SOMER, J.B. and SCHWARTZ, C.J.: Focal ^{3}H-cholesterol uptake in the pig aorta. Atherosclerosis 16: 377–388 (1972).

3   GERRITY, R.G.; RICHARDSON, M.; SOMER, J.B.; BELL, F.P., and SCHWARTZ, C.J.: Endothelial cell morphology in areas of in vivo Evans blue uptake in the young pig aorta. II. Ultrastructure of the intima. Am. J. Path. (in press).

4   FRY, D.L.: Responses of the arterial wall to certain physical factors; in Atherogenesis: initiating factors. Ciba Found. Symp., Vol. 12, pp. 93–102 (Elsevier, Amsterdam 1973).

5   STEFANOVICH, V. and GORE, I.: Cholesterol diet and permeability of rabbit aorta. Expl molec. Path. 14: 20–27 (1971).

6   BALINT, A.; VERESS, B., and JELLINEK, H.: Modifications of surface coat of aortic endothelial cells in hyperlipemic rats. Pathol. Eur. 9: 105–108 (1974).

Dr. R.G. GERRITY, Department of Atherosclerosis and Thrombosis Research, The Cleveland Clinic Foundation, Cleveland, OH 44106 (USA)

Prog. biochem. Pharmacol., vol. 14, pp. 138–152 (Karger, Basel 1977)

Studies on the Passage of Plasma Proteins Across Arterial Endothelium in Relation to Atherogenesis

K.W. WALTON and C.J. MORRIS

Department of Experimental Pathology, University of Birmingham, Birmingham

Previous work from this Department, using autologous total low density lipoproteins (VLDL and LDL) isotopically labelled in the protein moiety, established that these proteins can be identified in atherosclerotic lesions in the human [1] and in the lipid-fed rabbit [2]. It has similarly been shown by the technique of immunofluorescence, that not only the apolipoprotein B which is common to VLDL and LDL, but also apolipoprotein C, which is characteristic of lipoproteins larger in molecular size than LDL, can be demonstrated in plaques. In some individuals, the antigen characteristic of the variant lipoprotein known as Lp(à) lipoprotein was additionally demonstrated [3, 4].

The topographic distribution of the apolipoproteins thus delineated corresponded closely with that of extracellular lipid and cholesterol as shown by conventional histological methods. It was therefore concluded that the TLDL serve as the principal vehicles transporting serum lipids into the arterial intima and also into certain extravascular lesions found in association with hyperlipidaemia and severe atherosclerosis [5].

More recent work, involving the two-dimensional electrophoresis of the tissue fluid contained in samples of arterial intima into antiserum-containing gels, established that almost all the proteins of plasma enter the intimal connective tissue. But if intimal samples from areas affected by atherosclerosis are electrophoresed in this manner until no further plasma protein emerges, and the *same* intimal sample is then examined by immunofluorescence, it is possible to demonstrate a residual firmly bound fraction of LDL still present in the tissue. These observations were taken to indicate that the development of atherosclerotic lesions depends not only upon the entry of plasma proteins into areas of increased permeability, but also upon the selective binding at such sites of the lipoproteins to connective tissue components [6, 7].

In order to study in more detail the nature of the lipoproteins bound, and of the sites of their interaction with connective tissue elements, the immunoperoxidase technique has been employed at the electron microscope level. This communication is a summary of some of the results obtained. A more detailed account will appear elsewhere.

Materials and Methods

Tissues Examined

Material was taken at routine autopsies from 4 male cases and 1 female case of sudden death due to ischaemic heart disease. The male subjects ranged in age from 57 to 74, the woman was aged 39. Raised atherosclerotic lesions (including fibro-fatty plaques) originating in the aorta, basilar, coeliac axis and splenic arteries were examined. From 1 case (male aged 63) an area of the anterior cusp of the mitral valve showing lipid infiltration was also examined.

Histological Techniques

For examination by conventional histological techniques and by immunofluorescence the tissues were snap-frozen, sections cut, stained and examined using the staining methods, fluorescein-labelled antisera and the apparatus detailed in earlier communications [8, 9]. Adjacent portions of tissue were also examined by the immunoperoxidase techniques as detailed below.

Immunoperoxidase Method

Ammonium sulphate precipitated globulin fractions of sheep anti-human LDL (anti-apolipoprotein B) were conjugated to horseradish peroxidase (Sigma, type VI) by the periodate method [10] using 0.08 M periodate. The $F(ab)_2$ fraction (sub-component containing the antibody combining site) prepared by papain digestion of IgG isolated by diethylaminoethylcellulose chromatography of rabbit anti-LDL was similarly conjugated. In each case the final conjugate was purified by gelfiltration through a G-150 Sephadex column eluted with 0.15 M saline buffered at pH 7.4 with 0.02 M phosphate. The material from the first peak eluted was concentrated by ultrafiltration using a PM-10 filter (Amicon Corp., Lexington).

The tissues were reacted with the conjugate in one of two ways:

(i) Unfixed 6-μm frozen sections were reacted with the conjugate for 1 h at room temperature followed by extensive washing in phosphate-buffered saline (PBS). Sections were then fixed in 4 % glutaraldehyde in 0.1 M cacodylate buffer (pH 7.4) for 30 min, washed in 0.05 M Tris HCl buffer (pH 7.4) and peroxidase reactivity developed by the method of GRAHAM and KARNOVSKY [11]. Sections were washed in distilled water, post-osmicated in 2 % osmium tetroxide in distilled water, dehydrated and surface-embedded from the glass slide in SPURR's [12] resin. This method allowed electron microscope examination of sections adjacent to those treated by conventional histological and immunological techniques.

(ii) Small pieces (approximately 6 × 3 mm) of tissue were fixed for 1 h in 4 % paraformaldehyde in 0.1 M cacodylate buffer (pH 7.4) and washed in several changes of PBS. Thick sections (100 μm) were cut on a Porter-Blum TC-2 tissue chopper, the tissue being supported in 7 % agar. The thick sections were incubated with peroxidase conjugate for 4 h and subsequently treated as in (i). Control sections were treated with unlabelled antiserum but subsequently handled in exactly the same fashion as in (i) and (ii).

Ultra-thin sections were viewed in a Siemens Elmiskop 102 electron microscope at an accelerating voltage of 80 kV. Sections were usually viewed unstained but in some instances brief staining with methanolic uranyl acetate was employed. For light microscopy 6-μm frozen sections treated with peroxidase-labelled antibody and developed for peroxidase activity were examined unstained or counterstained with haematoxylin and eosin.

Results

In some of the arterial lesions examined, extracellular lipid, as revealed in sections 'stained' with oil red O, and examined by light microscopy, was present in the intima in two forms: (a) as material in the interstitial matrix, sometimes as pools of amorphous structureless lipid; (b) deposited apparently on the surface of collagen bundles. Lipid was also seen to be deposited on the internal elastic lamina, and in some instances to be involving the superficial media apparently on the surface of smooth muscle cells. Specific fluorescence was seen at all these sites in corresponding sections treated with fluorescein-labelled anti-LDL and a

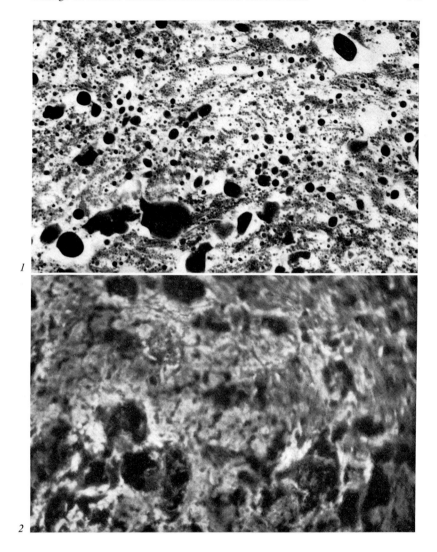

Fig. 1. Lipid pool ('atheroma') in depth of intima from plaque in splenic artery in man aged 74 showing lipid as droplets of varying size (black in picture, bright red in original) in interstitial tissue and on surface of collagen fibrils, as seen in light microscope. Oil red O, light green, haematoxylin. × 500.

Fig. 2. Corresponding field from adjacent section of same material as in figure 1, after treatment with fluorescein-labelled anti-LDL. Note more even distribution of specific fluorescence (greyish-white in picture, bright green in original) when viewed in ultraviolet/blue light. × 500.

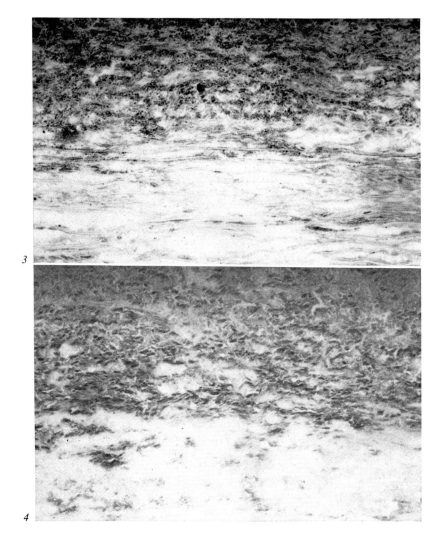

Fig. 3. Intimal/medial junction of fibro-fatty plaque from aorta of man aged 63, showing lipid droplets on surface of collagen in intima, aligned along elastic fibres in media and on surface of intimal smooth muscle cells (black in picture, bright red in original). Oil red O, light green, haematoxylin. × 4/3.

Fig. 4. Corresponding field from adjacent section of same material as in figure 3 after treatment with peroxidase-labelled F(ab)₂ fragment of anti-LDL. No counterstain. Note even distribution of reaction product (dark grey in picture, brown in original) on collagen in depth of intima and deposits on elastic fibres and on smooth muscle cells in media. × 4/3.

brown reaction product was evident in sections treated with peroxidase-labelled anti-LDL (fig. 1–4).

Lipoprotein Deposition in the Interstitial Matrix

When areas corresponding to those examined by light microscopy were treated with peroxidase-labelled antibody fractions and viewed in the electron microscope, areas showing interstitial lipid and lipoprotein deposition by light microscopy revealed large number of electron-dense spherical particles of varying size. The smallest of these, when examined at high magnification, were seen to be homogeneously covered by electron-dense material (the osmicated reaction product of diamino-benzidine with the peroxidase coupled to the antibody fraction), indicating that these were immunologically identifiable as material reacting with anti-LDL (anti-apolipoprotein B). In some instances, the plane of section was such as to show granules of electron-dense reaction product arranged in circles, as though surrounding a hollow sphere (fig. 5). The internal diameter of the spheres was found to vary between about 22 and 48 nm. This corresponds to the range of molecular diameters found for individual lipoprotein molecules when isolated and purified fractions of LDL, VLDL and intermediate lipoproteins are examined in the electron microscope [13].

In addition to immunologically reactive particles of this range of size, larger spherical structures, some of which bore partial or complete coating of reaction product, were seen. It was not possible to decide whether these were aggregates of LDL or VLDL or whether some were chylomicra.

Lipoprotein Deposition in Association with Collagen

In fibro-fatty arterial plaques, lipid (lipoprotein) deposition occurs in association with coarse (mature) collagen fibres and bundles. A similar distribution is frequently seen in relation to the collagen of the lamina propria of the anterior cusp of the mitral valve [9].

At these sites, when examined in the light microscope after treatment with oil red O, the strands of collagen appear to be coated by lipid droplets (fig. 6). The term 'peri-fibrous lipid' has been used to describe this appearance. The distribution in droplets is probably artefactual, being due to partial extraction of the lipid by the solvent in which the fat stain is dissolved [9, 16]. This is because when aqueous reagents such as labelled anti-LDL antibodies are applied to the same or corresponding

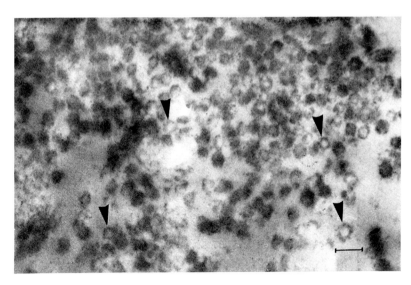

Fig. 5. Lipid pool in depth of intima from aortic plaque from man aged 74, after treatment with peroxidase-labelled anti-LDL and examined in electron microscope. Note circular structures of varying size in interstitial matrix, some uniformly coated and others surrounded by electron-dense reaction product (arrows). Scale marker: 100 nm. $\times$ 75,000.

sections, a closely similar distribution is seen but the labelled antibodies are bound evenly and smoothly to the collagen (fig. 7).

On examining corresponding areas in the electron microscope after treatment with either whole immunoglobulin antibody (anti-LDL) labelled with peroxidase, or even more markedly with the peroxidase-labelled $F(ab)_2$ fraction of anti-LDL (which can be envisaged as penetrating the tissue more effectively), a heavy deposit of electron-dense reaction product enclosing spherical particles is seen on the outer surface of bundles of collagen fibrils in the intima. However, smaller deposits of the reaction product are also seen within bundles, dispersed irregularly along the course of indidividual fibrils (fig. 8). Where bundles are cut rtansversely or tangentially, fibrils can be seen in cross-section to be surrounded by reaction product (fig. 9). The fibrils in the superficial and mid-parts of plaques usually resemble native (64–67 nm banded) collagen.

In some instances (as for example in an advanced fibro-fatty plaque from the aorta of a woman aged 39) polymorphic forms of collagen are observed in both the superficial and the deeper regions of the plaque and

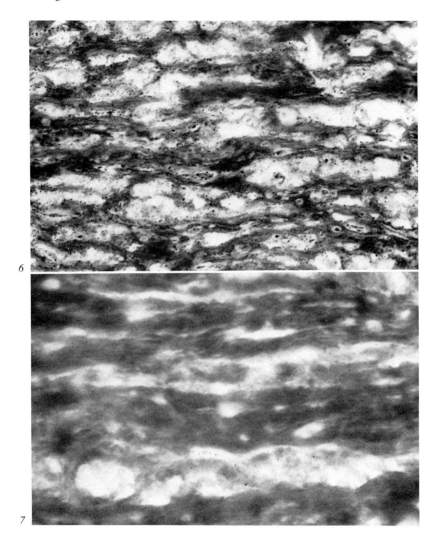

Fig. 6. Fibrotic area in depth of plaque at mouth of coeliac axis artery in man aged 74. Note lipid disposed as fine droplets (black in picture, bright red in original) in 'peri-fibrous' distribution on collagen. Light microscope. Oil red O, light green, haematoxylin. × 500.

Fig. 7. Corresponding field from adjacent section of same material as in figure 6 after treatment with peroxidase labelled anti-LDL. Note even distribution of reaction product (dark grey in picture, brown in original) on collagen strands. Light microscope. × 500.

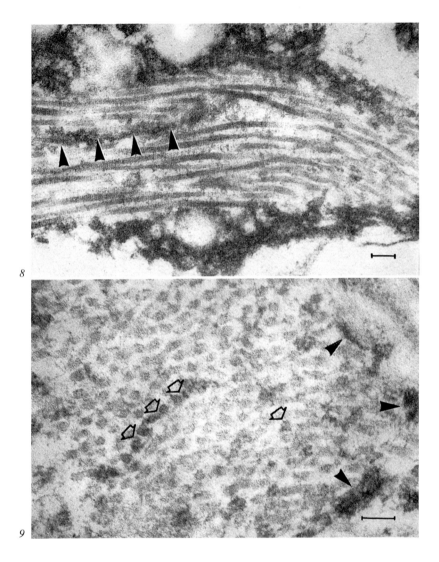

Fig. 8. Longitudinally disposed collagen bundle in lamina propria of anterior cusp of mitral valve from man aged 63. Tissue treated with peroxidase-labelled anti-LDL. Note electron-dense reaction product surrounding spheres of varying size which are applied to outer aspect of collagen bundle. But note similar structures along course of individual fibrils of native collagen within bundles. (arrows). Scale marker: 100 nm. × 60,000.

Fig. 9. Another collagen bundle, out transversely, from same material as in figure 8. Note electron-dense reaction product applied to outer aspect of bundle (solid arrows) and also applied to and surrounding individual collagen fibrils (open arrows). Scale marker: 100 nm. × 90,000.

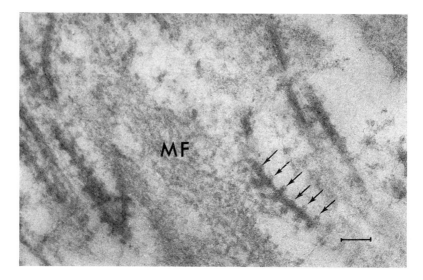

Fig. 10. Polymorphic forms of collagen in fibro-fatty atherosclerotic plaque from woman aged 39. Tissue treated with peroxidase-labelled anti-LDL. Note randomly disposed microfibrils (MF) and fibrous long-spacing collagen with electron-dense reaction product applied at regular periodicity (arrows) Scale marker: 200 nm. $\times$ 37,500.

at the intimal/medial junction. These take the forms of disorganised arrays of microfibrils lying in a structureless matrix and also of bundles apparently composed of fine fibrils with marked transverse striations at regular intervals. The latter resembles fibrous long spacing collagen (FLSC). In this instance the electron-dense reaction product is also disposed at regular intervals along the FLSC, being bound at the transverse bands at intervals of about 120 nm along these structures (fig. 10). The possible significance of this observation is discussed below.

Lipoprotein Deposition in Association with other
Connective Tissue Components

In arteries showing lipid (lipoprotein) deposition on the elastic laminae and in relation to smooth muscle cells in the superficial media in the light microscope, examination of corresponding sections treated with peroxidase-labelled immunoglobulin, or F(ab)$_2$ fragment, of anti-LDL in the electron microscope showed the presence of reaction product

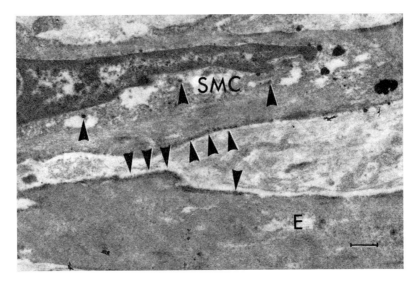

Fig. 11. Media underlying plaque in splenic artery from man aged 74 (adjacent section of same material as in figures 1 and 2) after treatment of section with peroxidase-labelled anti-LDL. Note electron-dense reaction product applied to surface membrane and within cytoplasm (arrows) of medial smooth muscle cell (SMC) and also to surface of adjacent elastin (E). Scale marker: 800 nm. × 9,000.

deposited on elastin, and upon the cytoplasmic membrane or within smooth muscle cells (fig. 11).

Discussion

In relation to the degree of altered permeability which occurs at the sites of atherosclerotic lesions, the results now reported support the inferences drawn from previous studies using immunofluorescence. These, which showed apolipoproteins C and Lp(a) to be identifiable in plaques [3, 4], led to the conclusion that lipoproteins larger in molecular size than LDL can permeate endothelium to participate in atherogenesis. This conclusion is now confirmed visually since apolipoprotein B is known to be present in both LDL and VLDL (and also in intermediate-sized lipoproteins) while the peroxidase-labelled antibody is now found to interact with spherical particles (molecules) with diameters corresponding to those of this range of lipoproteins. The present observations, made in plaques from the aorta, the splenic and coeliac arteries and a heart valve, thus confirm and extend similar findings reported for cerebral arteries [5].

In addition to lipoprotein thus identified in the interstitial matrix, the use of the immunoperoxidase technique has allowed the identification of the binding of these lipoproteins by connective tissue fibres such as collagen and elastin and their uptake into smooth muscle cells. Attention has previously been drawn [8, 9, 16] to the discrepancy between the disposal of lipoprotein taken up by large fat-filled cells in the intima, and that entering smooth muscle cells *in situ* in the media. Though lipid persists in intimal fat-filled cells, they show variable immunoreactivity to labelled anti-LDL suggesting that the protein moiety of the lipoprotein (site of antigenic reactivity) undergoes digestion by intracellular proteases in these cells. On the other hand, both lipid staining and immunological reactivity persist in fully differentiated smooth muscle cells in the media, suggesting that such cells are less capable of intracellular digestion of the lipoprotein. At the electron microscopic level, it was noticeable that the reaction product, which serves as the marker for the presence of the lipoprotein, in addition to being bound to the outer surface of the cell membrane, when intracellular, was either randomly distributed in the cytoplasm or perinuclear in position, but *not* closely associated with lysosomes or other organelles concerned with intracellular digestive processes.

With regard to native collagen of normal morphology, heavy deposits of lipoprotein were found on the outer surface of the bundles of fibrils forming the macroscopic collagen fibre, thus conforming with the 'perifibrous' distribution seen in the light microscope. But reaction product was also distributed in a perifibrillar fashion (fig. 8, 9). In relation to the microfibril's length, the distribution of the lipoprotein thus identified was often irregular and discontinuous. It has been shown by NAKAO and BASHEY [17] that native collagen fibrils bind ruthenium red particularly at certain periodicities (between the d and a_4 bands) suggesting the interaction of glycosaminoglycans or proteoglycans at these sites. Since these charged macromolecules have also been suggested to bind lipoproteins, it seems possible that this may be the molecular mechanism underlying the appearance now found and thus account for much of the 'bound' fraction of lipoprotein previously alluded to [6, 7].

This suggested mechanism is even more likely in relation to the interaction of the lipoprotein with FLSC. This 'abnormal' polymorphic form of collagen is known to be formed in an altered micro-environment in connective tissue in a number of pathological conditions [18, 19] though its occurrence has not, to our knowledge, previously been described in atherosclerotic plaques. Structural studies have suggested that its characteristic morphology arises from the occurrence of unpaired positively charged side chains in the amino acid sequence, which occur with a regular periodicity, becoming aligned in adjoining fibrils by intermolecular bridging by glycosaminoglycans interacting with these side chains [19]. The finding now of LDL interaction at these periodicities suggests that the glycosaminoglycans also bind lipoprotein. From the viewpoint of atherogenesis, the formation of FLSC in advanced plaques may be of significance since the tensile strength of this form of collagen is likely to be less than of 'normal' or native collagen so that its occurrence may be conductive to arterial dilation and other complications associated with reduced tensile strength of the arterial wall.

Summary

Previous studies using isotopically labelled lipoproteins or immunohistological characterisation of the apolipoproteins present in atherosclerotic lesions have suggested that lipoproteins varying in size from LDL to VLDL gain entry to the lesions. It has also been shown that a fraction of these lipoproteins is firmly bound to various constituents of the arterial wall. Using the immunoperoxidase technique at the electron microscopic level, it is now confirmed that spherical molecules specifically interacting with labelled anti-LDL (anti-apolipoprotein B) and of a range of molecular diameters corresponding to those of LDL to VLDL are identifiable in the interstitial matrix of lesions. The labelled antibodies also identified lipoprotein bound to elastin, within smooth muscle cells, and bound to collagen fibres. In advanced lesions lipoprotein was found to be bound not only to 'normal' (native) collagen fibrils but also with a characteristic periodicity to fibrous long-spacing collagen. The occurrence of this 'abnormal' form of collagen in plaques is now reported for the first time but its possible significance in relation to atherogenesis is discussed.

Acknowledgements

The assistance of Dr. I. HUNNEYBALL in preparing and purifying the F(ab)$_2$ fraction of rabbit IgG antibody with anti-human LDL activity is gratefully acknowledged.

References

1 WALTON, P.W.; SCOTT, P.J.; VERRIER JONES, J.; FLETCHER, R.F., and WHITEHEAD, T.P.: Studies on low-density lipoprotein turnover in relation to Atromid therapy. J. Atheroscler. Res. *3:* 396–414 (1963).

2 WALTON, K.W.; THOMAS, C., and DUNKERLEY, D.J.: The pathogenesis of xanthomata. J. Path. Bact. *109:* 271–289 (1973).

3 WALTON, K.W.: Identification of lipoproteins involved in human atherosclerosis; in SCHETTLER and WEIZEL Atherosclerosis III. Proc. 3rd Int. Symp., pp. 93–95 (Springer, Berlin 1974).

4 WALTON, K.W.; HITCHENS, J.; MAGNANI, H.N., and KHAN, M.: A study of methods of identification and estimation of Lp(a) lipoprotein and of its significance in health, hyperlipidaemia and atherosclerosis. Atherosclerosis *20:* 323–346 (1974).

5 WALTON, K.W.: Pathogenetic mechanisms in atherosclerosis. Am. J. Cardiol. *35:* 542–558 (1975).

6 WALTON, K.W. and BRADBY, G.V.H.: The significance of 'bound' and 'labile' fractions of low-density lipoprotein and fibrinogen in the arterial wall; in HAUST Proc. Int. Workshop, Conference on Atherosclerosis, London, Ont. 1975 (Plenum Press, New York, in press).

7 BRADBY, G.V.H. and WALTON, K.W.: Low-density lipoprotein binding in atherosclerotic intima (in preparation, 1977).

8 WALTON, K.W. and WILLIAMSON, N.: Histological and immunofluorescent studies on the evolution of the human atherosclerotic plaque. J. Atheroscler. Res. *8:* 599–624 (1968).

9 WALTON, K.W.; WILLIAMSON, N., and JOHNSON, A.G.: The pathogenesis of atherosclerosis of the mitral and aortic valves. J. Path. Bact. *101:* 205–220 (1970).

10 NAKANE, P.K. and KAWAOI, A.: Peroxidase-labelled antibody. A new method of conjugation. J. Histochem. Cytochem. *22:* 1084–1091 (1974).

11 GRAHAM, R.C. and KARNOVSKY, M.J.: The early stages of absorption of injected horseradish peroxidase in the proximal tubules of mouse kidney. Ultrastructural cytochemistry by a new technique. J. Histochem. Cytochem. *14:* 291–296 (1966).

12 SPURR, A.R.: A low viscosity epoxy resin embedding medium for electron microscopy. J. Ultrastruct. Res. *26:* 31–43 (1969).

13 FORTE, G.M.; NICHOLS, A.V., and GLASER, R.M.: Electron microscopy of human serum lipoproteins using negative staining. Chem. Phys. Lipids *2:* 326–408 (1968).

14 SMITH, E.B.; EVANS, P.H., and DOWNHAM, M.D.: Lipid in the aortic intima. The correlation of morphological and chemical characteristics. J. Atheroscler. Res. *7:* 171–186 (1967).

15 HOFF, H.F. and GAUBATZ, J.W.: Ultrastructural localization of plasma lipoproteins in human intracranial arteries. Virchows Arch. path. Anat. Histol. *369:* 111–121 (1975).

16   WALTON, K.W.; DUNKERLEY, D.J.; JOHNSON, A.G.; KHAN, M.K.; MORRIS, C.J., and WATTS, R.B.: Investigation by immunofluorescence of arterial lesions in rabbits on two different lipid supplements and treated with pyridinol carbamate. Atherosclerosis 23: 117–139 (1976).

17   NAKAO, K. and BASHEY, R.I.: Fine structure of collagen fibrils as revealed by Ruthenium red. Expl molec. Path. 17: 6–13 (1972).

18   BANFIELD, W.G.; LEE, C.K., and LEE, C.W.: Myocardial collagen of the fibrous long-spacing type. Archs Path. 95: 262–266 (1973).

19   DOYLE, B.B.; HUKINS, D.W.L.; HULMES, D.J.S.; MILLER, A., and WOODHEAD-GALLOWAY, J.: Collagen polymorphism. Its origin in the amino-acid sequence. J. molec. Biol. 91: 79–99 (1975).

Prof. Dr. K.W. WALTON, Department of Experimental Pathology, University of Birmingham, *Birmingham* (England)

Prog. biochem. Pharmacol., vol. 14, pp. 153–156 (Karger, Basel 1977)

Permeability in Atherosclerosis: a New Fluorescence Test with Trypan Blue in Green Light[1]

C.W.M. ADAMS

Department of Pathology, Guy's Hospital Medical School, London University, London

Much current work on arterial permeability is concerned with the lumenal endothelium, yet FELT [1960] pointed out that the endothelial surface is much greater in the vasa vasorum that in the main lumen. Over 50 years ago PETROFF [1922/23] found that intravenously injected trypan blue strains both the inner and outer surfaces of the rat aorta. We showed that more ^{125}I-labelled albumin enters the outer surface of the *normal* rabbit aorta than the inner [Adams *et al.*, 1968; ADAMS, 1971] but entry reverses in established atheroma [ADAMS *et al.*, 1970; ADAMS, 1971]. DUNCAN and BUCK [1961, 1962] found that the total entry of labelled albumin into the outer wall of the dog aorta was greater than or equal to that in the inner from the mid-thoracic aorta downwards.

Albumin influx has been shown to increase in atherosclerosis, as shown (i) with labelled albumin [ADAMS *et al.*, 1970; ADAMS, 1971; STEFANOVICH and GORE, 1971], (ii) by gross staining with trypan blue [FRIEDMAN and BYERS, 1963] and (iii) by following the entry of albumin-sized particles (VERESS *et al.*, 1970, 1972; KAROZUMI, 1975]. Recently we have followed albumin entry with a histological method for trypan blue, where even small amounts of the dye are demonstrated by red fluorescence in green light [ADAMS and BAYLISS, 1977]. Non-specific fluorescence is absent at this wavelength.

[1] Partly supported by a grant from the British Heart Foundation.

Methods

Albino rats were injected in a tail vein with a filtered 1 % solution of trypan blue (BDH) and were killed at intervals of 15 min to 24 h after injection. NZW rabbits were injected in a marginal ear vein with trypan blue and killed at intervals of 30 min to 24 h after injection; some were fed a cholesterol-enriched diet for 1–12 weeks.

Aortic sections were cut on the cryostat, post-fixed for 10 min in 5 % TCA–10 % formalin and then mounted in glycerine jelly. We used the Leitz Orthoplan fluorescence system No. 4 at 570 nm (see ADAMS and BAYLISS, 1977].

Results

In the rat more albumin-trypan blue complex entered the outer than the inner surface of the aorta (fig. 1). In the rabbit, the thoracic aorta showed greater entry into the outer surface than the inner or equal entry into both surfaces. The rabbit's aortic arch, however, showed rather greater entry from the inner than the outer surface.

Aortic elastic lamellae fluoresced strongly with trypan blue; the intensity of fluorescence indicated how much albumin had entered [see ADAMS and BAYLISS, 1977].

In cholesterol-fed rabbits, intimal fluorescence focally increased from

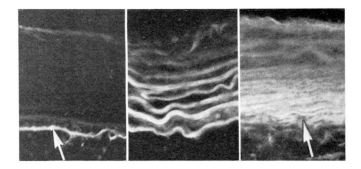

Fig. 1. Aortas from rats injected with trypan blue 15 min, 4 h and 24 h previously (left to right). Inner surface at top, outer at bottom. Note greater entry from outer surface (arrows). Red fluorescence at 570 nm. × 270.

the second week onwards after starting the diet, and these increases just preceded the appearance of lipid droplets in the endothelium.

Raised atheromatous plaques developed from 7 weeks onwards. Some stained strongly on naked eye examination and, correspondingly, showed intense histological fluorescence, but others were nearly unreactive. In spite of this variability, the zone surrounding these raised lesions frequently stained or fluoresced strongly.

Discussion

Much of the trypan blue-albumin complex appeared to enter the normal rat aorta and rabbit *thoracic* aorta from the outer surface. The entry from outside accords with our previous isotope findings [ADAMS *et al.*, 1968; ADAMS, 1971] and with DUNCAN and BUCK's [1961, 1962) findings in the dog's lower thoracic aorta. BELL *et al.* [1974] reported that albumin enters almost exclusively from the inner surface of the normal pig aorta, but BRATZLER *et al.* [1976] found entry from both surfaces of the normal rabbit aorta.

The results here confirm and extend previous studies to the effect that arterial permeability increases during the development of atherosclerosis (see above).

Increased fluorescence with trypan blue was observed before endothelial lipid droplets appeared and, likewise, the normal endothelium around raised lesions often showed increased fluorescence [see also FRIEDMAN and BYERS, 1963]. This is consistent with previous observations on increased permeability before lipid droplets or lesions appear [VERESS *et al.*, 1972; WRIGHT *et al.*, 1975].

The variability of fluorescence in the substance of plaques suggests that some continue to imbibe, whereas others become quiescent. The frequently increased permeability at the edge of plaques indicates that this zone may be a major site of growth and progression.

References

ADAMS, C.W.M.: Lipids, lipoproteins and atherosclerotic lesions. Proc. R. Soc. Med. 64: 902 (1971).
ADAMS, C.W.M. and BAYLISS, O.B.: Permeability of inner and outer layers of rat

and rabbit aortic wall: two new microscopic tests with trypan blue. Atherosclerosis *11:* 119 (1970).

ADAMS, C.W.M.; MORGAN, R.S., and BAYLISS, O.B.: The differential entry of
(^{125}I) albumin into mildly and severely atheromatous rabbit aortas. Atherosclerosis *11:* 119 (1970).

ADAMS, C.W.M.; VIRAG, S.; MORGAN, R.S., and ORTON, C.C.: Dissociation of (^{3}H)
cholesterol and ^{125}I-labelled plasma protein influx in normal and atheromatous rabbit, aorta. J. Atheroscler. Res. *8:* 679 (1968).

BELL, R.; ADAMSON, I., and SCHWARTZ, C.J.: Aortic endothelial permeability to
albumin: focal and regional patterns of uptake and transmural distribution of
[131]I-albumin in the young pig. Expl molec. Path. *20:* 57 (1974).

BRATZLER, R.L.; CHISOLM, G.M.; COLTON, C.K.; SMITH, K.A.; ZILVERSMIT, D.B.,
and LEES, R.S.: The distribution of labelled albumin across the rabbit thoracic
aorta *in vivo.* Circulation Res. (in press, 1976).

DUNCAN, L.E. and BUCK, K.: Passage of labelled albumin into canine aortic wall
in vivo and *in vitro.* Am. J. Physiol. *200:* 622 (1961).

DUNCAN, L.E. and BUCK, K.: Comparison of rates at which albumin enters walls of
small and large aortas. Am. J. Physiol. *203:* 1167 (1962).

FELT, V.: The role of the blood vessel wall in the pathogenesis of atherosclerosis.
Rev. Czech. Med. *6:* 126 (1960).

FRIEDMAN, M. and BYERS, S.: Endothelial permeability in atherosclerosis. Archs
Path. *76:* 99 (1963).

HECK, A.F.; HASUO, M.; FURUSE, M.; BROCK, M., and DIETZ, H.: Distribution of
serum protein in intracranial blood vessels of the cat. Atherosclerosis *23:*
227 (1976).

KUROZUMI, T.: Electronmicroscopic study on permeability of the aorta and basilar
artery of the rabbit – with special reference to the changes of permeability
by hypercholesteremia. Expl. molec. Path. *23:* 1 (1975).

PETROFF, J.R.: Über die Vitalfärbung der Gefässwandlungen. Beitr. path. Anat. *71:*
115 (1922/23).

STEFANOVICH, V. and GORE, I.: Cholesterol diet and permeability of rabbit aorta.
Expl molec. Path. *14:* 20 (1971).

VERESS, B.; BÁLINT, A., and JELLINEK, H.: Permeability of the aorta in hypercholesterolaemic rats. Electron microscopic observations. Acta morph. Acad.
Sci. hung. *20:* 199 (1972).

VERESS, B.; BÁLINT, A.; KÓCZÉ, A.; NAGY, Z., and JELLINEK, H.: Increasing aortic
permeability by atherogenic diet. Atherosclerosis *11:* 369 (1970).

WRIGHT, H.P.; EVANS, M., and GREEN, R.P.: Aortic endothelial mitosis and Evans
blue uptake in cholesterol-fed subscorbutic guinea pigs. Atherosclerosis *21:*
105 (1975).

Professor C.W.M. ADAMS, Department of Pathology, Guy's Hospital Medical
School, London University, *London* (England)

Prog. biochem. Pharmacol., vol. 14, pp. 157–160 (Karger, Basel 1977)

Time Course of Experimental Transmural Permeability Disturbance in the Aorta of Rats

Z. Detre, T. Kerényi and H. Jellinek

2nd Department of Pathology, Semmelweis Medical University, Budapest

Introduction

The concept that endothelial injury promotes atherosclerosis dates back to Virchow. Schürmann and McMahon were the first to observe that insudation and accumulation of plasma substances in the vascular wall due to increased permeability are important pathogenetic factors in the development of hypertensive vascular lesions. Interest has been increasingly focused on permeability disturbances induced by various experimental methods.

In order to elucidate the early alterations in the permeability of the aortic wall and the possible involvement of humoral and hemodynamic factors in this process, experimental hypertension was produced by complete ligature of the aorta between the origins of the renal arteries. This model permits the comparison of the aortic segments above and below the ligature in respect of the different blood pressure levels and hemodynamic stresses.

Material and Methods

The experiments were carried out on Wistar rats weighing 220–280 g. Two groups of controls were used. One was left untreated while the other was nephrectomized on the left side immediately after the ligature of the aorta, and the animals of this latter group were sacrificed on the 7th day following the operation. The animals of the experimental group were sacrificed at different points of time up to 3 weeks following the aortic ligature.

Colloidal iron (Ferrlecit) – given intravenously 2 h prior to sacrifice (1 ml/100 g BW) – was used as a tracer of transmural permeability alterations. A microanalytical method was developed to determine the colloidal iron content of the arterial wall in order to avoid subjective errors in the evaluation of histological sections due to the patchy distribution of lesions. The region of the ligature was excised and the aortic segments above and below the ligature were investigated separately. The iron content was referred to 1 mg dry weight of aortic tissue.

Results

As the left renal artery branches off distal to the right one, the ligature results in an ischemic atrophy of the left kidney with the typical features of the endocrine kidney and subsequent arterial hypertension.

Plasma renin activity increased significantly by the 7th day and showed a decline after the 3rd week. Blood pressure in the carotid and femoral arteries and iron content of the aortic segments are demonstrated on figures 1–4.

Fibrinoid arteriolar changes have already been observed at the 3rd day but the most serious lesions were detected 7 days after the coarctation. These necrotic arteriolar walls were positive with Prussian blue reaction following colloidal iron administration, indicating an increased arteriolar transmural permeability, while at the 3rd week when intimal proliferations media hypertrophy and periarteritis nodosa-like pictures were observed no Prussian blue positivity was detected.

Discussion

Our previous investigations on permeability of hypercholesteremic rat aortas together with the present results furnish additional data to the observation that permeability disturbance is the earliest manifestation of the aortic wall injury. The time course of the aortic permeability disturbance was the same in both the hypercholesteremic and hypertensive experimental models.

The same time course was detected in the small muscular arteries of rats suffering from experimental malignant hypertension. Of particular interest was the demonstration of parallelism in the permeability distur-

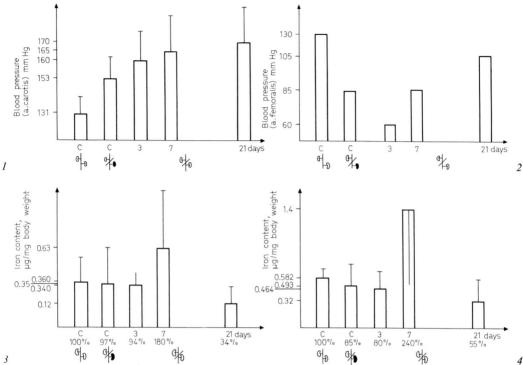

Fig. 1. The mean blood pressure in the carotid was significantly elevated on the 3rd day after coarctation and a continuous rise was present throughout the whole period of the experiment. In the control animals with coarctation and left side nephrectomy a moderate but nonsignificant rise in blood pressure was detected on the 7th day after operation, however, no effect was detectable on plasma renin activity.

Fig. 2. The mean blood pressure in the femoral artery having definitely fallen after coarctation shows a rise towards normal values and by the 3rd week it can be considered as normal. In the control animals with coarctation and left side nephrectomy the same tension was found as in the 7-day-old experimental group.

Fig. 3. The microanalytically evaluated iron content of the aortic specimen is related to the present permeability disturbance. In the aortic segment above the ligature, maximum permeability increase was detected 7 days after ligature and it decreased by the 3rd week, although blood pressure continues to increase in that period of the experiment.

Fig. 4. The same pattern of permeability disturbance was observed in the aortic segment below the ligature, where, following a low pressure phase normotension was detected at the 3rd week. The maximum iron content, thus the top of permeability increase, was on the 7th day and on the 3rd week the permeability was found to be lower than in the normal control. In spite of the fact that the tension in the femoral artery was the same in the 7-day-old experimental group as in the control animals with coarctation and left kidney excised, a significant difference in permeability levels existed between them.

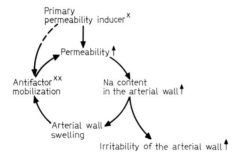

Fig. 5. R-A-S (primary permeability stimulator) and prostaglandins (antifactor) are antagonistic in respect of hypertension but may be synergistic in respect of the arterial wall permeability. Prostaglandins generated locally in the arterial wall might well be the common mediator of permeability disturbances in various experimental conditions. $\times$ = Hypercholesterolemia: triglycerides?, hypertension: R-A-S?, hypoxia; $\times\times$ = tension lowering factors (P.G.?).

bances in the two segments of the aorta, in spite of the significant difference between their tension values and consequently between their hemodynamic conditions. There is a number of data available suggesting that the R-A-S responsible for the renal hypertension can induce injuries of the arterial wall. It has been known that a primary permeability stimulator may cause directly or indirectly the appearance of certain antifactors (e.g. angiotensin-prostaglandins in renal hypertension). Certain antifactors like prostaglandins themselves are, however, also known to be strong permeability inducers. In that context the factors antagonistic in respect of hypertension may be synergistic in respect of the arterial wall permeability. Thus vascular permeability changes in hypertension can be regarded as due either to a direct injury caused by hypertension inducers, or to antihypertensive substances induced by the former, or to both.

Z. DETRE, 2nd Department of Pathology, Semmelweis Medical University, Üllői-ut 93, *1091 Budapest* (Hungary)

Prog. biochem. Pharmacol., vol. 14, pp. 161–163 (Karger, Basel 1977)

Arterial Permeability to Labeled Protein

U. Fuchs, M. Jobst, G. Gepp and D. Gottschild

Department of Experimental Pathology, Institute of Pathology, and Department of Nuclear Medicine, Clinic of Radiology, Karl Marx University, Leipzig

Introduction

A number of different tracers were used to determine the permeability of the vessel wall [a comprehensive survey is given in Jellinek, 1974]. The present authors have been using labeled albumin in an attempt to determine changes in permeability in some experimental models.

Material and Methods

^{131}J or ^{51}Cr-labeled human serum albumin was intravenously administered to a total of 74 rabbits. Following this, angiotensin II (3 $\mu g/kg$), serotonin (1.5 $\mu g/kg$), prostaglandin E_2 (20 $\mu g/kg$), and bradykinin (1.5 $\mu g/kg$) were administered intravenously and intracardially, respectively. The aorta was divided into 15 segments and was subsequently weighed. The number of pulses was determined in the scintillation counter. The permeability index was determined from the ratio of tissue activity to blood activity. Conventional scanning and transmission electron microscope investigations were also made.

Results

The permeability index, which was related to weight, showed a maximum in the aortic arch and in the abdominal aorta. The lowest values were found in the descending thoracic aorta. A short-term blood pressure increase brought about by angiotensin II was observed to increase the number of pulses over the aortic wall 4.3 times. Electron microscope examinations allowed to determine the presence of damaged endothelia and isolated parietal microthrombi. Serotonin, prostaglandin E_2, and bradykinin were found to increase the index of permeability. In the femoral artery, the permeability of the vessel wall showed a considerable increase after death. A comparison of various arteries indicated a particularly high permeability index in the coronary artery. High values were also found in the aortic and pulmonary valves of the heart.

Discussion

The pulse rates determined by us were found to be dependent upon the supply of albumin to, the discharge of albumin from, and the incorporation of albumin in the aortic wall. Important factors affecting the index of permeability are the wall tension (normal wall tension or tension increased by angiotensin), the surface-to-weight ratio of the aortic segments, and the structure of the intercellular junctions, which can be varied in individual portions of the vessel [HÜTTNER et al., 1973] and which can be altered experimentally. Angiotensin, serotonin, and bradykinin tend to dilate and open the intercellular junctions [CONSTANTINIDES, 1969], thus greatly facilitating the supply of albumin [FUCHS et al., 1974].

Summary

Labeled albumin, which was administered intravenously, was detected, with the use of a scintillation counter, in the aortic wall of rabbits. Relative to weight, the permeability index was highest in the aortic arch and abdominal aorta and lowest in the medial thoracic aorta. Angiotensin II and various mediators were found to increase the permeability of the aortic wall.

References

CONSTANTINIDES, P.: Ultrastructural injury of arterial endothelium. II. Effects of vasoactive amines. Archs Path. 88: 106–112 (1969).

FUCHS, U.; GEPP, G.; LÖBE, J.; HAUFFE, W., and RIETHLING, A.K.: Labelled serum albumin in the aortic wall after short-term blood pressure increase by angiotensin II. Arterial Wall 2: 187–199 (1974).

HÜTTNER, I.; BOUTET, M., and MORE, R.H.: Studies on protein passage through arterial endothelium. I. Structural correlates of permeability in rat arterial endothelium. Lab. Invest. 28: 672–677 (1973).

JELLINEK, H.: Arterial lesions and arteriosclerosis (Akadémiai Kiado, Budapest 1974).

U. FUCHS, MD, Department of Experimental Pathology, Institute of Pathology, Karl Marx University at Leipzig, Liebigstrasse 26, 701 Leipzig (GDR)

Prog. biochem. Pharmacol., vol. 14, pp. 164–170 (Karger, Basel 1977)

Scanning Electron Microscopy of Arterial Endothelium[1]

D.E. Bowyer, P.F. Davies, M.A. Reidy, T.B. Goode and E.S. Green

Department of Pathology (Head: Prof. P. Wildy), University of Cambridge, Cambridge

Introduction

Loss of endothelial integrity is important in initiation and development of atherosclerotic lesions [12]. Factors which determine integrity of endothelium are, however, poorly understood, although it is known that haemodynamic forces [7, 10] and toxaemia, such as endotoxaemia [11] are injurious.

One of the reasons for slow progress in the study of endothelial integrity lies in the technical difficulties for its assessment. Transmission electron microscopy is unsatisfactory because the amount of tissue sampled is small. This disadvantage is overcome by methods for viewing *en face,* such as cleared whole artery and Häutchen preparations, and the more recently established method of scanning electron microscopy (SEM), which allows observation of large areas of endothelium without removal. SEM is not, however, without its pitfalls and early studies paid too little attention to the possibility of artefacts. Three problems were outstanding:

(1) Staining. In some studies, failure to visualise endothelial cells *per se* gave erroneous concepts of the presence and position of individual cells. This is overcome by staining with silver salts [8].

(2) Fixation. In general arteries have been fixed at either atmospheric pressure or only briefly (e.g. for 15 min) at physiological pressure.

[1] We are grateful to May and Baker Ltd., Dagenham, Essex, for financial support of these studies.

This led to the misleading suggestion that endothelial cells are composed of folds and gullies, linked by bridges [13]. In reality this is caused by contraction of underlying elastic lamellae [3].

(3) Drying. Almost all studies have employed drying techniques which use organic solvents to remove water. This leads to loss of lipid and collapse of atherosclerotic lesions, giving the impression of a fragmented, even absent endothelium [1, 14].

In order to make SEM a more reliable method of endothelial integrity we have used staining, prolonged fixation under pressure [5] and air drying of tissue without organic solvents [6]. Our methods are now briefly described and illustrated.

Materials and Methods

Animals. The majority of studies were carried out in New Zealand White rabbits, mainly males, aged between 4 weeks and 1 year. Atherosclerotic lesions were induced by feeding a semi-synthetic diet containing 20 % w/w beef tallow and 0.2 % w/w cholesterol for up to 24 weeks. Two male cynomolgus monkeys *(Macaca irus),* 2 and 9 years old, were also studied.

Silver staining of aortas and prolonged fixation at physiological pressure. Heparin (1,000 IU/kg; Evans Medical Ltd., UK) was injected intravenously 2 min before death. Rabbits were killed by a blow on the neck. Cynomolgus monkeys were anaesthetised with 0.2 ml of Vetalar i.m. (Parke-Davis, Pontypool, UK) followed by Nembutal (Abbott Laboratories, UK) 6 mg/kg i.v. and killed by an overdose of Nembutal. A cannula was inserted in the ascending aorta and a femoral artery transected to allow outflow of solutions. By means of a 3-way tap, solutions were introduced from reservoirs at a pressure of 100 mm Hg as follows: (1) 50 ml of isotonic glucose (4.6 % w/v in 20mM HEPES buffer, pH 7.4) to wash out blood; (2) 50 ml of 0.2 % w/v silver nitrate in 4.2 % w/v glucose in 20 mM HEPES buffer, pH 7.4 which was held in the artery for about 30 sec; (3) a further 50 ml of isotonic glucose; (4) phosphate buffered formalin fixative. This was 2 % formalin (i.e. 0.8 % w/v formaldehyde and 0.2 % v/v methanol) in 16 mM phosphate buffer, pH 7.4 (total tonicity 390 mosm, of which the phosphate buffer vehicle contributed 40 mosm). The artery was fixed at 100 mm Hg for 12–16 h. Such prolonged fixation at physiological pressure is absolutely critical for proper fixation and flattening of the elastic lamellae. Pressure fixation for a few minutes is inadequate.

Drying and SEM. Arteries were excised, opened and pinned onto a board covered with aluminium foil, washed with deionised water for 30 min and then dried in air, without prior solvent dehydration, in a desiccator over silica gel for 3 days. Segments were coated for SEM with up to 30 mm of gold in a sputtering unit (Polaron Ltd., Watford, UK) and viewed in a Stereoscan S600 at 15 kV.

Results

Normal rabbits. (1) Areas away from branches of normal rabbit aorta showed complete layers of endothelial cells outlined by silver (fig. 1). (2) At branches, the area of the aorta distal to flow dividers always showed poor staining. Cells on the dividers were intact in 4-week-old animals, but were disrupted in older ones. Areas of poor silver staining and cellular erosion increased with age. (3) The shape of normal cells depended on their location. On the posterior wall they were long and narrow (60–80 × 10 μm), being aligned with flow lines. In the aortic arch they were hexagonal (30 × 30 μm) having a less well defined orientation. (4) Brightly stained (argyrophilic) areas were frequently found in 4-week-old animals (fig. 2) and to a lesser extent in older ones. (5) In animals brought into the Department and held for only a few days before study, a high incidence of bizarre cell shapes and argyrophilic areas were found.

Atherosclerotic rabbits during development of lesions. (1) After 3 weeks of diet (plasma cholesterol concentrations 567 mg/100 ml) most of the endothelium was normal, but argyrophilic cells and areas of enlarged, poorly staining cells were found. (2) After 6 weeks (plasma cholesterol 1,247 mg/100 ml) small lesions were visible as focal swellings. They were always covered with endothelium, which was, however, composed of large cells and was poorly stained (fig. 3). (3) After 12, 20 or 24 weeks (plasma cholesterol 1,305, 1,984, 2,401 mg/100 ml) larger lesions were seen and were always endothelialised.

Young cynomolgus monkey, aged 2 years. (1) Large areas of intact endothelium. (2) Poor staining of flow dividers. (3) Shape changes of endothelium related to flow patterns (fig. 4). (4) Argyrophilic areas were occasionally found on flow dividers. Small bodies, about 1 μm in diameter, were always associated with them (fig. 5).

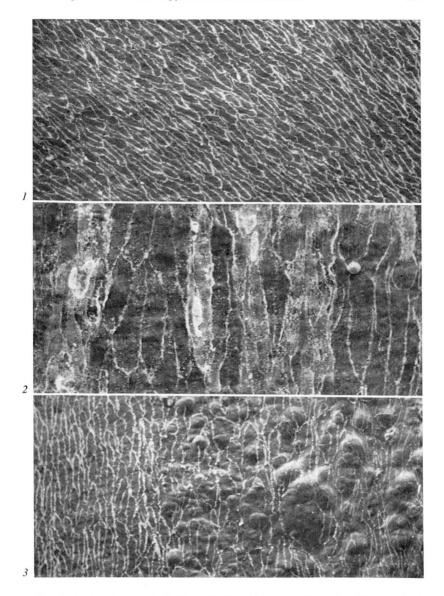

Fig. 1. Aorta of normal, Redfern strain rabbit aged 12 weeks. Silver stained, air dried. SEM. × 210.

Fig. 2. Argyrophilic cells in aorta of a normal rabbit aged 4 weeks. Silver stained, air dried. SEM. × 420.

Fig. 3. Atherosclerotic lesion in a rabbit fed an atherogenic diet for 12 weeks. Silver stained, air dried. SEM. × 210.

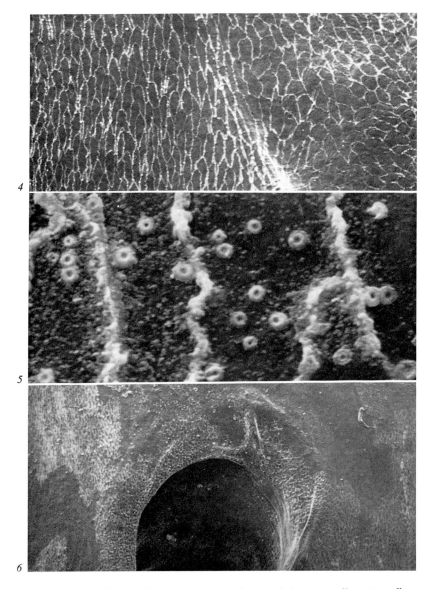

Fig. 4. Aorta of normal cynomolgus monkey aged 2 years, adjacent to flow divider of intercostal ostium. Aorta runs top to bottom on the left and entrance to branch is towards the right. Cells are aligned in the direction of flow and change orientation abruptly on flow divider. Silver stained, air dried. SEM. $\times$ 210.

Fig. 5. Small bodies, possibly platelets (diameter about 1 μm) associated with argyrophilic cells in cynomolgus monkey. Silver stained, air dried. SEM. $\times$ 4,200.

Fig. 6. Entrance to an intercostal branch of a cynomolgus monkey aged 9 years, showing large areas of endothelial desquamation. Silver stained, air dried. SEM. $\times$ 50.

Old cynomolgus monkey, aged 9 years. (1) Large areas appeared denuded of endothelium (fig. 6). (2) Many argyrophilic cells were seen and always had attached bodies resembling platelets.

Discussion

The proper assessment of tissue morphology by SEM demands careful control of artefacts of tissue preparation. GARBASCH and CHRISTENSEN [8] first recognised that silver staining provided an unambiguous demonstration of endothelial cells in SEM. Our results now indicate that prolonged fixation at physiological pressure and avoidance of loss of lipids, especially from atherosclerotic lesions, further improves realistic assessment. Following prolonged pressure fixation, the endothelium appears as a flattened sheet of cells which probably represents the arrangement *in vivo,* a conclusion supported by recent observations of CLARK and GLAGOV [4].

Investigation of aortas of normal rabbits and cynomolgus monkeys has revealed large areas of confluent normal cells the shape of which depends on blood flow patterns. In normal animals, areas associated with high shear stress showed poor silver staining and erosion of cells [10] and these correspond with regions which, in the rabbit, develop induced arrow-head sudanophilic lesions. Argyrophilic areas, as described by CHRISTENSEN [2] using SEM were also seen. These may be agonal or regenerating cells, or indeed an area from which endothelial cells have been lost. In rabbits studied soon after transport to the Department there was a high frequency of bizarre endothelial cell outlines and argyrophilic areas, suggesting that stress associated with transfer to a new environment may affect endothelial structure. In cynomolgus monkeys, small bodies, which were biconcave disks, were always associated with argyrophilic areas. Observation of cynomolgus monkey platelets prepared under the same conditions of staining and fixation suggested these were platelets. In an old monkey the large areas denuded of endothelium never had associated platelet-like bodies or platelet aggregates, as might have been expected, but the reasons are not obvious.

With respect to atherosclerotic arteries, our early observations using drying with organic solvents after silver staining suggested that lesions lacked endothelium and the surface was disrupted, as reported by others [1, 14]. When, however, tissue was air dried as described, without application of organic solvents, endothelium over lesions was found to be intact [6, 9]. A potential disadvantage of air drying is that fine structural detail is lost, but this was not an important consideration in assessing cellular integrity. Shrinkage of tissue did not appear to occur, because the cells in the neighbourhood of lesions were normal size, whilst those over lesions were somewhat larger.

Using the technique described above we are now investigating the factors which may delay the repair of endothelium following injury.

References

1   BRUIJN, W.C. DE and MOURIK, W. VAN: Virchows Arch. Abt. A. Path. Anat. *365:* 23–40 (1975).
2   CHRISTENSEN, C.B.: Virchows Arch. Abt. A. Path. Anat. *363:* 33–46 (1974).
3   CHRISTENSEN, B.C. and GARBASCH, C.: Angiologica *9:* 15–26 (1972).
4   CLARK, J.M. and GLAGOV, S.: Br. J. exp. Path. *57:* 129–135 (1976).
5   DAVIES, P.F. and BOWYER, D.E.: Atherosclerosis *21:* 463–469 (1975).
6   DAVIES, P.F.; REIDY, M.A.; GOODE, T.B., and BOWYER, D.E.: Atherosclerosis *25:* 125–130 (1976).
7   FRY, D.L.: in SCHEINBERG Cerebrovascular diseases, pp. 77ff (Raven Press, New York 1976).
8   GARBASCH, C. and CHRISTENSEN, B.C.: Angiologica *7:* 365–373 (1970).
9   GOODE, T.B.; DAVIES, P.F.; REIDY, M.A., and BOWYER, D.E.: Atherosclerosis *27:* 235–251 (1977).
10 REIDY, M.A. and BOWYER, D.E.: Atherosclerosis *26:* 181–194 (1977).
11 REIDY, M.A. and BOWYER, D.E.: Atherosclerosis *26:* 319–328 (1977).
12 ROSS, R. and GLOMSET, J.A.: New Engl. J. Med. *295:* 369–377, 420–425 (1976).
13 SHIMAMOTO, T.: in SHIMAMOTO and NUMANO Atherogenesis I, pp. 5–27 (Excerpta Medica, Amsterdam 1969).
14 WEBER, G.; FABRINI, P.; CAPACCIOLI, E., and RESI, L.: Atherosclerosis *22:* 565–572 (1975).

Dr. D.E. BOWYER, Department of Pathology, University of Cambridge, *Cambridge CB2 1QP* (England)

Prog. biochem. Pharmacol., vol. 14, pp. 171–174 (Karger, Basel 1977)

Surface Characteristics of
Human Atherosclerotic Lesions

B. Veress, Z. Saródy, J. Csengody and H. Jellinek

2nd Department of Pathology and 3rd Department of Surgery,
Semmelweis Medical University, Budapest

Introduction

Scanning electron microscopy (SEM) was applied to the study of
vascular lesions in the late 60s. The data, however, due to the technical
difficulties and to differences in the preparative methods in various
laboratories, are still controversial and can hardly be compared, including
the finer details even of the normal endothelium. In the light of recent
observations of Christensen and Garbarsch [1972], de Bruijn and van
Mourik [1975], Clark and Glagov [1976], Davies *et al.* [1976], and
Reidy and Bowyer [1977] it seems that some of the features described
earlier are artefacts. In the present paper we describe the surface alterations observed in human atherosclerotic lesions with comparison of conventional vacuum and the critical point drying.

Material and Methods

The femoral arteries were removed from five patients prior to the
amputation of the leg. The specimens were fixed in 1.5 % glutaraldehyde,
dehydrated in alcohol and prepared for coating by means of either vacuum
drying or of the critical point device. The parts of the arteries appearing
normal on gross inspection were used for comparison.

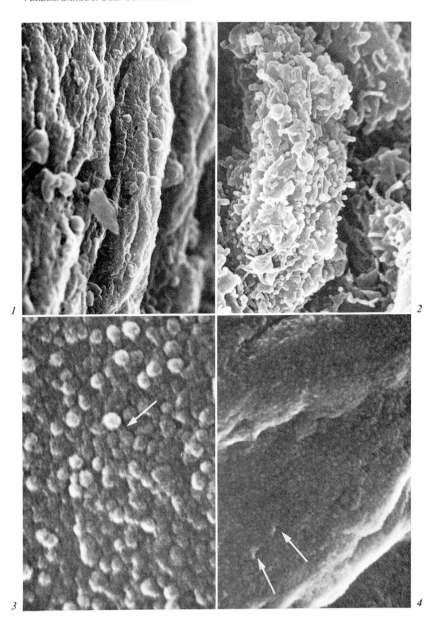

Fig. 1. Vacuum drying. × 2,600.
Fig. 2. Critical point drying. × 1,800.
Fig. 3. Vacuum drying. × 53,000.
Fig. 4. Critical point drying. × 53,000.

Results

Two pathological phenomena could be seen in our material: (1) thrombus formation; and (2) alteration of the intima.

In two out of five arteries thrombus formation was present. The longitudinal furrows were masked by a thick fibrin coat, RBCs, platelets and white blood cells. In other regions over the plaques there were round-shaped particles, spheres of 1.2 μm in diameter attached to or immersed into the endothelial surface (fig. 1). Sometimes crater-like depressions were seen on the surface of the intima.

As regards the intimal alterations, two types of atherosclerotic lesions could be differentiated in the human vessels. The *elevated* type of lesions exhibited folds and furrows, however, covered by apparently smaller endothelial cells with very marked bulging of their nuclear areas. The other, so-called 'in the level' type showed a more or less *flat* surface only with occasional bulging of individual cells.

With higher magnification, the surfaces of the normal-looking cells were smooth while those of cells from atherosclerotic regions were villous-granular in appearance or exhibited membranous folds and ruffles (fig. 2).

At the highest magnification examined the smooth-looking surface of normal endothelium prepared by vacuum-drying revealed a surface resembling that of tightly packed small villi with small artificial cracks between them (fig. 3). When the critical point device was applied the bundling of the villi did not occur and the surface resembled that of a fine velvet tissue. Here and there small, roughly circular villous-less spots were also recognizable, representing probably the orifices of pinocytic vesicles (fig. 4). The endothelial cells from atherosclerotic plaques revealed similar fine surface organization but exhibited large folds, villous projections and ruffles.

Discussion

We may interpret the results presented as follows: at this phase of our observations several phenomena (spheres, nature of some of the cells, craters) cannot be explained based upon their SEM appearance only.

The low power SEM micrographs revealed the presence of both flat and elevated lesions in human material similar to those described in atherosclerosis of various animals [DE BRUIJN and VAN MOURIK, 1975]. At the moment it is not possible to decide whether these lesions represent genuinely different types of pathologic processes or whether they are just different phases of one and the same process.

The presence of microthrombi may be considered as an evidence for their probable importance in initiating the development of atherosclerotic lesions and may also complicate the late phase.

It seems that the arrangement and structure of the endothelial cell membrane was much better preserved by the method of critical point drying than by vacuum drying. Regarding the velvet-like appearance of the cell membrane and its possible change in different conditions further, very thorough studies are necessary.

The fairly characteristic changes of the endothelial surface in the plaque areas, the ruffles and villous projections in particular, may represent either the extensive bleb formation of dying cells or the enhanced membrane activity of damaged cells.

References

BRUIJN, W.C. DE and MOURIK, W. VAN: Scanning electron microscopic observations of endothelial changes in experimentally induced atheromatosis of rabbit aortas. Virchows Arch. path. Anat. Physiol. *365:* 23–40 (1975).

CHRISTENSEN, B.C. and GARBARSCH, C.: A scanning electron microscopic (SEM) study on the endothelium of the normal rabbit aorta. Angiologica *9:* 15–26 (1972).

CLARK, J.M. and GLAGOV, S.: Luminal surface of distended arteries by scanning electron microscopy: eliminating configurational and technical artefacts. Br. J. exp. Path. *57:* 129–135 (1976).

DAVIES, P.F.; REIDY, M.A.; GOODE, T.B., and BOWYER, D.E.: Scanning electron microscopy in the evaluation of endothelial integrity of the fatty lesion in atherosclerosis. Atherosclerosis *25:* 125–130 (1976).

REIDY, M.A. and BOWYER, D.E.: Scanning electron microscopy: morphology of aortic endothelium following injury by endotoxin and during subsequent repair. Atherosclerosis *26:* 319–328 (1977).

Dr. B. VERESS, 2nd Department of Pathology and 3rd Department of Surgery, Semmelweis Medical University, *Budapest* (Hungary)

Prog. biochem. Pharmacol., vol. 14, pp. 175–181 (Karger, Basel 1977)

Scanning Electron Microscopy of Aortic Endothelium Following Injury by Endotoxin and During Subsequent Repair

M.A. Reidy[1] and D.E. Bowyer

Department of Biophysics, University of Western Ontario, London, Ont., and Department of Pathology, University of Cambridge, Cambridge

It is widely held that disturbance in the integrity of arterial endothelium can lead to the development of atherosclerosis since both injury to endothelial cells or a change in their permeability will permit an enhanced entry of plasma constituents into the arterial wall [8]. The consequence of this action may result in platelet adherence, a proliferation and migration of medial smooth muscle cells into the intima [15] and possibly lipid accumulation [2].

In order to study the effects of endothelial cell injury, various techniques have been used to damage the luminal surface of arteries [6]. These methods are usually mechanical, such as a Fogarthy catheter [5, 11] or a metal scraper [1, 12] and, while they are very successful in causing endothelial injury, they can often bring about considerable medial damage which has been shown to influence endothelial regeneration [17]. In order, therefore, to study the effects of endothelial injury we sought a method which injured endothelial cells with a minimal effect on the media.

It has been known for some time that endotoxin derived from certain gram-negative bacteria have the ability to act on the endothelial surface and bring about widespread endothelial desquamation. It is still unclear as to how endotoxin acts, and while platelets have been implicated as mediators [3], some workers consider that the toxin acts directly on the endothelial cells [10]. In these studies rabbits arteries were injured by administration of a single intravenous injection of endotoxin (200 μg/kg body weight) derived from *Serratia marcescens*. These animals were killed 1 h, 14 and 28 days later. Their aortas were prepared for scanning elec-

---

[1] Ontario Heart Foundation Fellow.

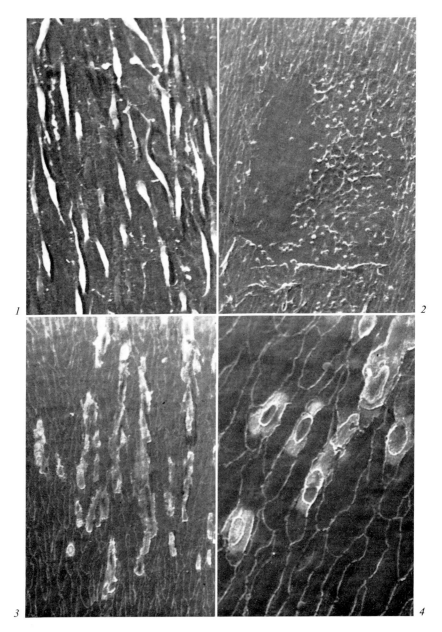

Fig. 1. Rabbit aorta 1 h after administration of endotoxin. Silver stained. SEM.
× 460.

tron microscopy (SEM) by staining with buffered 0.2 % $AgNO_3$ and fixation at physiological press for at least 12 h. Silver nitrate is a well-known stain for endothelial cell boundaries and fixation at physiological pressure ensures that the elastic fibres were fixed in their *in vivo* state, thus minimising formation of artefacts [7, 13]. The specimens were then coated with gold and viewed by SEM in a Cambridge S600 Stereoscan at a beam voltage of 15 kV.

1 h after endotoxin administration (fig. 1) the endothelial cells were spindle-shaped in appearance and seemed curled up. These cells were similar to injured endothelial cells reported in other studies. In other areas of these aortas (fig. 2) the endothelium was found to have been removed und platelets were seen adhering to the exposed subendothelium. Normal endothelial cells surrounded these areas. In the aortas from animals killed 14 days after endotoxin administration a few spindle cells were seen on the aortic surface and large numbers of cells and small bodies with brightly stained boundaries were present. Giant cells with well stained cell boundaries were also observed in these vessels. 28 days after endotoxin injection no spindle-shaped cells were present and instead the aortas are covered with rows of endothelial cells which were heavily stained with silver (fig. 3). These cells were similar in shape and size to the normal endothelial cells and their surface appeared bright and granular when viewed by SEM. The extent of silver staining varied between cells, in some the entire surface was heavily stained while in others only parts of the cell, for example the area associated with the nucleus, was stained (fig. 4). Argyrophilic cells were also occasionally observed in the 14-day animals. Giant cells were also present in 28-day aortas but unlike those previously shown, their entire surface was heavily stained with silver. Another interesting finding in these arteries was that argyrophilic cells were often found clustered around denuded regions. Figure 5 shows a region without endothelial cover and no adhering platelets. The endothelial cells bordering this area were intensely stained with silver, whilst the cells further away from the denuded zone were normal, both in silver staining and size. A further feature of these cells was that a large number

---

Fig. 2. As in figure 1, showing platelet adherence on an area denuded of endothelium. Silver stained. SEM. × 230.

Fig. 3. Rabbit aorta 28 days after administration of endotoxin showing argyrophilic cells. Silver stained. SEM. × 230.

Fig. 4. As in figure 3. Silver stained. SEM. × 460.

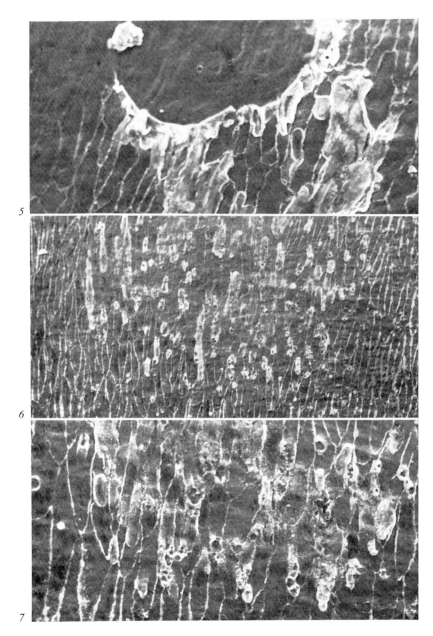

Fig. 5. Rabbit aorta, 28 days after administration of endotoxin, showing a denuded area without platelets. Silver stained. SEM. $\times$ 460.

of stomata were often present in areas showing no obvious signs of damage.

In a second experiment it was decided to influence the formation of these argyrophilic cells by feeding a diet containing 0.2 % cholesterol and 20 % beef tallow to animals given endotoxin. Rabbits were fed this diet for 2 weeks and then given a single intravenous injection of endotoxin as before. They were then fed the diet for a further 2 or 4 weeks, after which time they were killed and their aortas prepared for SEM.

2 weeks after injury by endotoxin no argyrophilic cells were observed and the aortas contained rows of irregularly shaped cells or small bodies with heavily silver-stained borders. No large giant cells were seen in these vessels. 4 weeks after toxin administration many argyrophilic cells were present (fig. 6). These cells, however, were different from those previously reported in this study, in that their surfaces were irregular and contained pits and small craters (fig. 7). Normally stained endothelial cells with no visible changes in their surface morphology were seen elsewhere in these vessels.

These results show that endotoxin causes widespread endothelial injury and some time after the initial injury, certain endothelial cells become avidly stained with silver. These argyrophilic cells were seen 14 days and, more noticeably, 28 days after injury and were often located on the borders of denuded zones. These findings have led us to suggest that these cells are young or possibly regenerating endothelial cells which are more permeable to silver salts [14]. Endothelial regeneration is known to occur several days after endotoxin administration [9] and similarly stained cells have been observed in arteries several days after injury by noradrenaline [4]. Furthermore, in a Häutchen study POOLE et al. [12] observed silver granules in dividing endothelial cells. Recently we have observed similar argyrophilic cells in the aortas of 1-week-old animals where the endothelium is known to be actively dividing as judged by its high mitotic index [16].

The morphology of the argyrophilic cells was altered by feeding a diet producing hypercholesterolaemia while no changes were observed in the surrounding normal silver-stained endothelial cells. Thus, if argyrophilic

Fig. 6. Rabbit aorta, 28 days after administration of endotoxin in a hypercholesterolaemic animal, showing argyrophilic cells. Silver stained. SEM. × 230.

Fig. 7. As in figure 6, showing pits and craters on the surface of argyrophilic cells. Silver stained. SEM. × 460.

cells are indeed young or regenerating then they may be more susceptible to noxious agents such as a raised plasma cholesterol, than are the normal older cells. These findings suggest, therefore, that atherogenic agents may act not only by injuring the arterial cells directly, but by modifying endothelial repair.

References

1   BJÖRKERUD, S.: Reaction of the aortic wall of the rabbit after superficial longitudinal, mechanical trauma. Virchows Arch. Abt. A. Path. Anat. *347:* 197–210 (1969).

2   BJÖRKERUD, S. and BONDJERS, G.: Arterial repair and atherosclerosis after mechanical injury. Part 5: Tissue response after induction of a large superficial transverse injury. Atherosclerosis *18:* 235–255 (1973).

3   BROWN, D.L. and LACHMANN, P.J.: The behaviour of complement and platelets in letal endotoxin shock in rabbits. Int. Archs Allergy appl. Immun. *45:* 193–205 (1973).

4   CHRISTENSEN, C.B.: Repair in arterial tissue. A scanning electron microscopic study on the endothelium of the rabbit thoracic aorta following noradrenaline in toxic doses. Virchows Arch. Abt. A. Path. Anat. *363:* 33–46 (1974).

5   CHRISTENSEN, B.C. and GARBASCH, C.: Repair of arterial tissue. A scanning electron microscopic and light microscopic study of the endothelium of rabbit thoracic aorta, following a single dilation injury. Virchows Arch. Abt. A. Path. Anat. *360:* 93–106 (1973).

6   CONSTANTINIDES, P.: In Experimental atherosclerosis (Elsevier, Amsterdam 1965).

7   DAVIES, P.F. and BOWYER, D.E.: Scanning electron microscopy: arterial endothelial integrity after fixation at physiological pressure. Atherosclerosis *21:* 463–469 (1975).

8   FRY, D.L.: Responses of the arterial wall to certain physical factors; in Atherogenesis: initiating factors. Ciba Found. Symp., No. 12 (Elsevier, Amsterdam 1973).

9   GAYNOR, E.: Increased mitotic activity in rabbit endothelium after endotoxin. An autoradiographic study. Lab. Invest. *24:* 318–320 (1971).

10 GAYNOR, E.; BOUVIER, C.A., and SPAET, T.H.: Vascular lesions: possible pathogenic basis of the generalised Schwartzman reaction. Science *170:* 986–988 (1970).

11 HELIN, P.; LORENZEN, I.; GARBARSCH, C., and MATTHIESSEN, M.E.: Repair in arterial tissue: morphological and biochemical changes in rabbit aorta after a single dilatation injury. Circulation Res. *29:* 542–554 (1971).

12 POOLE, J.C.F.; SANDERS, A.G., and FLOREY, H.W.: The regeneration of aortic endothelium. J. Path. Bact. *75:* 133–143 (1958).

13 REIDY, M.A. and BOWYER, D.E.: Scanning electron microscopy of arteries: the morphology of aortic endothelium in haemodynamically stressed areas associated with branches. Atherosclerosis 26: 181–194 (1977).

14 REIDY, M.A. and BOWYER, D.E.: Scanning electron microscopy: morphology of aortic endothelium following injury by endotoxin and during subsequent repair. Atherosclerosis 26: 319–328 (1977).

15 ROSS, R. and GLOMSET, J.A.: The pathogenesis of atherosclerosis. New Engl. J. Med. 295: 369–377 (1976).

16 SADE, R.M.; FOLKMANN, J., and COTTRAN, R.S.: DNA synthesis in endothelium of aortic segments in vitro. Expl Cell Res. 74: 297–306 (1972).

17 SCHWARTZ, S.M.; STEMERMAN, M.B., and BENDITT, E.P.: The aortic intima. II. Repair of the aortic lining after mechanical denudation. Am. J. Path. 81: 15–31 (1975).

Dr. M.A. REIDY, University of Western Ontario, London, Ont. (Canada)

Prog. biochem. Pharmacol., vol. 14, pp. 182–184 (Karger, Basel 1977)

Scanning Electron Microscopy of the Aorta

U. Fuchs

Department of Experimental Pathology, Institute of Pathology,
Karl Marx University, Leipzig

Introduction

The normal and pathologically altered inner surface of the aorta has been examined, by scanning electron microscopy, under different conditions. The objective of this study was to determine the normal relief and its change caused by a short-time increase of blood pressure and arteriosclerosis.

Material and Methods

Cholesterol was administered to rabbits for 12–18 weeks, the amount of cholesterol administered varying between 45 and 84 g. To other rabbits, 3–10 μg/kg of angiotensin II was intravenously administered once or five times. In the latter case, injections were made at 10-min intervals. Also examined were untreated control animals and arteriosclerotic aortae obtained from man. Specimens were prepared by a method suitable for scanning electron microscopy. The intercellular junctions were coated with silver. Furthermore, transmission and light microscope studies were made.

Results

The folds of the inner surface of the endothelium are produced by shrinkage of the vessel wall during fixing and drying. They are longer than the endothelia, involving not only the endothelium, but also deeper portions of the vessel wall. The folds are close to, but not always touching, each other. The surface of the flat areas lying between them is rather rough. The normal folded relief ends at the foot of the arteriosclerotic plaques. Here, small and irregular wavy formations can be observed. Loss of endothelia results in the elastic windowed lamella becoming apparent. Narrower folds, parietal microthrombi, filaments of fibrin, amorphous and granular material, and adherent mononuclear leukocytes can be observed after a short-time increase in blood pressure brought about by angiotensin II. A continuous endovasal film of fibrin could not be observed.

Discussion

The folds do not represent the endothelia, as has already been reported by GARBASCH and COLLATZ CHRISTENSEN [1970]. In arteriosclerotic beds the consistency of the inner aortic layers is different from that in the normal vessel wall, and this results in a different texture of the surface being observed here [FUCHS, 1972]. Damage to endothelia leads to amorphous accumulations of blood plasma, which probably contain fragments of the glycocalyx, of fibrin, thrombocytes, and mononuclear leukocytes [WEBER and TOSI, 1971; WEBER et al., 1973; FUCHS et al., 1974; GEPP, 1974].

Summary

The folds of the intimal surface do not represent the endothelia. Rather, they are produced by tissue shrinkage occurring during preparation, with the shrinking process proceeding in the arteriosclerotic bed differing from that in the normal vessel wall. Consequently, the surface appearance, or texture, of arteriosclerotic beds is different from that of the normal vessel wall. Administration of angiotensin results in the deposition of parietal microthrombi and fibrin filaments as well as in the adhesion of mononuclear leukocytes to the inner coat of the vessel.

References

FUCHS, U.: Das innere Relief der normalen und der arteriosklerotischen Aorta im Rasterelektronenmikroskop. Exp. Path. 7: 45–59 (1972).

FUCHS, U.; GEPP, G.; LÖBE, J.; HAUFFE, W., and RIETHLING, A.K.: Labelled serum albumin in the aortic wall after short-term blood pressure increase by angiotensin II. Arterial Wall 2: 187–199 (1974).

GARBASCH, C. and COLLATZ CHRISTENSEN, B.: Scanning electron microscopy of aortic endothelial cell boundaries after staining with silver nitrate. Angiologica 7: 365–373 (1970).

GEPP, G.: Das innere Relief der Aorta im Rasterelektronenmikroskop; Med. Dipl. Arbeit, Leipzig (1974).

WEBER, G.; FABBRINI, P., and RESI, L.: On the presence of a concanavalin-A reactive coat over the endothelial aortic surface and its modifications during early experimental cholesterol atherogenesis in rabbits. Virchows Arch. Abt. A Path. Anat. 359: 299–307 (1973).

WEBER, G. and TOSI, C.: Observations with the scanning microscope on the development of cholesterol aortic arteriosclerosis in the guinea pig. Virchows Arch. Abt. A Path. Anat. 353: 325–332 (1971).

U. FUCHS, MD, Department of Experimental Pathology, Institute of Pathology, Karl Marx University at Leipzig, Liebigstrasse 26, 701 Leipzig (GDR)

Prog. biochem. Pharmacol., vol. 14, pp. 185–186 (Karger, Basel 1977)

Processing with Arterial Tissues for SEM Examinations

G. WEBER

Department of Pathology, University of Siena, Siena

All the participants of the SEM session have agreed on the opportunity of proposing a 'common method' of processing arterial tissues for SEM examinations. The author has been kindly invited to write some introductory remarks. Through underlining the usefulness of such a proposal in helping to achieve better results and a fruitful comparison of results obtained in different laboratories, attention has to be recalled to the fact that a too rigid standardization of methods may actually pose limits on further developmental research. At any rate, some further points deserve also a careful cautious consideration. For people working, for instance, on the endothelial surface coat, the 'common method' has to be modified to allow the employment of con A. Con A, as is well known, has to be acting on pieces of tissues still living or very shortly fixed [BERNHARD and AVRAMEAS, 1971] or even used by perfusion with phytohemagglutinin and horseradish peroxidase in unfixed material [as recently proposed by STEIN et al., 1976]. Those working with the regional differences of the surface coat of endothelial cells (as evidenced for instance in pigs by Evans blue injections) will not make easily use of fixation by perfusion, because after fixation by perfusion the different regional patterns (so-called 'blue' and 'white' areas) may be inapparent [SCHWARTZ, 1975]. Prolonged pressure-fixation after perfusion of living animals cannot be used when biochemical analytical procedures on tissues are to be programmed or tissue cultures have to be prepared. Not to speak of the effects of different enzymatic actions upon the surface coat that cannot obviously be studied unless fresh tissues are available. Moreover, pressure-fixation procedures, which may result useful in normal tissues, have still to be subjected to further critical studies because we have to learn still more on possible different resistance of areas unaffected by lesions nearby areas affected by lesions: and different lesions ('gelatinous' vs. SMC-'hyperplastic') could be affected in different ways by such 'pressure-fixation' procedures. On the contrary, further improvements of the technique may also be required if SEM observation of intimal surface is to be compared with TEM observation of the same tissue [KELLY *et al.*, 1973; WICKHAM and WORTHEN, 1973; ROBERTSON and McKALEN, 1975].

SEM and TEM comparative observations are so often needed in fact by the pathologist to distinguish for instance between surface modifications due to endothelial lesions or to subendothelial pathological processes which could give place to similar surface aspects by SEM. Finally it must also be reminded here that the human pathologist, while bringing forward basic studies on animal models, aims to study, by SEM and TEM, also human material such as for instance the heart coronaries or the brain arteries. As the application of the 'common method' here proposed is almost unconceivable on human material, such material will have maybe to be examined after fixation by immersion, simply taking care that the pieces have been distended over cardboard.

References

BERNHARD, W. and AVRAMEAS, S.: Expl Cell Res. *64:* 232 (1971).
KELLY, R.O.; DEKKER, R.A.F., and BLUEMINK, J.G.: J. Ultrastruct. Res. *45:* 254 (1973).
ROBERTSON, A.L. and McKALEN, A.: 33rd Ann. Proc. Electron Microscopy Soc. Am., Las Vegas 1975.
SCHWARTZ, C.J.: Int. Workshop Conf. on Atherosclerosis, London Ont. 1975.
STEIN, O.; CHAJEK, T., and STEIN, Y.: Lab. Invest. *35:* 103 (1976).
WICKHAM, M.G. and WORTHEN, D.M.: Stain Technol. *48:* 63 (1973).

Dr. G. WEBER, Department of Pathology, University of Siena, *Siena* (Italy)

Prog. biochem. Pharmacol., vol. 14, pp. 187–188 (Karger, Basel 1977)

Methodological Aspects of Arterial Wall SEM

Anna Kádár and B. Veress

2nd Department of Pathology and 2nd Central Laboratory for Electron Microscopy, Semmelweis Medical University, Budapest

In our opinion the morphological investigations including light microscopy, electron microscopy and scanning electron microscopy are based on 'standardized artefacts'. The problem is that for the electron microscope and especially for the scanning electron microscope our techniques are not yet standardized, mainly because these instruments are very young in the field of biological research. Therefore, we should agree on one preparation method for investigating arterial endothelium which would be suggested to be used in every laboratory as a control method beside using their own techniques.

We agree basically with Dr. Gerrity's ideas which he listed during the discussion. Every laboratory has to develop their its method adapted to the type of experiment, to the experimental animals or to human material. It is extremely important to pay attention to every minor detail too.

Dr. Bowyer's method of pressure fixation and silver staining seems to be suitable for certain experimental conditions. Certainly a different method should be developed as a standard method for preparation of human material.

For this reason we would suggest – as a standard method for comparison – for investigation of *experimental animals* the pressure fixation with or without silver staining, and air drying without any prior dehydration with organic solvents.

For *human material* we would suggest immersion fixation with or without silver staining and air drying without any pre-or dehydration with organic solvents.

The normal controls both in experimental animals and in human material should be after the pressure or immersion fixation, dried in a critical point dryer too with CO_2 with a prior dehydration with organic solvents (beside the above mentioned methods).

It is suggested that these methods should be used in every laboratory working on arterial luminal surfaces in addition to their own techniques. This would enable us to compare our results and may help to come to a conclusion which would create a basic preparation method for scanning electron microscopy as it had been created for transmission electron microscopy, i.e. the Karnovsky method, as the Reynold's method, or the embedding methods.

Dr. A. KÁDÁR, 2nd Department of Pathology and 2nd Central Laboratory for Electron Microscopy, Semmelweis Medical University, *Budapest* (Hungary)

Prog. biochem. Pharmacol., vol. 14, pp. 189–191 (Karger, Basel 1977)

Recommended Preparation Method for SEM in the Rabbit Aorta

K. Kjeldsen and H.K. Thomsen

Rigshospitalet, University Hospital, Department of Clinical Chemistry, Copenhagen

Anesthesia

It is important that the animal is alive when one starts the perfusion and that the heart is still beating. We therefore use either a blow on the head or intraperitoneal Nembutal anesthesia.

Perfusion and Fixation in situ

We open both abdomen and thorax rapidly and insert a large-bore cannula in the left ventricle of the heart. Infusion of fixative should always be made *with* the blood stream and not against it. The pressure should be measured both at the point of inflow (ca. 100 mm Hg) and at the point of outflow (ca. 90 mm Hg), which with our technique is somewhere in the lower part of the iliac artery. The fixative should be 37° C, oxygenated and freshly filtered through charcoal in order to get rid of aldehyde polymerization products.

We usually start the perfusion with about 100 ml of heparinated Ringer solution (1,000 IU) in order to wash out blood remnants. As a rule we use for the aorta 2 % glutaraldehyde + 2 % formaldehyde (prepared from paraformaldehyde) in 0.1 M sodium cacodylate buffer with 0.05 M calcium chloride (pH 7.4). The final osmolality is close to 900 mosm. The osmolality should always be checked with an osmometer. For the perfusion we now use 1 liter of fixative for each animal. The period of fixation is about 1 h.

Removal of the Aorta and Cutting of Specimens

After *in situ* perfusion the aorta should be carefully removed without stretching or bending the vessel. Postfixation at room temperature in the same fixative for 24 h. Thereafter, the aorta should be placed *in situ* and opened along both sides with scissors which are not pointed. Cutting out of specimens should only be done with razor blades. Both the opening and the cutting should be performed on wax in a Petrimdish with the vessel immersed in the same fixative and the specimens should thereafter only be handled with wooden sticks on the adventitial side. Osmification for 2 h in 2 % osmium tetroxide at room temperature, washing in cacodylate buffer and through graded solutions of acetone to pure acetone. It is important that the acetone is 100 %. Extra drying is often necessary.

Drying Procedure

For drying we recommend 'The Critical Point' drying. It is essential to have control of both pressure and temperature. If possible, the drying procedure should not be done step-wise, but continuously.

Mounting of Specimens on Stubs

When the specimens are mounted on stubs, we use double-adhesive tape. If silver-dag is used to secure contact, this should be used sparingly and must be completely dry before the specimens are placed in the coater. Otherwise, escaping acetone remnants may cause artefacts in the specimens since the silver-collodium is dissolved in acetone.

Coating Procedure

Immediately after the drying process the specimens should be moved to the coater and coated with gold by DC sputtering. We use argon and a distance to the specimens of about 10 cm. The procedure should be as short as possible and the gold coat as thin as possible (about 100 Å) in order not to mask delicate surface structures (the surface should look grey and not golden). Immediately after the coating procedure the specimens should be moved to the SEM. If it is not possible to scan the specimens the same day, they should be kept in vacuum in the coater and *not* in a vacutainer. Otherwise one will find small cracks in the surface, due to differences in pressure and humidity.

Electron Microscopy

During the microscopy the lowest possible beam energy should be used in order to avoid damage of the specimen. At present we use 7.5 kV. 'Spot-size' should of course be adjusted accordingly. We also find it worthwhile to use a camera with good lenses and a large negative (e.g. Hasselblad).

After microscopy the specimens should be discarded, since deterioration seems to start immediately if they are kept in a vacutainer.

Dr. K. KJELDSEN, Department of Clinical Chemistry, Rigshospitalet, University Hospital, *DK-2100 Copenhagen* (Denmark)

Prog. biochem. Pharmacol., vol. 14, pp. 192–195 (Karger, Basel 1977)

SEM and the Surface Coat

Discussion on Reliable Assessment of Endothelial Morphology of Arteries by SEM

D. E. BOWYER

Department of Pathology, University of Cambridge, Cambridge

Although SEM offers a number of advantages over other *en face* techniques for observation of arterial endothelium, e.g. direct observation of the endothelium without removal, early results were difficult to interpret because of artefacts introduced during tissue preparation. In attempts to help workers to avoid artefacts, the meeting agreed to try to find a consensus of opinion of the necessary methods for proper tissue preparation. It was agreed, however, that although these techniques should provide a sound base-line for possible interpretation of SEM of arteries, it would be undesirable to recommend a single standard method since this might only serve to inhibit further improvements in methodology.

Handling of Tissue in Animal
1. Anaesthetic may cause alterations to endothelial cells (EC); neuroleptic analgesics (e.g. Hypnorm) and diazepam used for premedication reduce the required dose of anaesthetic
2. Anticoagulants – inject heparin (1,000 iu/kg) 2 min before killing

General Consideration for Solutions for Infusion
1. Should be isotonic; it should be more accurate to calculate tonicity from weighed amounts of solutes than measurement by osmometer, but measurement of final solution by osmometer checks for errors
2. pH 7.4
3. Temperature 37° C or room temperature; 37° C may decrease fixation time
4. Glucose may be necessary for EC survival, but long exposure of cells in culture to glucose-enriched media causes shape changes
5. Possibly add anticoagulant, e.g. heparin
6. Possibly oxygenate – air/5 % CO_2, not pure oxygen

Method of Introduction of Solutions
1. Use clean tubes and containers
2. Possibly measure animals blood pressure; remember BP altered by anaesthesia
3. Introduce catheter into circulation under anaesthesia or as soon as possible after killing
4. Do not touch or otherwise disturb artery to be examined
5. If thoracotomy is required do not section intercostal arteries which would cause loss of fluids – use rib retractors
6. Maintain the correct pressure of solutions; where a number of solutions are to be infused, use reservoirs at the correct pressure and change between solution by Y junctions so pressure and flow rate never change; avoid air in solution lines
7. Restrict flow rate of solutions to physiological levels with adjustable clamp on the outflow artery; high flow rates may detach adherent cells from endothelium

Silver Staining
1. If silver nitrate is used, blood should be washed from artery with a buffered isotonic solution without chloride ions, e.g. 4.6 % w/v glucose in 20 mM HEPES buffer pH 7.4
2. Silver nitrate solution must be prepared immediately before use and protected from light by covering the container with aluminium foil
3. Silver nitrate solution should be buffered isotonic, e.g. 0.2 % w/v silver nitrate in 4.2 % w/v glucose in 20 mM HEPES buffer pH 7.4 and held in artery for a carefully defined time; silver precipitates spoil preparations if blood is not properly washed out, or if exposure to silver salts is prolonged
4. Silver stain is washed out by more isotonic buffered glucose
5. Silver staining destroys semi-permeable properties of cell membrane and therefore prevents cell blebbing if subsequent fixative is hypotonic; it may, however, destroy microvilli and subcellular architecture
6. Silver proteinate does not precipitate silver halides in presence of physiological salt solutions

Composition of Fixatives
1. The vehicle should be a buffer which is itself isotonic, e.g. 120 mM phosphate buffer, pH 7.4; aldehydes make no contribution to the *effective* tonicity
2. If combined TEM and SEM is required fixative should possibly contain glucose or sucrose as well as buffer salts, to give required isotonicity in order better to preserve subcellular organelles
3. Low concentrations of aldehydes may be used if fixation is prolonged, e.g. total concentration 2 %
4. Formalin contains methanol and is a bad fixative for TEM, although perfectly satisfactory for SEM after silver nitrate staining; paraformaldehyde is preferred
5. Post-fixation of pressure-fixed tissue with osmium salts may be important

for TEM; notice that in fixed tissue, which has not been treated with silver salts, osmium stains EC boundaries weakly thus revealing cells; osmium also stains lipid droplets

Fixation

1. Fixation is intended not only to preserve tissue from autolysis but to *fix* (stabilise) the relative position of the components such as elastic lamellae in the way in which one wishes to see them; this is usually in the positions and dimensions they would have *in vivo*
2. To fix elastic lamellae as they would be *in vivo* under physiological pressure it is imperative to fix at pressure for a prolonged period; for small arteries 6 h may suffice, but 12 h is a safe time (time depends also on temperature of fixative)
3. Fixation of arteries *in situ* in whole animal minimises damage to artery; volume of fixative required is only about 3 times blood volume of animal, provided there are no leaks from severed blood vessels
4. Pressure of fixation should be set so that the diameter of the fixed artery is similar to that *in vivo;* a pressure equivalent to systolic may cause dilation because fixation destroys the normal resilience of elastica and collagen; diastolic pressure is good value but pressure should be increased if, after 12 h fixation, elastic lamellae and hence endothelium appear folded

Removal of tissue from Animal

1. Tissue must be handled very carefully by adventitia, using fine forceps with plastic-covered tips
2. The artery should be opened with fine scissors with rounded tips, e.g. strabismus scissors
3. When segments are cut for mounting on stubs, a very sharp scalpel should be used; some people prefer a razor-blade because it has a finer edge
4. Prolonged post-fixation with osmium tetroxide may give a stronger, harder tissue
5. It is advisable to gently dissect adipose tissue from adventitia, otherwise lipid may be deposited on the endothelium during dehydration in solvents
6. Tissue should be washed in two changes of deionised water for 15 min each, to remove fixative

Dehydration

1. Various approaches are
    None, i.e. replica
    Freeze-drying either in a freeze drier or on a cold-stage in the microscope
    Dehydrate with solvent, then critical point dry (CPD)
    Dehydrate with solvent, then dry in air
    Dry in air
2. For preservation of surface fine-structural detail CPD is essential
3. Techniques which use organic solvents remove lipid and may cause artefacts in atherosclerotic lesions; this applies to CPD

4. With solvent dehydration a graded series of solvents should be used, e.g. ethanol – 30, 50, 70, 80, 90, 95, 100 % with 15 min in each; some people recommend longer times in each and two changes of each, especially for thick or large specimens

5. Final solvents should themselves be dried, e.g. by molecular sieve

6. With CPD, freon 16 is not a good transition fluid because of volatility; with CO_2 the system must be flushed well, preferably using two changes of CO_2

7. For CPD use a good bomb with thermostatted jacket and ensure that the temperature for loading the bomb is low enough to prevent boiling of liquid; pressure readings in the bomb will not be correct if liquid CO_2 covers the opening to the pressure gauge

8. Air drying will produce damage to microvilli, but allows excellent assessment of endothelial integrity of arteries which have been silver-stained and fixed for a prolonged period at physiological pressure; little shrinkage occurs

9. After drying keep specimen dry in a desiccator over fresh silica gel or better phosphorus pentoxide; if the desiccator is evacuated, vent via a drying tube

10. Tissue may deteriorate if left for more than a day or so even in a desiccator; coat and view as soon as possible

Mounting on Stubs, Coating and Viewing

1. Silver dag paint is excellent, but may ooze through branches and obscure endothelium

2. Sputter-coating gives a more even coat than vacuum evaporation; keep coating time to a minimum to prevent heating; 1 min will usually deposit a sufficient layer of gold

3. View as soon as possible; if necessary store coated stub in an evacuated desiccator and vent to dry air or inert gas

4. Use a low beam voltage to avoid burning specimen; the lower the beam voltage the thinner the coating of metal required; at any beam voltage the intensity of the incident beam on a unit area of tissue will depend on the adjustment of the condenser lenses (so-called spot size); a small spot may burn the tissue

5. If a stationary spot or single line scan is used to set exposure levels for photography, this should be done at the edge of the field to avoid possibility of burn marks on the area of interest

---

Dr. D.E. Bowyer, Department of Pathology, University of Cambridge, *Cambridge CB2 1QP* (England)

Prog. biochem. Pharmacol., vol. 14, pp. 196–202 (Karger, Basel 1977)

Some Remarks on Arterial Tissue Preparation for SEM

H. Stachelberger, H. Redl, F. Ring and H. Sinzinger

Department of Botany and Technical Microscopy, 2nd Department of Internal Medicine and Department of Physiology, University of Vienna, Vienna

The SEM offers a great number of advantages over other methods for studying the vessel surface. However, it is very difficult to interpret results, especially about pathological structures in human material. For example, the different processing with experimental animal and human material does not allow to obtain comparable results of the investigated material.

During the special session about scanning electron microscopy and surface coat all participants agreed in discussing the necessary tissue preparation methods for SEM. The discussed techniques and methods should serve as a base in interpretation of appearance and findings of arterial tissue in SEM [Boyde, 1976: 'Do's and don'ts in biological specimen preparation']. It is not the aim of the contributions to propose a common method for working with arterial samples. This would only prohibit further methodological evaluation and experience in the future.

The main problem is what one wants to study. To preserve a fine structural surface detail requires a careful use of fixatives. Under the same conditions a true-to-life demonstration of microvilli is not possible.

All participants further agreed to deliver in the future a more detailed description of methods and techniques used. This is necessary to allow a comparison of all the results obtained by different tissue and different examination of research groups. This requirement was also made some years ago by Boyde and Vesely [1972] and by Brunk et al. [1975].

A. Handling of Arterial Tissue in Animals
[in complete agreement with BOWYER, this volume]

B. Considerations for Infusion
[in complete agreement with BOWYER, this volume]

C. Solutions for Fixation

1. Effective Osmolarity

The question if the effective osmolarity is given only by the buffer solution or solution and fixative is not quite clear answered. SQUIER *et al.* [1976] was able to show with quantitative methods the osmotic efficacy of glutaraldehyde on erythrocytes. Therefore it is important to describe the osmolarity of the buffer as well as the osmolarity of the fixative.

2. Selection of Buffer

Cacodylate, veronal and triethanolamine buffer should be used instead of phosphate buffer for a better preservation of membranes. In the presence of Ca^{++} phosphate buffer can produce precipitates. The adding of Ca^{++} and (or) Mg^{++} is important to maintain the membrane lipids [MITCHELL, 1969].

The best concentration of buffer is 0.05–0.1 M; the solution should contain 1–3 mM Ca^{++} with glucose or saccharose (isotonic). Hypotonic solutions are producing vesicles within the cells. Bursting of those vesicles may lead to crater formation. This has been shown in cinematographic studies by BRUNK *et al.* [1975] – compare GREGORIUS and RAND [1975] and CLARK and GLAGOV [1976].

3. Fixative

Carefully cleaned glutaraldehyde (ampules) – 1.5–2 % or a combination with formaldehyde prepared from paraformaldehyde. Aldehydes are only inducing a cross-linking of proteins. Therefore a postfixation of the lipids with OsO_4 solution must follow to prevent the wash-out of lipids (95 %) [STEIN and STEIN, 1971].

4. Commendable Composition after BRUNK et al. [1975]

2 % glutaraldehyde in 0.1 M Na-cacodylate-HCl buffer with 0.1 M saccharose, pH 7.2; osmolarity of buffer 300 mosm, osmolarity 510 mosm, adding 1–3 mM Ca^{++}.

D. Perfusion and Fixation

A great number of investigators showed that perfusion fixation is better to preserve a true-to-life fixation of arterial tissue. It is favorable to rinse the vessel (Ringer lactate $+$ 1 $^0/_0$ saccharose) to clean the endothelium of adhering blood cells.

1. Sites for Introducing Catheter Into the Circulation
[compare BOWYER, this volume]
BUSS and HOLLWEG [1977] are drawing attention to the importance of a physiological flow rate.

2. Perfusion Pressure
To keep a constant pressure and flow we are using a perfusion apparatus with two reservoirs, a three-way-cock and a pressure control [ROSE, 1975]. During perfusion air bubbles should be avoided. We use a continuous flow (mean value between systolic and diastolic pressure). There are many reports about the influence of pressure fixation on the 'longitudinal relief'. CLARK and GLAGOV [1976] reported that this relief is produced by too low pressure fixation ($\leq$ 80 mm Hg). In contrary, BUSS and HOLLWEG [1971] found the same relief using 200 mm Hg only to a smaller amount. These folds are dependent on the internal elastic membrane and probably on the contractility of the smooth muscle cells in part [SUNAGA et al., 1973].

3. Perfusion and Fixation Time
The blood vessels are rinsed by the threefold amount of blood volume and after this immediately fixed. There are different opinions about the fixation time. BOWYER [personal commun., 1977] is fixing for 6–12 h at a physiological pressure. We use the scheme after BUSS et al. [1976] and BUSS and HOLLWEG [1977]: a short perfusion fixation for about 15 min followed by a diffusion fixation in the same solution (4° C, 2–24 h), washing in buffer solution, postfixation in OsO_4 (1–2 h, 4° C).

E. Staining Procedures

Compare BOWYER [this volume], COLLATZ-CHRISTENSEN and GARBASCH [1972], GARBASCH and COLLATZ-CHRISTENSEN [1970], DENEE et al. [1977] and MUNGER [1977].

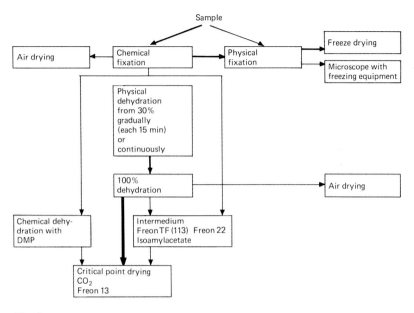

Fig. 1.

F. Dehydration (fig. 1)

After osmium fixation the samples should be sufficiently rinsed either with isotonic buffer solution or with aqua destillata (osmotic problem). Recent results by BOYDE *et al.* [1977] showed that the volume of the samples increases about 30 % during first dehydration step (30 % solution), without any difference between washing and not washing. In each special case one has to decide to wash or not.

1. Physical Dehydration

As solvents ethanol, acetone and others can be used. The dehydration can be performed gradually every 15 min (fig. 1) or more practically continuously by using a gradient mixer. This method was introduced in our laboratorium as routine method to prevent turbulences as seen in the automatic dehydration apparatus. We use isotonic glucose [BOYDE *et al.,* 1977] or the fixation solutions to produce the low percentage dehydration medium. This prevents part of the described volume alterations.

2. Chemical Dehydration [MULLER and JACK, 1975]

The water content of the tissue is removed by 2,2-dimethoxypropane (DMP) (fig. 1); the usefulness of this method is not yet clear. KAHN et al. [1977] reported no significant difference to common dehydration methods; BOYDE et al. [1977] found a significantly increased shrinkage in comparison to physical dehydration.

G. Drying

1. Air Drying

Strong damages on small structures. Surface alterations can be seen; we do not use it.

2. Freeze Drying

Should be used in all cases as control to critical point drying (CPD). SCHNEIDER [1976] reported about a shrinkage during CPD of 43 % (diameter of lymphocytes), BOYDE et al. [1977] found a volume reduction of 62 %. After freeze-etching, BOYDE et al. [1977] reported only a linear shrinkage of 4.5 %.

3. CPD

The most common drying method. Since the results of LEWIS et al. [1975] and COHEN [1977] showed the miscibility of ethanol and fl.CO_2 the use of isoamylacetate as intermedium is no longer necessary.

Some remarks on the use of CPD: (a) there should be a window; (b) there should be a gradual exchange of fluids (by a valve on the ground or by exhausting from the ground); (c) convection should be prevented by low heating rates; stirring mechanisms should be avoided; optimal heating rate 1° C/min; (d) the cylinder should be filled only to 75 % to avoid bursting during heating; (e) the maximal temperature should be exceeded 10° C (because of resistant solvents); the return to atmospheric pressure should be slowly (about 15 min) to prevent condensation due to adiabatic cooling; storing of samples in an exsiccator; sputtering as soon as possible.

H. Sputtering (conditions used in our Laboratory)

A thin continuous coating has more advantages than not coating the surface of arterial tissue specimen. An alternative way is described by

MUNGER [1977] using various impregnation techniques (OTO method). Its use can be of interest for the purpose of controlling of coated material but is not yet a routine method.

Some guidelines for the usage of sputtering devices:

(a) Reconstruction of a sputtering device for 'trioden' sputtering [INGRAM et al., 1976] or use of permanent magnet in a DC apparatus (Balzers-device) [compare PANAYI et al., 1977].

(b) Use of high voltage (4kV), low current (5 mA), a long distance between target and sample, a very clean vacuum (0.05 Torr argon).

(c) With this method a coat of about 100 Å/min can be deposited. The thickness of the coat should be controlled.

(d) Cooling of the specimen is not important (isolation), a target cooling should be provided.

(e) Au/Pd is the most favorable (data from our laboratory) type: selfmade in Balzers BAF 310 with magnet; 4 kV; 0.05 Torr argon (diffusion pump); 100 Å/min (measured with quartz crystal thin film monitor); 1 min = 100 Å; Au/Pd, 60/40; heating from of the specimen room temperature to 48° C with thermistor; without target cooling; within 1 minute >200° C; distance target to sample 4 cm.

In comparison: BUSS and HOLLWEG [1977]: Au; 8 mA; 0.12 Torr; 10–12 min.

It is very important to define the thickness of the coat. In SEM only this is made visible.

I. Mounting

The arterial tissue samples should be mounted with silver paint (not using double adhesive tape). It is favorable to surround the observation area tight with silver paint (not too liquid!) to guarantee stability and contact.

References

BOWYER, D.E.: SEM and the Surface Coat. Prog. biochem. Pharmacol., vol. 14, pp. 192–195 (Karger, Basel/New York 1977).
BOWYER, D.E.: personal commun. (1977).
BOYDE, A.: IITRI/SEM, p. 683 (1976).
BOYDE, A.; BAILEY, E.; JONES, S.J., and TAMARIN, A.: IITRI/SEM, p. 507 (1977).
BOYDE, A. and VESELY, P.: IITRI/SEM, p. 265 (1972).

BRUNK, U.; BELL, P.; COLLING, P.; FORSBY, N., and FREDRIKSON, B.A.: IITRI/SEM, p. 379 (1975).

BUSS, H. and HOLLWEG, H.G.: IITRI/SEM, p. 467 (1977).

BUSS, H.; KLOSE, J.P., and HOLLWEG, H.G.: IITRI/SEM, p. 217 (1976).

CLARK, J.M. and GLAGOV, S.: Br. J. exp. Path. 57: 129 (1976).

COHEN, A.L.: IITRI/SEM, p. 525 (1977).

COLLATZ-CHRISTENSEN, B. and GARBASCH, C.: Angiologica 9: 15 (1972).

DENEE, P.B.; FREDERICKSON, R.G., and POPE, R.S.: IITRI/SEM, p. 83 (1977).

GARBASCH, C. and COLLATZ-CHRISTENSEN, B.: Angiologica 7: 365 (1970).

GREGORIUS, F.K. and RAND, R.W.: Surg. Neurol. 4: 252 (1975).

INGRAM, P.; MOROSOFF, N.; POPE, L.; ALLEN, F., and TISCHER, C.: IITRI/SEM, p. 75 (1976).

LEWIS, E.R.; JACKSON, L., and SCOTT, T.: IITRI/SEM, p. 317 (1975).

KAHN, L.E.; FROMMES, S.P., and CANCILLA, P.A.: IITRI/SEM, p. 501 (1977).

MITCHELL, C.D.: J. Cell Biol. 40: 869 (1969).

MUNGER, B.L.: IITRI/SEM, p. 481 (1977).

MULLER, L. and JACK, T.: J. Histochem. Cytochem. 23: 107 (1975).

PANAYI, P.N.; CHESHIRE, D.C., and ECHLIN, P.: IITRI/SEM, p. 463 (1977).

ROSE, G.L.: Experientia 31: 998 (1975).

SCHNEIDER, G.B.: Am. J. Anat. 146: 93 (1976).

SQUIER, C.A.; HART, J.S., and CHURCHLAND, A.: Histochemistry 48: 7 (1976).

STEIN, O. and STEIN, Y.: Adv. Lipid. Res. 9: 1 (1971).

SUNAGA, T.; SHIMAMOTO, T., and NELSON, E.: IITRI/SEM, p. 459 (1973).

H. SINZINGER, Department of Physiology, University of Vienna, Schwarzspanier-strasse 17, *1090 Vienna* (Austria)

Prog. biochem. Pharmacol., vol. 14, pp. 203–207 (Karger, Basel 1977)

Early Permeability Changes in Human Atherosclerotic Lesions [1]

M. Daria Haust

Departments of Pathology, Paediatrics and Clinical Neurological Sciences, University of Western Ontario and Children's Psychiatric Research Institute, London, Ont.

Introduction

The relation of focal, arterial intimal edema to the atherosclerotic plaque, a concept introduced early in this century by German pathologists [7, 10, 11], has not been universally recognized on the North American continent. Only a few pathologists have been attempting during the last two decades to draw the attention to these early atherosclerotic lesions [2, 5, 6, 8, 9].

In an attempt at studying the sequential changes of intimal components subsequent to the episode of insudation which results in focal edema, electron microscopic examination of these lesions was carried out. The purpose of this communication is to summarize briefly the preliminary results of these morphological studies.

Material and Methods

Gelatinous elevations, i.e. grossly visible lesions representing focal, arterial intimal edema, were removed at the postmortem examination from aortae of children ranging in age from 1 $1/2$ to 14 years. The present preliminary studies are based on examination of ten representative blocks of tissues. These were prefixed in glutaraldehyde, postfixed in osmium tetroxide and embedded in Epon-812, and the thin sections were stained

[1] Supported by grants MT-1037 from The Medical Research Council and T.3-11 from the Ontario Heart Foundation, Toronto, Canada.

on copper grids, by uranyl acetate and lead citrate. All procedures were carried out by established routine techniques for electron microscopy. The sections were examined in a Philips-300 electron microscope.

Results

Small gelatinous elevations usually represented an edema ($=$ insudate) in the superficial intima; the edema was largely serous in nature as indicated by the presence of finely floccular and filamentous substance, and by lack of fibrin in the dilated, interfibrillary extracellular spaces (fig. 1). The individual collagen fibrils retained their structural integrity even when they were widely separated from each other by the edema fluid. On the other hand, elastic tissue elements appeared to have lost their microfibrillar component, particularly in the more superficial intimal layers. In the deeper layers the elastic tissue was permeated in addition, by small unstructured bodies of various electron density; these were associated with remnants of membranous arrays and an electron-lucent substance. The bodies were similar to those generally interpreted as representing lipids.

In larger lesions the edema seemed to permeate the basal lamina of the intimal smooth muscle cells. The basal lamina often was broadened and separated from the cellular bodies. In the latter event the involved extensions of the smooth muscle cells were electro-lucent and swollen and the change was interpreted as an intracellular edema. In gelatinous elevations containing a largely serous edema, neither changes of the overlying endothelium, nor necrosis of the intimal smooth muscle cells were apparent.

Lesions containing edema that was serofibrinous in nature showed, in addition to the (accentuated) above features, varying amounts of fibrin

Fig. 1. Electron microscopy of a gelatinous lesion in aortic intima. The endothelium (top) shows no degenerative changes. The fine, flocculofilamentous intercellular substance indicating insudate (edema) permeates elastic tissue elements (bottom). A few small osmiophilic bodies are also present in the latter. $\times 11,700$. *Inset* Numerous osmiophilic bodies (lipids) permeate elastic tissue in another area of the same lesion. $\times 7,500$.

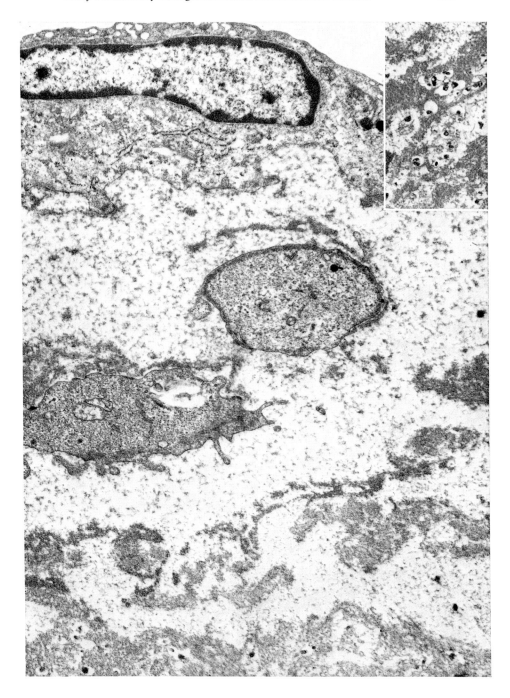

clumps and bands in the extracellular space. The overlying endothelium was swollen and its intercellular junctions straight and short; the usual cellular overlapping and junctional interdigitations were largely absent. Necrosis of intimal smooth muscle cells was not evident, but the small number of blocks examined to-date does not permit a definitive statement on the subject.

Discussion

Present studies are an extension of the previously reported observations by electron microscopy [3, 4] and further substantiate the evidence [1] that specific tissue changes underlie the lesions grossly discernible as gelatinous elevations. The edema fluid appears to permeate (selectively?) the elastic tissue elements, 'obliterating' their microfibrillar component and effecting elastolysis.

The observed intracellular edema of smooth muscle cells, that follows (or accompanies?) the separation of the basal lamina from their bodies, is a degenerative and thus a reversible process. It is therefore reasonable to state that a gelatinous elevation containing only a serous insudate may be reversible, particularly in view of the lack of apparent alterations of the overlying endothelium. The changes observed in the endothelium in lesions containing a serofibrinous insudate, the presence of fibrin in the intima, and the more severe changes of the elastic tissue and the smooth muscle cells, make a return to the 'status quo' improbable. Detailed interpretation of these and other features observed must await, however, further work.

Summary

Electron microscopy of aortic gelatinous elevations (one form of the earliest atherosclerotic lesion) in children and young subjects indicates that the alterations of the intimal components depend upon the nature and extent of the insudate. The entering insudate permeates the elastic tissue elements with ensuing elastolysis, and separates the basal lamina from the smooth muscle cells with resultant intracellular edema. Edema and shortening of the junctional appositions of endothelium is evident, in addition, in the presence of fibrinous insudate.

References

1   DOERR, W.: Perfusionstheorie der Arteriosklerose; in BARGMANN und DOERR Zwanglose Abhandlungen aus dem Gebiet der normalen und pathologischen Anatomie, Heft 13 (Thieme, Stuttgart 1963).

2   HAUST, M.D.: The role of plasma proteins in arteriosclerosis; thesis Queen's University, Kingston, Ont. (1959).

3   HAUST, M.D.: The morphogenesis and fate of potential and early atherosclerotic lesions in man. Hum. Path. 2: 1–29 (1971).

4   HAUST, M.D.: Pediatrics and atherosclerosis; in BOLANDE and ROSENBERG Perspectives in pediatric pathology (Year Book, Chicago, in press 1977).

5   HAUST, M.D. and MORE, R.H.: Morphologic evidence and significance of permeation in the genesis of arteriosclerosis. Circulation 16: 496 (1957).

6   HAUST, M.D.; MORE, R.H., and MOVAT, H.Z.: The mechanism of fibrosis in arteriosclerosis. Am. J. Path. 35: 265–273 (1959).

7   MEYER, W.W.: Die Bedeutung der Eiweissablagerungen in der Histogenese arteriosklerotischer Intima-Veränderungen der Aorta. Virchows Arch. path. Anat. 316: 268–316 (1949).

8   MORE, R.H. and HAUST, M.D.: Atherogenesis and plasma constituents. Am. J. Path. 38: 527–537 (1961).

9   MOVAT, H.Z.; HAUST, M.D., and MORE, R.H.: The morphologic elements in the early lesions of arteriosclerosis. Am. J. Path. 35: 93–101 (1959).

10 RIBBERT, H.: Über die Genese der arteriosklerotischen Veränderungen der Intima. Verh. dt. path. Ges. 8: 162–177 (1904).

11 RÖSSLE, R.: Über die serösen Entzündungen der Organe. Virchows Arch. path. Anat. 311: 252–284 (1944).

Dr. M.D. HAUST, Departments of Pathology, Paediatrics and Clinical Neurological Sciences, University of Western Ontario and Children's Psychiatric Research Institute, London, Ont. (Canada)

Prog. biochem. Pharmacol., vol. 14, pp. 208–212 (Karger, Basel 1977)

Surface Changes after Various Types of Endothelial Injury

Harry Jellinek[1]

2nd Department of Pathology, Semmelweis Medical University, Budapest

Using horseradish peroxidase as tracer we have found that already after 1 min of hypoxia and 5 min of recirculation the endothelial cells exhibited signs of marked damage. In the normal vessels horseradish peroxidase binds only to the interendothelial junctions while in the damaged vessel it appeared also in the necrotizing endothelial cells.

In such short-term experiments we observed among the normal endothelial cells also some horseradish peroxidase filled, dark, damaged ones. To exclude the possibility that the latter represented just some cells in the final phase of the normal cell turnover, the experiment was performed also on another model.

The previously described method of acidpainting was applied. The appearance in the endothelial cells of intravenously administered colloidal iron was detected by the Prussian blue reaction within the first hour following acid treatment (fig. 1). The presence of iron was readily detected after 1 h of recirculation (fig. 2).

Lipofundin and colloidal iron were simultaneously administered after 1 min of hypoxia and 5 min of recirculation. In this experiment the endothelial cells were found to have vanished from the intimal surface and the colloidal iron was present at the surface of the denuded elastica. Lipofundin chylomicron with or without iron was also seen at the luminal surface of the elastica (fig. 3).

In a series of experiments we studied the effect of hypoxia of 1, 2 or 5 min duration after 15, 20 or 60 min of recirculation. The severity of the

[1] Technical coworker: Andrea Vicenty; operations: Iringo Németh, Teréz Zombori; EM engineer: Z. Saródy; photo assistants: Emöke Kádár, Katalin Kovács.

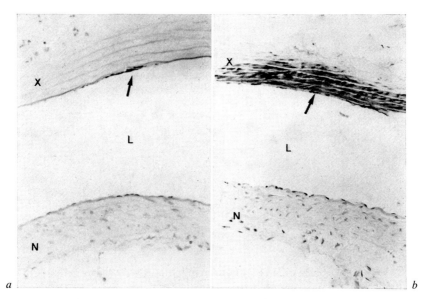

Fig. 1. a The large amount of colloidal iron accumulated in the necrotized endothelial cells of an acid-painted aorta recirculated for 1 h is intensively stained by Prussian blue. *b* After 48 h iron is accumulated in the entire vessel wall. L = Lumen; X = acid-painted area; N = normal area.

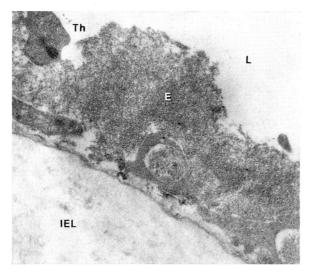

Fig. 2. The necrotized endothelial cell (E) from a vessel hypoxied for 1 h and recirculated for 1 h is completely filled with iron granules. L = Lumen; IEL = internal elastic lamina; Th = thrombocyte.

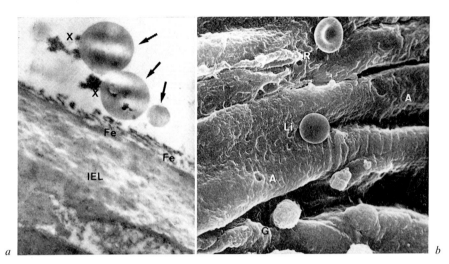

Fig. 3. a Transmission electron micrograph of a vessel hypoxied for 1 min and recirculated for 5 min. A Lipofundin chylomicron is shown (→) with occasional iron granules on its surface (X). Iron (Fe) is present also at the surface of the endothelium-deprived elastic lamina. The preparation was contrasted only with uranylacetate. *b* Scanning electron micrograph. On the relatively undamaged aortic intimal surface (A) a red blood cell (R), a leukocyte (G) and a Lipofundin chylomicron (Li) are shown.

damage appeared to depend essentially on the duration of hypoxia. In all experiments described the vessel damages were studied also by scanning electron microscopy.

In the *hypoxia experiments* described earlier [ELEMÉR *et al.*, 1976] the first change detectable by SEM was the formation of endothelial protrusions and craters. In addition to this we have seen also focal necrosis of the endothelial cells and the appearance of thrombocytes in the necrotic foci. In other completely denuded areas of the intima the presence of phagocytes was observed. As a result of increased rate of mitosis the denuded area became successively covered by endothelial cells. These regeneration phenomena are quite marred already after 40 h following hypoxia. After 10 days the damaged areas are fully covered by new cells.

Acid-painted mural specimens were also examined by scanning electron microscopy. The normal undulating structure disappeared first, in the early stage of the change, and subsequently complete deterioration of the intima took place in less injured areas until by 12–24 days a newly formed layer of endothelial tissue appeared in the intimal area.

The superficial changes found in vascular wall injury inflicted by painting with acid were in every respect similar to those occurring in experimental hypoxia [ELEMÉR et al., 1976].

The superficial changes were also compared to those occurring in *experimental hypertension.* According to the previously used experimental rat hypertension model [JELLINEK et al., 1969], renal hypertension was induced in 12 rats by the method of Lörincz and Gorácz. The animals were killed 5, 9, 12, 17 and 21 days after the intervention and their aorta was examined as described in the foregoing.

The undelating mural structure became damaged also under such conditions, having been replaced by cell debris, red blood cells, leukocytes and cell detritus. The endothelial cells localizing in the marginal zones extended processes with the obvious tendency of initiating cell growth above the deteriorating areas.

It follows that the superficial changes, above all the injury of the endothelium, bear the primary responsibility for the increase of vascular permeability, which allows for the entrance of colloidal iron and Lipofundin into the endothelium and deeper seated layers, to judge from light and electron microscopic evidence.

References

CHRISTENSEN, B.C. and GARBARSCH, C.: Repair in arterial tissue. A scanning electron-microscopic (SEM) and light-microscopic study on the endothelium of rabbit thoracic aorta following a single dilatation injury. Virchows Arch. Abt. A Path. Anat. *360:* 93–106 (1973).

ELEMÉR, G.; KERÉNYI, T., and JELLINEK, H.: Effect of temporary hypoxia on permeability of rat aorta. Pathol. Eur. *10:* 123–128 (1975).

ELEMÉR, G.; KERÉNYI, T., and JELLINEK, H.: Scanning (SEM) and transmission (TEM) electron-microscopic studies on post-ischemic endothelial lesions following recirculation. Atherosclerosis *24:* 219–232 (1976).

FROST, H.: Investigations into the pathogenesis of arteriosclerosis. Drug prophylaxis; in SHIMAMOTO Atherogenesis II, pp. 32–51 (Excerpta Medica, Amsterdam 1972).

JELLINEK, H.: Arterial lesions and arteriosclerosis (Plenum Press/Akadémiai Kiadó, Budapest 1974).

JELLINEK, H. und ELEMÉR, G.: Die Transportstörungen der Arterienwand als Initialfaktor der zellulären Reaktion. Atherogenese *1:* 1–20 (1976).

NELSON, E.; SUNAGA, T.; SHIMAMOTO, T.; KAWAMURA, T.; RENNELS, M.L., and HEBEL, R.: Ischemic carotid endothelium. Archs. Path. *99:* 125–132 (1975).

WEBER, G.; FABBRINI, P., and RESI, L.: On the presence of a concanavalin-A reactive coat over the endothelial aortic surface and its modifications during early experimental cholesterol atherogenesis in rabbits. Virchows Arch. Abt. A. Path. Anat. *359:* 299–307 (1973).

WEBER, G.; FABBRINI, P., and RESI, L.: Scanning and transmission electron microscopy observations on the surface lining of aortic intimal plaques in rabbits on a hypercholesterolic diet. Virchows Arch. Abt. A. Path. Histol. *364:* 325–331 (1974).

Dr. H. JELLINEK, Professor of Pathology, 2nd Department of Pathology, Semmelweis Medical University, *Budapest* (Hungary)

Prog. biochem. Pharmacol., vol. 14, pp. 213–219 (Karger, Basel 1977)

Endothelial Cell Injury in Early Mild Hypercholesterolemia

Ross G. Gerrity and Colin J. Schwartz

Department of Atherosclerosis and Thrombosis Research, The Cleveland Clinic Foundation, Cleveland, Ohio

Introduction

Areas of spontaneously occurring enhanced permeability to ^{131}I-albumin and ^{131}I-fibrinogen [1] in the pig aorta are readily demarcated by their uptake of the protein-binding azo dye, Evans blue. Such areas also exhibit differences in endothelial cell morphology [2], and increased susceptibility to endotoxin-induced endothelial injury [3]. The present study was undertaken to examine the earliest alterations in endothelial structure which occur in experimental hypercholesterolemia, particularly with reference to areas of enhanced endothelial permeability and susceptibility to injury.

Materials and Methods

12 male Yorkshire-Landrace pigs, 6 weeks of age, were fed a chow diet supplemented with 19.5 % lard and either 0.5 or 1.5 % cholesterol, and 6 control pigs were fed commercial chow diet. Animals were killed at 2, 4 and 6 weeks after diet initiation, and blood samples were taken prior to killing for serum cholesterol determination and lipoprotein studies. The animals were injected with Evans blue 3 h prior to sacrifice, and perfusion-fixed with glutaraldehyde. Samples of aorta from areas of dye uptake and areas devoid of dye uptake were post-fixed in OsO_4. Some blocks from each site were stained with ruthenium red. All samples were dehydrated in ethanol, and samples for TEM were embedded in

Spurr's resin, sectioned, and stained with uranium and lead salts prior to viewing. SEM samples were critical-point dried from CO_2, and coated with gold.

Results

Serum total cholesterol levels in control animals ranged from 80 to 120 mg/dl over the 6-week feeding period. Pigs fed the 0.5 % cholesterol diet or the 1.5 % cholesterol diet showed a graded mild hypercholesterolemia, averaging 190 and 275 mg/dl, respectively, 6 weeks after diet initiation.

Light microscopic studies on areas of greater permeability as demarcated by their uptake of Evans blue (blue areas) and on areas of no dye uptake (white areas) from cholesterol/lard-fed pigs and controls are summarized in table I. Results from the two test diets have been pooled. In this series of preliminary studies, leukocytes were found adherent to the endothelium in 85 % of blocks observed from blue areas of cholesterol/lard-fed pigs, as compared to 68 % in white areas from the same animals, and 11 % in combined blue and white areas from control animals. A similar pattern was also found in the number of blocks showing leukocytic cells in the subendothelial space (SES). Moreover, the occurrence of leukocytes adherent to the endothelium or in the SES was asso-

Table I. Hypercholesterolemia-induced endothelial injury in the Evans blue model[1]

Site	Adherent leukocytes	Leukocytic cells in SES	Endothelial injury
Control blue and white[2]	11	4	0
Hypercholesterolemic[3] blue	85	58	5
white	68	27	5

[1] Preliminary data derived from 12 hypercholesterolemic and 6 control pigs examined at 2, 4 and 6 weeks after diet initiation.

[2] Figures represent percentage of blocks from 150 blocks total.

[3] Figures represent percentage of blocks from 145 blocks each of blue and white areas.

ciated with recognizable light microscopic endothelial injury in only 5 % of the blocks examined.

This latter finding was confirmed by transmission electron microscopy. In most instances leukocytes were adherent to endothelium which was normal in its ultrastructural appearance, with well-defined endoplasmic reticulum, mitochondria, vesicles, and intact plasma and nuclear membranes (fig. 1, 2). The luminal surface of endothelial cells, as viewed by scanning electron microscopy, showed no abnormalities in areas adjacent to adherent leukocytes (fig. 3). In some instances, leukocytes were attached to sites where the endothelium was extremely thin and tenuous (fig. 4). Blood-derived cells were frequently seen in the SES underlying such sites, and occasionally extended through endothelial junctions into the lumen (fig. 5).

Endothelial cells in cholesterol/lard-fed pigs exhibit numerous lysosomes which were not seen as frequently in control animals. In addition, the endothelial cytoplasm of cholesterol/lard-fed animals contained large numbers of filaments, which often appeared to run in tracts through the cell, and merged with dense bodies on the plasma membrane of the abluminal and junctional aspects of the cell (fig. 2). In samples from cholesterol/lard-fed pigs which had been stained with ruthenium red, individual endothelial cells were frequently found which exhibited marked cytoplasmic uptake of this stain, while adjoining cells did not. Moreover, most endothelial cells underlying adherent leukocytes exhibited cytoplasmic uptake of ruthenium red, although they appeared otherwise ultrastructurally normal (fig. 6).

Discussion

These preliminary results indicate that alterations to the aortic endothelium in pigs occur as early as 2 weeks after the initiation of a hypercholesterolemic diet in the absence of lipid accumulation or lesion formation. These changes involve an increase in lysosomal bodies, which has also been reported in arterial smooth muscle cells, experimental hypertension [4], and the formation of numerous cytoplasmic filaments. Leukocyte involvement with the endothelium occurs at a very early stage. Whether this interaction is the result of, or results in, endothelial injury is uncertain, but the possibility that endothelial injury is initiated by leukocytes and/or platelets [5] cannot be excluded. The cytoplasmic up-

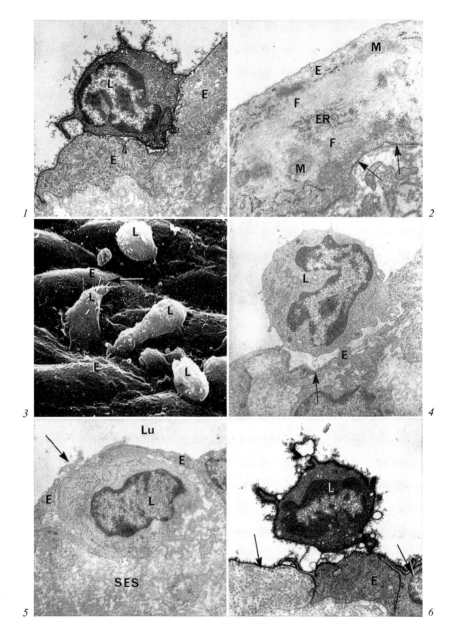

Fig. 1. Electron micrograph of leukocyte (L) adherent to endothelium (E) from a white area in the aortic arch of a pig fed 0.5 % cholesterol/lard diet for 6 weeks. Endothelium is normal in appearance. Ruthenium red stain. ×5,600.

take of ruthenium red by individual endothelial cells, particularly those underlying leukocytes, is of twofold interest. It suggests that early endothelial injury may involve alterations of membrane function resulting in increased permeability, which has previously been associated with atherosclerosis [6]. The relationship of these findings to the enhanced permeability areas of the Evans blue model is as yet uncertain, except that other studies have demonstrated increased endothelial cell turnover in blue areas [7], and a significantly greater number of injured cells which also exhibit cytoplasmic staining with ruthenium red [2]. Secondly, it suggests that such cellular injury may not be manifest in overt structural alteration, since most of these cells appear structurally normal. As such, it points out that one might not, or should not, expect to consistently find distinct morphological correlates for a functional disturbance, and that ultrastructural alterations may be inadequate as criteria for defining certain forms of cellular injury. The occurrence of endothelial alterations associated with leukocytic cells in the very early stages of hypercholesterolemia has implications in terms of later lesion formation, in that such cells may be a source of foam cells in the lesion. Alternatively, they may initiate localized immune responses in the intima, or differentiate to form pseudoendothelial or smooth muscle-like cells. Secondly, the observed cytoplasmic uptake of ruthenium red is suggestive of permeability changes

---

Fig. 2. Endothelial cell (E) cytoplasm from a blue area in the aorta of a pig fed 0.5 % cholesterol/lard diet for 6 weeks. Cytoplasmic filaments (F) run in tracts through the cell, and dense bodies (arrows) are visible on abluminal plasma membrane. Mitochondria (M) and endoplasmic reticulum (ER) are normal in appearance. ×14,000.

Fig. 3. Scanning electron micrograph of a white area from a pig fed 1.5 % cholesterol/lard for 4 weeks. Several leukocytes (L) are adherent to endothelial (E) surface, and extensions from the leukocytes (arrow) are visible. ×4,200.

Fig. 4. Leukocyte (L) adherent to thin, tenuous endothelium (E) in the region of an intercellular junction (arrow), from a blue area in a pig fed 0.5 % cholesterol/lard for 6 weeks. ×5,600.

Fig. 5. Leukocyte (L) lying in subendothelial space (SES), but extending through an intercellular junction (arrow) between two endothelial cells (E) into the lumen (Lu). From a blue area in a pig fed 0.5 % cholesterol/lard for 2 weeks. ×5,600.

Fig. 6. Leukocyte (L) adherent to an endothelial cell (E) which is normal in appearance, but which has taken up ruthenium red in its cytoplasm. Adjacent endothelial cells (arrows) are not stained. From a white area in a pig fed 0.5 % cholesterol/lard for 2 weeks. Ruthenium red stain. ×4,200.

or membrane breakdown which could facilitate the influx of lipoproteins or factors influencing growth and proliferation of intimal-medial cells.

Summary

Hypercholesterolemia was induced in 6-week-old male swine by feeding them a chow diet supplemented with lard and cholesterol. Aortic samples from areas of spontaneously-differing permeability to proteins, as demarcated by their uptake of Evans blue dye, were prepared and examined using light microscopy and scanning and transmission electron microscopy. At 2, 4, and 6 weeks after diet initiation, cholesterol/lard-fed animals demonstrated leukocyte adhesion to aortic endothelium in both greater (blue) and lesser (white) permeability areas, being greater in the former. Endothelial cells underlying leukocytes were generally normal in ultrastructural appearance, but showed cytoplasmic uptake of ruthenium red. Endothelial cells in cholesterol/lard-fed animals contained more lysosomes and cytoplasmic filaments than seen in control animals. Blood-derived cells were more frequently seen in the intima of cholesterol/lard-fed animals, and were often observed associated with intercellular junctions in the endothelium.

References

1   BELL, F.P.; ADAMSON, I.L.; GALLUS, A.S., and SCHWARTZ, C.J.: Endothelial permeability. Focal and regional patterns of ^{131}I-albumin and ^{131}I-fibrinogen uptake and transmural distribution in the pig aorta; in SCHETTLER and WEIZEL Atherosclerosis III. Proc. 3rd Int. Symp. (Springer, Berlin 1973).

2   GERRITY, R.G.; RICHARDSON, M.; SOMER, J.B.; BELL, F.P., and SCHWARTZ, C.J.: Endothelial cell morphology in areas of in vivo Evans blue uptake in the young pig aorta. II. Ultrastructure of the intima. Am. J. Path. (in press).

3   GERRITY, R.G.; RICHARDSON, M.; CAPLAN, B.A.; CADE, J.F.; HIRSH, J., and SCHWARTZ, C.J.: Endotoxin-induced vascular endothelial injury and repair. II. Focal injury, en face morphology, ^{3}H-thymidine uptake and circulating endothelial cells in the dog. Expl molec. Path. 24: 59–69 (1976).

4   WOLINSKY, H.; GOLDFISCHER, S.; SCHILLER, B., and KASAK, L.E.: Lysosomes in aortic smooth muscle cells. Effects of hypertension. Am. J. Path. 73: 727–732 (1973).

5   JØRGENSEN, L.; PACKHAM, M.A.; ROWSELL, H.C., and MUSTARD, J.F.: Deposition of formed elements of blood on the intima and signs of intimal injury in the aorta of rabbits, pig and man. Lab. Invest. 27: 341–348 (1972).

6   STEFANOVICH, V. and GORE, I.: Cholesterol diet and permeability of rabbit aorta. Expl molec. Path. *14:* 20–29 (1971).

7   CAPLAN, B.A. and SCHWARTZ, C.J.: Increased endothelial cell turnover in areas of *in vivo* Evans blue uptake in the pig aorta. Atherosclerosis *17:* 401–417 (1973).

Dr. R.G. GERRITY, Department of Atherosclerosis and Thrombosis Research, The Cleveland Clinic Foundation, *Cleveland, OH 44106* (USA)

Prog. biochem. Pharmacol., vol. 14, pp. 220–224 (Karger, Basel 1977)

Spontaneous Endothelial Cell Injury in the Intimal Cushions of Atherosclerotic Pigeons[1]

J.C. Lewis, V. Fuster and B.A. Kottke

Mayo Clinic and Foundation, Rochester, Minn.

As was presented in the Workshop on the Arterial Smooth Muscle Cells, the White Carneau pigeon develops spontaneous atherosclerotic lesions in an intimal cushion on the aorta which is located near the origin of the celiac branch with an incidence of nearly 100 %. Biochemical evidence of cholesterol accumulation is present by 12 months of age. By 3 years of age, gross yellow lesions in this area are readily apparent in nearly all birds. None of these changes are seen in the atherosclerosis-resistant Show Racer bird which lives in the same environment, eats the same cholesterol-free diet and has similar levels of serum cholesterol and triglycerides with a similar lipoprotein profile on electrophoresis.

Information along several lines suggests that, as with other commonly studied laboratory species, thrombosis plays an important role in the genesis of arterial lesions in the While Carneau pigeon. Since studies by Ross et al. [1974] have demonstrated the role of a platelet-derived factor, having many physical chemical properties similar to platelet factor 4, in stimulation of smooth muscle proliferation, Fuster et al. [1977] have measured the levels of platelet factor 4-like activity in the serum of birds from both species at multiple ages. While at 3 months of age the levels of platelet factor 4-like activity are similar in both breeds, the levels of this factor decrease and are barely detectable in 12- and 36-month-old Show Racer pigeons. In contrast the levels of platelet factor 4 increase 1.5- to 2-fold in the susceptible White Carneau breed at 12–36 months of age.

[1] Supported by a SCOR (Specialized Center of Research) grant, HL 14196, from the National Heart, Lung and Blood Institute.

Table I. Effect on platelet factor 4-like activity in thrombocyte-rich plasma (TRP) and thrombocyte-poor plasma (TPP) when thrombocytes were damaged by Triton-X or by clotting

Pigeon (1 year)	Platelet factor 4, units			
	TRP Triton-X	TRP serum	TPP Triton-X	TPP serum
Atherosclerosis susceptible	1.96	1.33	0	0
Atherosclerosis resistant	0	0	0	0

Either treatment of thrombocyte-enriched plasma from birds having lesions with Triton-X or allowing the plasma to clot resulted in the release of measurable amounts of the platelet factor 4-like activity (table I). No activity was detectable when thrombocyte-poor plasma was subjected to similar treatments. This clearly indicates a thrombocyte origin for the elevated activity in White Carneau pigeons.

Since chemical characterization has been completed for neither the substance(s) responsible for the platelet factor 4-like activity in the pigeon nor for the platelet protein implicated by Ross *et al.* [1974] in smooth muscle proliferation, their relationship is not clearly established. It furthermore remains to be determined whether or not the increase in serum platelet factor 4-like activity in the White Carneau pigeon is genetically determined or if it is a secondary manifestation of the atherogenic process.

The nucleated avian thrombocyte has many of the physiological and hemostatic functions associated with mammalian platelets. They aggregate *in vitro* in the presence of collagen, thrombin or relatively low concentrations of 5-hydroxytryptamine [BELAMARICH, 1973] and they take part in the formation of hemostatic plugs following vessel injury (fig. 1). Ultrastructural studies of pigeon thrombocytes have revealed the presence of multiple cytoplasmic vacuoles [LEWIS *et al.,* 1976]. One of these vacuoles, the large principal vacuole, is closely apposed to the nuclear envelope and contains a dense granule resembling the reserpine-sensitive amine storage site described in other avian thrombocytes [KURUMA *et al.,* 1970]. It is assumed, although unproven, that the contents of this large principal vacuole are extruded from the thrombocyte subsequent to activation in a

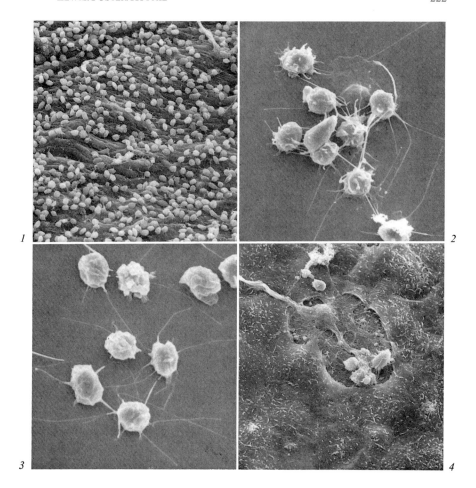

Fig. 1. Pigeon thrombocytes adherent to the luminal surface of the aorta following *in vitro* endothelial damage. This adhesion is primary to hemostasis.

Fig. 2. Show Racer thrombocytes on glass. A cluster of thrombocytes and one flattened leukocyte are shown.

Fig. 3. White Carneau thrombocytes are singly adherent to the glass surface.

Fig. 4. Aorta from a 1-year-old White Carneau pigeon. The area shown, from the celiac bifurcation, has an extensive crater in the endothelium exposing the subendothelial fibrils.

manner analogous to the 'release reaction' described for mammalian platelets. The secondary vacuole system consists of multiple small vacuoles randomly positioned throughout the cytoplasm. Although this vacuolar system resembles ultrastructurally the open channel system of the mammalian platelet, it does not stain with either ruthenium red or lanthanum hydroxide, suggesting that the cisternae are not continuous with the extracellular medium.

Thrombocytes from White Carneau and Show Racer pigeons were found to be identical when studied by routine scanning and transmission electron microscopy; however, significant differences were noted between the breeds when scanning microscopy was used to study thrombocytes adherent to glass surfaces [LEWIS *et al.*, 1976]. Under conditions employed in our laboratory thrombocytes from the Show Racer and from young White Carneau pigeons formed aggregates (fig. 2) on the glass surface, whereas thrombocytes from White Carneau pigeons older than 1 year were singly adherent through the extension of a few slender pseudopods (fig. 3). The underlying cause of this adhesiveness distinction is unknown, but several possibilities exist. Among these are: (1) inherent differences between the breads are expressed during thrombogenesis only in older White Carneau birds; (2) factor(s) affecting circulating thrombocytes are present only in the plasma of birds with lesions; and (3) thrombocytes from White Carneau pigeons with lesions are refractory to glass adhesion due to stimulation occurring in circulation.

Consistent with these thrombocyte alterations are observations of the lesion-prone area made with scanning electron microscopy. Perfusion of aortas at arterial pressure with buffered 2.5 % glutaraldehyde, resulted in the preparation of intact vessel segments from a point below the celiac bifurcation to areas 15 mm cephalad to the origin of the branch. This segment included the vestigial ligament, openings of the intercostal arteries and the intimal cushion associated with the celiac origin. Birds from 5 weeks to 3 years of age have been studied. Ruffling of endothelial cell plasma membranes on the luminal surface in the intimal cushion area was found in both breeds at 5 weeks of age. In some of the 5-week-old White Carneau pigeons and in most of the older White Carneau pigeons studied this alteration was extended to include pitting of endothelial cell membranes and endothelial desquamation resulting in the appearance of craters on the luminal surface (fig. 4). Frequently large numbers of thrombocytes and leukocytes were adherent to the damaged areas [LEWIS and KOTTKE, in press]. It is important to note that these changes were localized primarily to the intimal cushion area with endothelium on either side of the cushion having a normal morphology. Furthermore, analogous alterations have not been observed to date in the Show Racer breed.

Summary

Since endothelial damage precedes sterol accumulation, platelet factor 4-like activity elevations and alterations in thrombocyte adhesiveness, it clearly is one of the earliest events in the pathogenesis of spontaneous pigeon atherosclerosis. Although the relationships among endothelial damage and the other events have not been elucidated, it is conceivable that products released from thrombocytes subsequent to adhesion on damaged endothelium may trigger other localized changes in the intimal cushion area and lead to the progression of atherosclerosis.

References

BELAMARICH, F.A.: Aggregation of duck thrombocytes by 5-hydroxytryptamine. Microvasc. Res. 6: 229–234 (1973).

FUSTER, V.; LEWIS, J.C.; KOTTKE, B.A.; RUIZ, C.E., and BOWIE, E.J.W.: Platelet factor 4-like activity in the initial stages of atherosclerosis in pigeons. Thromb. Res. 10: 169–172 (1977).

KURUMA, I.; OKADA, T.; KALAOKA, K., and SORIMACHI, M.: Ultrastructural observation of 5-hydroxytryptamine-storing granules in the domestic fowl thrombocytes. Z. Zellforsch. mikrosk. Anat. 108: 268–281 (1970).

LEWIS, J.C.; FUSTER, V., and KOTTKE, B.A.: Thrombocytes in atherosclerosis-resistant and atherosclerosis-susceptible breeds of pigeon: a comparative ultrastructural study. Expl molec. Path. 25: 332–343 (1976).

LEWIS, J.C. and KOTTKE, B.A.: Endothelial damage and thrombocyte adhesion in pigeon atherosclerosis. Science (in press).

ROSS, R.; GLOMSET, J.; KARIYA, B., and HARKER, L.A.: A platelet-dependent serum factor that stimulates the proliferation of arterial smooth muscle cells in vitro. Proc. natn. Acad. Sci. USA 71: 1207–1210 (1974).

J.C. LEWIS, PhD, Mayo Clinic and Foundation, 200 First Street, SW., Rochester, MN 55901 (USA)

Prog. biochem. Pharmacol., vol. 14, pp. 225–233 (Karger, Basel 1977)

Immunologic Arterial Injury in Atherogenesis[1]

C.R. Minick, D.R. Alonso and L. Rankin

Department of Pathology, Cornell University Medical College, New York, N.Y.

Introduction

Experimental and clinicopathologic evidence indicates that injury to the arterial wall is fundamental in the pathogenesis of athero-arteriosclerosis. Arterial injury, the resulting necrosis, inflammation, intimal hyperplasia, endothelial regeneration and other features of repair may favor deposition of blood-borne lipid at the site of injury and thereby lead to athero-arteriosclerosis [1, 2, 8, 9, 12–15, 18, 19]. Therefore, it is essential to our understanding of human arteriosclerosis to determine the etiologic factors causing arterial injury, the mechanism of injury, and the sequence of local reactive changes that may result from the injury.

There is considerable clinicopathologic evidence to indicate that injury, and in particular immunologic injury, may be important in the development of arteriosclerosis in man [2, 17, 20–24]. For several years, we have investigated the possibility that immunologic arterial injury may be a primary causative factor in athero-arteriosclerosis. Results of these experiments have clearly demonstrated that the synergy of immunologic injury to arteries and hypercholesterolemia can lead to atherosclerosis in rabbits [1, 8, 12–14]. In many instances the arterial lesions bear close resemblance to those seen in human arteriosclerosis.

It is the purpose of this communication to report on the results of these experiments and to discuss some of the mechanisms that may be important in the genesis of immunologically mediated arterial injury.

[1] Supported by grant from The Cross Foundation and research grants HL-01803, HL-18828, and HL-19109 from the National Heart, Lung, and Blood Institute of the National Institutes of Health.

Materials and Methods

Immunologic injury to arteries was induced in rabbits by repeated intravenous injections of foreign serum protein or by graft rejection induced in heterotopically placed cardiac allografts [1, 12]. Hypercholesterolemia was induced by feeding cholesterol-supplemented, or semi-synthetic lipid-rich, cholesterol-poor diets. Total serum cholesterols, and, in some instances, serum phospholipids and triglycerides were estimated as described previously [13].

Aortas, pulmonary arteries, and cardiac valves were examined grossly at the time of autopsy, and visible atherosclerotic lesions were quantitated. Hearts were cut into approximately 12 blocks, and sections of coronary arteries in each block were examined microscopically. In some experiments, sections of splenic, gastric, mesenteric, femoral, subclavian, hepatic, renal, carotid, cerebral, and pulmonary arteries and aortas were also examined microscopically. Arterial lesions were tabulated as to the size of artery involved and histologic character of lesions.

Selected blocks of tissue were prepared for transmission electron microscopy by standard techniques. Portions of arteries were also prepared for scanning microscopy. Rabbits were perfused with 1 % glutaraldehyde in Sorensen's phosphate buffer at 90 mm Hg for 40 min. Blocks of tissue were then fixed in 1 % glutaraldehyde for 1 h and washed in phosphate-buffered saline and postfixed in 1 % osmium tetroxide in Millonig's phosphate buffer. After washing in phosphate buffer and distilled water, they were dehydrated sequentially, first in a graded series of alcohols and then in a graded series of amyl acetate solutions in alcohol. Blocks of tissue were then critical-point dried in carbon dioxide at a pressure of 1,300 lb/in^2 and a temperature of 39–41° C.

Results

Results of our initial experiments in rabbits indicated that the synergy of immunologic arterial injury resulting from either repeated injections of foreign serum protein or graft rejection and hypercholesterolemia led to fatty-proliferative arterial lesions which involved large, medium, and small coronary arteries [1, 12]. Many of these fatty-proliferative arterial lesions bore striking resemblance to some stages of human athero-arteriosclerosis (fig. 1). Immunologic arterial injury alone led to fibromuscular proliferative intimal thickening in large, medium and small coronary arteries. Many of these latter arterial lesions resembled fibromuscular intimal thickening in man's arteries, which is called diffuse, or progressive intimal thickening [7, 10, 16]. Hypercholesterolemia alone led to predominantly fatty lesions with little proliferative change that were found primarily in small intramyocardial coronary arteries. The fatty lesions bore little resemblance to human atherosclerosis.

In our initial experiments, rabbits were fed a cholesterol supplement that resulted in an average serum cholesterol between 500 and 700 mg %, and their arteries were subjected to intense immunologic injury induced over a short period of time. It appeared reasonable to suggest that atherosclerosis that even more closely resembled that which occurs in man could be induced in rabbits by more chronic arterial injury in combination with a semi-synthetic, lipid-rich, cholesterol-poor diet that results in a concentration of serum cholesterol of the same magnitude as that in man. In long-term experiments, chronic atherosclerosis, which bore striking similarity to that in man was induced in rabbits by the combined action of foreign serum protein injected repeatedly at 4- to 8-week intervals and semi-synthetic, lipid-rich, cholesterol-poor diets fed for as long as 17 months [13]. These semi-synthetic lipid-rich diets resulted in an increase of serum cholesterol concentration from the normal range of 50–80 mg % to values that averaged between 200 and 250 mg %. Among the characteristics which these rabbit arterial lesions shared with human atherosclerosis were lipid-filled foam cells clustered deep in the intima, fatty hyaline change with little or no elastification, necrosis with pooled lipid deep in the intima, and cholesterol clefts deep in the intima and media with overlying fibromuscular caps or jackets, vascularization, occasional focal calcification of the intima, and, rarely, an overlying thrombus (fig. 2).

It could not be determined in experiments described above whether lipid had accumulated only acutely at sites of recent immunologic injury to arteries or whether fibromuscular intimal thickening, which resulted from immunologic injury during previous weeks or months had preferentially accumulated lipid and led to atherosclerosis. In subsequent experiments sites of immunologic arterial injury were allowed to heal for 40–80 days prior to the induction of hypercholesterolemia.

In these latter experiments, we were able to demonstrate in rabbits that immunologically induced arterial intimal thickening without evident lipid later accumulated lipid preferentially and evolved as atherosclerosis

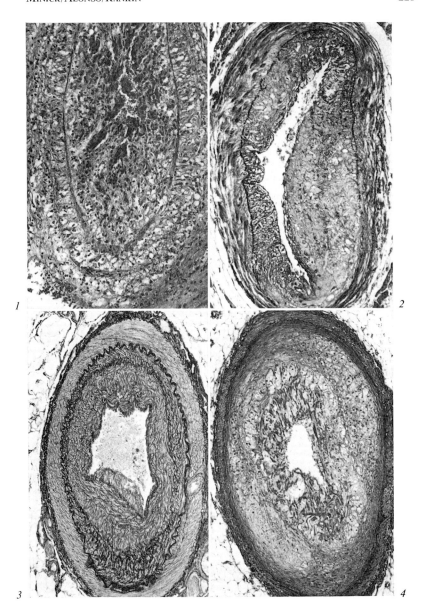

Fig. 1. Major coronary artery of cardiac allograft that functioned for 10 days. Lumen is occluded by proliferative intimal thickening containing many foam cells. Weigert-HE. × 96.

Fig. 2. Coronary atherosclerosis with areas of necrosis containing atheromatous gruel in a rabbit that received repeated injections of foreign serum protein and was (fig. 3, 4) [8]. The results of these experiments support the hypothesis that, in man, sites of fibromuscular intimal thickening that result from one or several instances of arterial injury may continue to have increased avidity for lipid for weeks, months, or even years after the initial injury.

Discussion

In summary, results of these experiments indicate that the synergy of immunologic arterial injury and lipid-rich diets induced arterial lesions in rabbits that in several important respects resemble athero-arteriosclerosis in man. First, immunologic response to foreign antigens occurs commonly in human populations. Second, the degree of hypercholesterolemia necessary to induce these rabbit lesions is of the same order of magnitude as that of adult humans in the United States. Third, arterial lesions induced by repeated injections of foreign serum protein in rabbits concomitantly fed a lipid-rich diet are histologically very similar to those of human arteriosclerosis. Fourth, marked involvement of the major coronary arteries is often a prominent feature of atherosclerosis both in man and in rabbits that received the lipid-rich diet and repeated injections of foreign serum protein. Finally, as in atherosclerosis in man, arterial lesions characterized by fibromuscular intimal thickening without appreciable lipid are a part of the spectrum of lesions in these rabbits. Like in man, there is evidence in rabbits to indicate that areas of intimal hyperplasia may later preferentially accumulate lipid and evolve as atherosclerosis.

Because the arterial lesions, induced in rabbits of these experiments bear such close resemblance to human atherosclerosis, it is especially important to study the early lesions in the rabbits to learn more about the pathogenesis of atherosclerosis in man. Recent evidence obtained by scanning and transmission electron microscopy in our laboratory indicates

---

fed semi-synthetic lipid-rich diet. Weigert-HE. × 210. From MINICK and MURPHY [13] by permission.

Fig. 3. Musculoelastic intimal thickening in a mesenteric artery of a rabbit. Arterial change is characteristic of those seen in rabbits fed diets low in lipid and injected with foreign serum protein. Weigert-HE. × 120. From HARDIN *et al.* [8] by permission.

Fig. 4. Atherosclerotic change in mesenteric artery similar to that illustrated in figure 3. Weigert-HE. × 78. From HARDIN *et al.* [8] by permission.

that endothelial injury and platelet interaction with the arterial wall are early features common to both arterial lesions resulting from immune complex disease and graft rejection [1, 14]. In both instances endothelial damage and loss precede the intimal thickening and lipid accumulation. Thus, these findings are in harmony with a rapidly growing body of evidence which supports the hypothesis that vascular injury, and, in particular, endothelial injury resulting from diverse etiologies may be an early event in the pathogenesis of atherosclerosis [18]. This hypothesis is based on the premise that normal endothelium acts as a barrier to a substance(s) in the blood that, upon exposure to vascular smooth muscle, promotes smooth muscle proliferation in the media and migration of proliferating smooth muscle cells into the intima where they contribute to fibromuscular intimal thickening [18].

The mechanism of immunological endothelial injury is complex and in some instances poorly understood. In immune complex disease, one of the animal models of immunologic arterial injury used in these experiments, there is strong evidence to indicate that the deposition of immune complexes and ensuing reactive changes in the arterial wall results from changes in endothelial permeability triggered by release of vasoactive amines from platelets and leukocytes. Release of these substances in turn results from reactions of antigen-antibody complexes and complement with platelets or binding of antigen to homocytotropic antibody on leukocytes and release of vasoactive amines or release of a factor from leukocytes, platelet activating factor, which then acts on platelets [4, 5]. Endothelial necrosis and sloughing would then be secondary to the necrosis and reactive changes occurring in the underlying arterial wall.

There is strong indirect evidence to support the above hypothesis. Colloidal carbon accumulates in arteries of animals with immune complex disease, which indicates increased permeability of endothelium to this macromolecule. Moreover, antihistamines and platelet depletion will result in a striking reduction in the incidence of arterial lesions that result from immune complex disease [4, 5]. Results of preliminary experiments reported from our laboratory have furnished direct evidence that endothelial injury is an important early event in vascular injury due to immune complex disease [14].

Immunopharmacologic mechanisms similar to those described in immune complex disease may also be important in increasing endothelial permeability in atopy. In these IgE-mediated responses, the reaction of antigen with homocytotropic antibody on leukocytes leads to release of vasoactive amines or of a platelet activating factor which aggregates platelets and leads to release of various vasoactive amines [4]. These vasoactive substances are known to lead to increased vascular permeability in the microcirculation as a result of contraction of endothelial cells. Since endothelial cells in some large musculoelastic and muscular arteries also contain contractile proteins, it is reasonable to suggest that these endothelial cells may react in a similar way [3]. In this manner, large circulating macromolecules such as lipoproteins and even antigen-antibody complexes resulting from other immune reactions could gain access to the arterial wall and lead to arterial injury.

In graft arteriosclerosis arterial injury is thought to be a result of either an Arthus-like reaction mediated by cytotoxic antibodies directed against cell antigens or a result of cellular immunity mediated by lymphocytes, presumably due to lymphokines [6]. Both of these mechanisms may be operating simultaneously in many instances. Immunologic arterial injury due to viral infections or those resulting from autoantibodies could also be mediated by mechanisms similar to those in graft rejection or immune complexes as described above.

Mechanisms outlined above may be important in the genesis of arterial injury resulting from immune responses to a variety of antigens including those in infecting microorganisms, vaccines, blood derivatives containing foreign antigens, antibiotics and other drugs, tobacco, foodstuffs and antigens derived from ones own tissues. In all of these instances, immunologic reaction to these and other antigens may lead to repeated or persistent immunologic injury and reactive changes in the arterial wall that could favor lipid deposition and lead to atherosclerosis.

References

1   ALONSO, D.R.; STAREK, P.K., and MINICK, C.R.: Studies on the pathogenesis of athero-arteriosclerosis induced in rabbit cardiac allografts by the synergy of graft rejection and hypercholesterolemia. Am. J. Path. (in press, 1977).

2   ANITSCHKOW, N.N.: Experimental arteriosclerosis in animals; in COWDRY Arteriosclerosis. A survey of the problem, pp. 271–322 (Macmillan, New York 1933).

3   BECKER, C.G.: Contractile and relaxing proteins of smooth muscle and platelets: their presence in endothelium. Ann. N.Y. Acad. Sci. *257:* 78–86 (1976).

4   BENVENISTE, J.; HENSON, P.M., and COCHRANE, C.G.: A possible role for IgE in immune complex disease; in ISHIZAKA and DAYTON The biological role of

the immunoglobulin E system, pp. 187–208 (US Dept. of Health, Education and Welfare, Washington 1972).

5   COCHRANE, C.G. and KOFFLER, D.: Immune complex disease in experimental animals and man. Adv. Immunol. 9: 185–264 (1972).

6   FOKER, J.E. and NAJARIAN, J.S.: The pathobiology of organ rejection; in NAJARIAN and SIMMONS Transplantation, pp. 122–145 (Lea & Febiger, Philadelphia 1972).

7   FRENCH, J.E.: Atherosclerosis in relation to structure function of the arterial intima; in EPSTEIN and RICHTER International review of experimental pathology; vol. 5, pp. 253–353 (Academic Press, London 1966).

8   HARDIN, N.J.; MINICK, C.R., and MURPHY, G.E.: Experimental induction of atherosclerosis by the synergy of allergic injury to arteries and lipid-rich diet. III. The role of earlier acquired fibromuscular intimal thickening in the pathogenesis of later developing atherosclerosis. Am. J. Path. 73: 301–326 (1973).

9   HASS, G.L.: Observations on vascular structure in relation to human and experimental arteriosclerosis; in Symposium on atherosclerosis, pp. 24–32 (National Academy of Sciences, Washington 1955).

10 GEER, J.C. and HAUST, M.D.: Smooth muscle cells in atherosclerosis; in POLLOCK, SIMMS and KIRK Monographs in atherosclerosis, vol. 2, pp. 39–59 (Karger, Basel 1972).

11 HAUST, M.D.: Arteriosclerosis; in BRUNSON and GALL Concepts of disease. A textbook of pathology, pp. 451–487 (Macmillan, New York 1971).

12 MINICK, C.R.; MURPHY, G.E., and CAMPBELL, W.G., jr.: Experimental induction of athero-arteriosclerosis by the synergy of allergic injury to arteries and lipid-rich diet. I. Effect of repeated injections of horse serum in rabbits fed a dietary cholesterol supplement. J. exp. Med. 124: 635–652 (1966).

13 MINICK, C.R. and MURPHY, G.E.: Experimental induction of athero-arteriosclerosis by the synergy of allergic injury to arteries and lipid-rich diet. II. Effect of repeatedly injected foreign protein in rabbits fed a lipid-rich, cholesterol-poor diet. Am. J. Path. 73: 265–300 (1973).

14 MINICK, C.R.: Immunologic arterial injury in atherogenesis. Ann. N.Y. Acad. Sci. 275: 210–227 (1976).

15 MINICK, C.R.; STEMERMAN, M.B., and INSULL, W., jr.: Effect of regenerated endothelium on lipid accumulation in arterial wall. Proc. natn. Acad. Sci. USA (in press, 1977).

16 MOVAT, H.Z.; MORE, R.H., and HAUST, M.D.: The diffuse intimal thickening of the human aorta with aging. Am. J. Path. 34: 1023–1031 (1958).

17 MURPHY, G.E.: Observations indicating that rheumatic injury to coronary arteries leads in some cases to precocious or later developing athero-arteriosclerosis of these arteries: a microscopic study of coronary arteries in infants, children, adolescents and adults with rheumatic heart disease (unpublished).

18 ROSS, R. and GLOMSET, J.A.: The pathogenesis of atherosclerosis. New Engl. J. Med. 295: 369–376, 420–425 (1976).

19 ROSS, R. and HARKER, L.: Hyperlipidemia and atherosclerosis: chronic hyperlipidemia initiates and maintains lesions by endothelial cell desquamation and lipid accumulation. Science 193: 1094–1100 (1976).

20 RIDER, A.K.; COPELAND, J.C.; HUNT, S.A.; MASON, J.; SPECTER, M.J.; WINKLE, R.A.; BIEBER, C.P.; BILLINGHAM, M.E.; DORY, E.; GRIEPP, R.B.; SCHROEDER, J.S.; STINSON, E.B.; HARRISON, D.C., and SHUMWAY, N.E.: The status of cardiac transplantation. Circulation *52:* 531–539 (1975).

21 SAPHIR, O.: Inflammatory factors in arteriosclerosis; in BLUMENTHAL Cowdry's arteriosclerosis, pp. 415–440 (Thomas, Springfield 1967).

22 TSAKRAKLIDES, V.G.; BLEIDEN, L.C., and EDWARDS, J.E.: Coronary atherosclerosis and myocardial infarction associated with systemic lupus erythematosus. Am. Heart J. *87:* 637–641 (1974).

23 ZEEK, P.: Studies in atherosclerosis. I. Conditions in childhood which predispose to the early development of atherosclerosis. Am. J. med. Sci. *184:* 350–356 (1932).

24 ZEEK, P.: Studies in atherosclerosis. II. Atheroma and its sequelae in rheumatic heart disease. Am. J. med. Sci. *184:* 356–364 (1932).

Dr. C.R. MINICK, Department of Pathology, Cornell University Medical College, *New York, N.Y.* (USA)

Prog. biochem. Pharmacol., vol. 14, pp. 234–240 (Karger, Basel 1977)

Smooth Muscle and Endothelial Cell Deaths in Atherogenesis Studied by Autoradiography[1]

W.A. Thomas, H. Imai, R.A. Florentin, J.M. Reiner and R. F. Scott

Albany Medical College, Albany, N.Y.

Arterial cell births and deaths go hand in hand in atherogenesis. In the early stages, when lesions are relatively thin, deaths appear to occur in scattered individual cells or in small foci. The cell fragments rapidly disintergrate and do not accumulate to a significant degree. Thus the early lesions consist largely of proliferating smooth muscle cells (SMC) and their biosynthetic products such as collagen and glycosaminoglycans. In advanced stages, when lesions are thick, the necrotic material accumulates to form the masses of lipid-rich partially calcified necrotic debris which we designate as atheromatous deposits.

As we described earlier in this volume, quantitative methods for study of arterial cell births in experimental animals have been developed and have been used to a limited extent in a number of laboratories for several years. Development of quantitative methods for study of arterial cell deaths has proved to be much more difficult.

In Albany we have used two approaches for quantitative studies of arterial SMC deaths in experimental animals. One involves the counting of dead cells by electron microscopy (EM). The other involves [³H]-thymidine autoradiography. Most of this presentation deals with the latter but we would like to begin by summarizing the EM approach and a few of the results.

The EM criteria that we have used for cell death include the traditional ones of pyknosis, karyorrhexis, karyolysis, and cell disintegration. The number of dead cells is expressed as a percentage of the total

[1] Supported by the USPHS NHLBI.

Table I. Average frequency per 100 nucleated SMC of cells judged by EM to be dead in aortas of control and experimental rabbits

Group	n	Dead cells
Controls	15	0.6
Fresh USP cholesterol, 1 g/kg	5	4.6**
Old USP cholesterol, 1 g/kg	5	8.3**
Fresh USP cholesterol, 250 mg/kg	3	1.7*
Cholesterol purified via dibromination, 250 mg/kg	4	1.6*
Concentrate of autoxidation products, 250 mg/kg	7	12.9**
Concentrate of autoxidation products, 10 mg/kg	4	2.8**

* $p < 0.05$, ** $p < 0.01$ for difference from controls.

cells in the same area. Counts are made without the observer knowing whether the specimen came from a control or from a treated animal.

Thus far we have carried out quantitative studies of dead arterial SMC with the EM method only in a period prior to development of overt lesions. In young swine we reported in 1970 [IMAI *et al.,* 1970] that the percentage of dead cells increases about 2-fold within 3 days after beginning an hyperlipidemic (HD) diet. This is the same time at which we begin to find increased mitotic activity [FLORENTIN *et al.,* 1969].

More recently we have been using the EM approach with rabbits to determine the toxicity for arterial SMC of autoxidation products of cholesterol as compared to highly purified cholestetrol [IMAI *et al.,* 1976]. With a 24-hour *in vivo* bioassay, we have found that a single oral dose of a concentrate of cholesterol oxidation products (and possibly other impurities) prepared from commercial cholesterol, produces arterial SMC deaths at dose levels where highly purified cholesterol has virtually no effect (table I). This result raises the possibility that the arterial SMC deaths associated with atherogenesis are more closely related to one or more cholesterol oxidation products than to cholesterol *per se.* We are now proceeding to investigate individual cholesterol oxidation products.

Although useful for comparative studies, the EM approach does not give us actual rates of cell death. The finding of recognizable dead SMC depends not only on the death rate but also on the speed with which the dead cell components are degraded and removed.

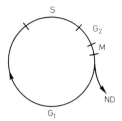

Fig. 1. Cell cycle. M = Mitosis, ND = nondividers, G_1 = the gap between M and S, S = DNA synthesis, G_2 = the gap between S and M, G_0 is ignored.

In 1976 we serendipitously discovered an autoradiographic method for obtaining quantitative information on arterial SMC deaths for at least one part of the cell cycle [Thomas *et al.*, 1976]. A diagram of the cell cycle is presented in figure 1. We were studying SMC birth rates in moderately advanced aortic lesions in swine by the dilution-of-label method described by us earlier in this volume. Lesions were produced by first denuding the endothelial cells (EC) with a ballon catheter and then feeding an HL diet. The swine were fed the HL diet for 60 days and then were injected with [³H]-thymidine. One-third of them were sacrificed 2 h later to provide pulse labelling indices and baseline grain number distributions. The remainder were continued on the HL diet, with half of these sacrificed 7 days later and the other half 37 days later. The primary objective was to determine whether there was a subset of lesion SMC with a cycle time of less than 7 days which might divide so frequently as to be 'lost' from view as labelled cells by 37 days. With each division, half of the isotopic label goes with each daughter cell and this is reflected in autoradiographs by halving of grain number counts.

We did not obtain conclusive evidence for a subset of SMC with a cycle time of less than 7 days. However, we did make some unexpected observations that are of considerable interest.

The unexpected observations relate to changes in labelling indices between 60 and 67 days. With a substantial proportion of labelled cells dividing and producing two labelled daughters, the total number of labelled cells should increase between 60 and 67 days. In assessing labelling indices, allowance must be made for several modifying factors, but these can be mathematically evaluated from autoradiographic grain number distributions at 60 days; and the expected labelling index at 67 days can be calculated.

Table II. Cell death rates in advanced lesions; labelling indices observed at 2 h and 7 days compared with labelling indices calculated on three bases

	Media		Lesions	
	2 h (n=3)	7 days (n=6)	2 h (n=3)	7 days (n=6)
Observed, %	0.50[1]	0.81	2.05	1.22
Predicted, %				
With zero deaths		0.73		2.42
With random deaths		0.73		2.42
With 60 % perimitotic deaths		0.33		1.22

[1] Labelling index.

The observed and predicted labelling indices from this experiment are shown in the top part of table II. The expected increase was found in the normal media; but in the lesions not only did we fail to observe the expected increase by 67 days but there was actually a significant lowering. The only reasonable explanation for this result is that substantial deaths have occurred among the labelled cells that were out of proportion to random deaths that probably occurred in the total cell population. During the 7-day interval the labelled cells were, in relation to the cell cycle, either in S, G_2, M, or early G_1 (fig. 1). For convenience we have referred to this portion of the cell cycle as the perimitotic period. The unlabelled cells, with the exception of the small number that entered S during the 7 days, would have been in G_1 or were nondividers (ND).

We can actually calculate the proportion of labelled cells that have died in the perimitotic period by determining the proportion necessary to obtain the labelling indices observed at 67 days. Results of this type of calculation are shown at the bottom of table II. The results suggest that more than half of the labelled cells had died. Thus this was a period of 'no growth' in the lesions as far as cells were concerned.

Histologic inspection showed foci of lipid-rich necrotic debris in many of the lesions, consistent with multiple cell deaths. The 7-day interval is too short to tell much about lesion growth; but the swine in this experiment that were kept alive for 30 more days (total of 97 days on HL diet) showed only minimal lesion growth in the 60- to 97-day interval.

Table III. Apparent arrest in G_2 of some SMC and short cycle times of others in moderately advanced lesions (70–100 days)

Group	Number of divisions				Total
	0 (G_2)	1	2	3	0–3
EH diet + EC denudation, %	65	5	5	25	100

More data are needed before we can place high perimitotic death rates in perspective as they relate to atherogenesis. We suspect that in the life history of a lesion there are some periods in which births exceed deaths and others in which deaths exceed births. Obviously, if the lesion is to continue to grow in terms of cells, the net result must favor births. In order to obtain regression in terms of cells, we would like to have the balance favor cell deaths.

In a more recent experiment (results of which are as yet unpublished) we studied by autoradiography the period 70–100 days on HL diet in swine subjected to balloon-EC-denudation at the outset. For unknown reasons the lesions appeared to grow much faster in this experiment than in the previous one; and apparently there were far fewer perimitotic cell deaths. Approximately 65 % of the labelled lesion SMC appeared to remain in G_2 for the entire 70- to 100-day period (table III). Most of the remainder not only went through the expected initial division following DNA synthesis but also through two more divisions; and their number was sufficient to account for the observed increase in cell numbers. Total cell cycle time for these rapid dividers was 11–14 days. Relationships among perimitotic deaths, G_2 arrest, and emergence of a dividing SMC population with a short cycle time are not known. They all suggest that profound changes are taking place in the population of SMC nuclei during atherogenesis.

EC deaths in atherogenesis are much easier to quantify than SMC deaths because of the monolayer nature of the endothelium. In spite of this, very few quantitative studies have been carried out. In the late 1960s we noted in several studies at Albany [FLORENTIN *et al.*, 1969], that mitotic and [3H]-thymidine labelling indices [THOMAS *et al.*, 1968] were increased in aortic EC of HL diet-fed swine to about the same extent as in SMC. Since the increases in the number of divisions for EC were not accompanied by piling up of EC, this result almost certainly reflects increased rate of loss of EC from the surface, probably (but not necessarily) because of EC deaths.

We have now devised a more direct way to study EC loss (? death), and had hoped to have completed a study by the time of this conference. Unfortunately this was not possible. However, we have completed enough of the study to demonstrate the feasibility of the method. Since the method of itself should be of some interest, we shall describe it here in brief.

In the experiment in progress, 15 young mash-fed swine (8–10 kg) were injected with [^{3}H]-thymidine at the outset. They continued on the commercial mash diet for 15 days to allow time for salvage labelling to be completed. 5 were then sacrificed to serve as a baseline group. Another 5 were given an atherogenic HL diet for the following 60 days and 5 were kept on mash for the same period. At 60 days these 10 were sacrificed.

The abdominal aorta from celiac axis to the trifurcation was obtained from each animal and fixed intact in formalin. Standardized sections were taken in such a fashion that the total EC for each abdominal aorta could be calculated. Autoradiographs were made and labelling indices and grain numbers per labelled nucleus are being determined. With appro-

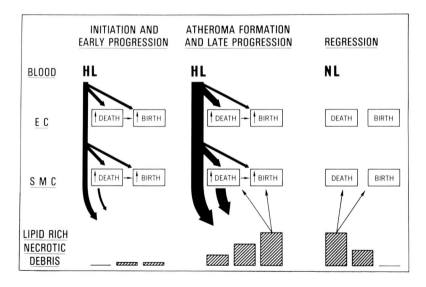

Fig. 2. Atherosclerosis.

priate mathematical treatment we can calculate how many labelled cells are present at zero time and at 60 days. We can also determine the number of divisions that have taken place in the interval and can predict what the terminal labelling index should have been with no loss of labelled EC in the 60-day interval. Comparison of this predicted value with the observed labelling index at 60 days will allow us to determine the number of labelled EC that have been lost from the surface by death or otherwise.

In conclusion we would like to present a diagram (fig. 2) adapted from Virchow that illustrates our current hypotheses regarding the role of arterial EC and SMC deaths in initiation, progression, and regression of atherosclerotic lesions. If the hypotheses are valid, arterial cell deaths play a key role in all phases.

References

FLORENTIN, R.A.; NAM, S.C.; LEE, K.T.; LEE, K.J., and THOMAS, W.A.: Increased mitotic activity in aortas of swine after three years of cholesterol feeding. Archs Path. *88:* 463–469 (1969).

IMAI, H.; LEE, S.K., and PASTORI, S.J.: Degeneration of arterial smooth muscle cells. Ultrastructural study of smooth muscle cell death in control and cholesterol-fed animals. Virchows Arch. path. Anat. Physiol. *350:* 183–204 (1970).

IMAI, H.; WERTHESSEN, N.T.; TAYLOR, C.B., and LEE, K.T.: Angiotoxicity and atherosclerosis due to contaminants of USP-grade cholesterol. Archs Path. Lab. Med. *100:* 565–572 (1976).

THOMAS, W.A.; FLORENTIN, R.A.; NAM, S.L.; KIM, D.N.; JONES, R.M., and LEE, K.T.: Preproliferative phase of atherosclerosis in swine fed cholesterol. Archs Path. *86:* 621–643 (1968).

THOMAS, W.A.; REINER, J.M.; FLORENTIN, R.A.; LEE, K.T., and LEE, W.M.: Population dynamics of arterial smooth muscle cells. V. Cell proliferation and cell death during initial 3 months in atherosclerotic lesions induced in swine by hypercholesterolemic diet and intimal trauma. Expl molec. Path. *24:* 360–374 (1976).

Dr. W.A. THOMAS, Albany Medical College, *Albany, N.Y.* (USA)

Prog. biochem. Pharmacol., vol. 14, pp. 241–247 (Karger, Basel 1977)

Arterial Cell Injury and Cell Death in Hypercholesterolemia and after Reduction of High Serum Cholesterol Levels[1]

H.C. STARY

Department of Pathology, Louisiana State University School of Medicine, New Orleans, La.

Introduction

Hypercholesterolemia is associated with arterial cell proliferation and cell death. Advanced atherosclerotic lesions, in addition to having a thickened and hypercellular intima, also have a soft core of cell debris and lipid derived from many generations of lipid-containing cells that have diet. Light microscopic observations by ANITSCHKOW [1] of regressing lesions showed that the hypercellularity of lesions can decrease by the disappearance of foam cells. Those observations were confirmed by electron microscopy [2, 13, 22]. Later we reported that the mode of foam cell disappearance is by cell death [18]. The present paper deals with the extent of smooth muscle and macrophage death in progressing and in regressing atherosclerotic lesions. The extent of endothelial cell death will be described elsewhere. Cell injury and cell death in normal control animals were also studied to serve as a baseline.

Methods

The design of the experiments on which these observations were based has been described elsewhere in detail [18]. Briefly, 53 mature, male rhesus monkeys, divided into 12 groups, were given a high-cholesterol diet (commercial diet supplemented with butter, beef tallow, casein, cholesterol, vitamins, and water) for 12 weeks. At the end of that period,

[1] Supported by USPHS NIH, grant HL 08974.

one group was killed to determine the extent and nature of the atherosclerotic lesions induced with the diet. The high-cholesterol diet was then
changed to low-cholesterol food (unsupplemented commercial diet), and
the remaining groups were killed after 2, 3, 4, 8, 12, 16, 24, 32, 40, 64
and 128 weeks. In addition, the experiments included 11 control monkeys
divided into four groups that received only low-cholesterol food for
varying periods. Tissue for electron microscopy was taken from the
proximal left coronary artery as described previously [17], and from
three standard sites in the thoracic and one standard site in the abdominal
segment of the aorta. The tissues were fixed in buffered osmium tetroxide,
and embedded in the epoxy resin Maraglas. Fine sections were stained
with lead citrate and uranyl acetate.

Results

General Observations

Control animals given only low-cholesterol food had mean serum
cholesterol levels in the range of 110–165 mg/dl. The aortic and coronary
artery intima of all control animals contained smooth muscle cells that
formed cushions at arterial forks, or diffuse intimal thickening. In addition
to smooth muscle cells, single isolated macrophages with or without lipid
inclusions occurred in the intima, but rarely. Monkeys on the high-
cholesterol diet had mean serum cholesterol levels in the range of
230–640 mg/dl during the 12-week period on the diet. The diet induced
intimal lesions in the aorta and coronary arteries, more severe in segments
with intimal cushions. In addition to intimal smooth muscle cells, lesions
now contained a considerable proportion of intimal macrophages, macrophage-derived foam cells, and eosinophil and neutrophil granulocytes.
Substitution of low-cholesterol food after the 12-week period on the high-
cholesterol diet caused a return of elevated serum cholesterol levels to
normal within 4–8 weeks in most animals. The increased intimal cellularity of the lesions began to decrease soon after serum cholesterol levels
had returned to normal, and by 24 weeks after diet change, intimal cellularity had returned to near normal.

Cell Injury

Evidence of cell injury was of two morphologically distinct types
and occurred in arterial smooth muscle cells under all dietary conditions.

One type consisted of edematous swelling of peripheral parts of the cell cytoplasm and formation of rounded projections that assumed the appearance of blebs or vesicles of the plasma membrane. Cytoplasm sequestered in vesicles showed partial or complete dissolution of cytoplasmic structures. Vesicles were sometimes attached to the remainder of the cell by only a thin stalk and many seemed to have completely separated from the main body of the cell. Dissolution of isolated vesicles was frequent. Vesiculation of the cell surface occurred in both intimal and medial smooth muscle cells of normocholesterolemic control animals. Its incidence increased in the smooth muscle cells of experimental lesions, where occasionally it was also observed in macrophages. In regressing lesions the incidence was not much increased over that of control animals.

The second type of cell damage evidence observed in arterial cells was that of autophagy. Autophagy consisted of enclosure of portions of cytoplasm, such as islands of myofilaments or mitochondria, in a thick, intensely osmiophilic membrane. Cytoplasmic components within the membrane frequently were disintegrated, and membranes became multilaminated and collapsed to form coarsely wrinkled residual bodies. When residual bodies occurred in normocholesterolemic animals, they were only one or two per cell, and rarely had almost the entire cytoplasm converted to numerous autophagosome-derived residual bodies. In control animals, autophagy occurred more frequently in medial than intimal cells, and more often in older animals. In the lesions of hypercholesterolemic animals, an increased number of cells showed evidence of autophagy, the cytoplasm being more frequently nearly filled with residual bodies. Cells with this type of evidence of cytoplasmic injury also contained variable numbers of lipid droplets. After reduction of high serum cholesterol levels, cells filled with autophagosome residuals were no longer observed. Such cells might have disintegrated earlier. The smooth muscle cells of regressing lesions, however, did still contain some evidence of increased autophagy.

Cell Death

Our morphologic criteria for cell death were either nuclear changes, such as shrinkage (pyknosis) or fragmentation (karyorrhexis), or dissolution of the plasma membrane and release of organelles and intracellular lipid inclusions into the extracellular space. Nuclear evidence of cell death was less frequent than rupture of the plasma membrane. In normocholesterolemic animals cell death was rare. In hypercholesterolemic animals, on the other hand, cell death was frequent in intimal lesions. Intimal smooth muscle cells, macrophages, and granulocytes were necrotic. The majority of necrotic cells in each lesion were macrophage-derived foam cells. Cell death was usually, but not inevitably, associated with a high content of lipid droplets in the cells. Dead smooth muscle cells sometimes contained few lipid droplets but numerous autophago-somes as evidence of preceding cell damage; sometimes dead smooth muscle cells contained no cytoplasmic inclusions of any type. After reduction of high serum cholesterol to normal levels, cell death continued in intimal lesions but was largely limited to macrophage-derived foam cells. Death of smooth muscle cells with or without lipid became infrequent. Death of macrophage-derived foam cells was frequent for the first 24 weeks after the diet was changed, that is, for about 16 weeks after high serum cholesterol levels had returned to normal. At that point few foam cells remained in intimal lesions and the cellularity of the intima approached that of normal control animals. Cell death was only sporadic at late regression periods. It remained more frequent in the isolated persisting macrophages than in intimal smooth muscle cells. Although infrequent in the minimal residual lesions found in late regression periods, cell death was still more frequent than in control animals that had never received a high-cholesterol diet and that were of comparable age.

Comment

Cell Injury

We have distinguished two distinct morphological expressions of cell injury: plasma membrane vesiculation, and autophagy of intracytoplasmic structures. Plasma membrane vesiculation was previously described in intimal and medial smooth muscle cells of normal animals [6, 8, 17, 19]. Careful perfusion techniques applied to the coronary arteries indicate that vesiculation is not an artifact [8, 15]. Plasma membrane vesiculation similar to that observed in arterial cells had been noted in a multitude of cell types undergoing various injuries [9, 10, 20]. In arterial cells the incidence is increased in mechanical injury [5], with increasing age [23], and in hypercholesterolemia [11, 22, 24]. The term 'ghost body' was applied to plasma membrane vesiculation by SCOTT et al. [11]. In time-lapse movies plasma membrane vesiculation is seen to be reversible in its early stages in some cell types [21].

Autophagy is the property of cells to digest portions of their own cytoplasm. The end products of autophagy were residual bodies composed of coarse lamellae. We have evidence that residual bodies derived through autophagy can be expelled from smooth muscle cells *in toto*. A similar observation was made by ERICSSON *et al.* [3], and the expelling process was called defecation. Residual bodies derived through autophagy can be distinguished from those derived through heterophagy of lipid droplets, which is described elsewhere in this volume [14].

Cell Death

Evidence of cell death in the aorta of normal animals has been reported by others [4, 7]. In the normal animals studied in the experiment reported here arterial cell death was extremely rare. Evidence of an extremely low rate of cell turnover in normal arteries is supported by radioautographic studies. Pulse labeling of normal rabbits with tritiated thymidine showed an average of only three labeled smooth muscle cells per 5-μm section of the entire length of the aorta [16]. Cell death was greatly increased in the atherosclerotic lesions of hypercholesterolemic animals. The high rate of cell death explains why the size of athero-sclerotic lesions does not fully reflect the high proliferative activity indicated by tritiated thymidine radioautography. With multiple injections of the tracer, 25 % of the cells of intimal lesions became labeled after 36 h [16]. With such extremely rapid cell proliferation lesions would rapidly become occlusive were cell death not to occur. Under our experimental conditions intimal macrophages proliferated faster than smooth muscle cells, and they also were the cell type that was dead more often. The type of cell that proliferates preferentially probably depends, to some extent, on the experimental manipulation that has occurred. Traditionally, cell death and accumulation of debris from necrotic cells is associated with advanced lesions. The present findings indicate that cell death is already frequent in early lesions. Death of macrophage-derived foam cells continued after the high-cholesterol diet was changed to normal food, while the cellularity of lesions was regressing. The occa-sional presence of a foam cell in an interendothelial junction has prompted some observers to speculate that cells can emigrate from lesions into the bloodstream, presumably to die in some distant graveyard. Our observa-tions in regressing lesions indicate that emigration of cells, if it occurs at all, is not the major cause of the decrease in cellularity. Smooth muscle cell death was rare in regressing lesions. The discrepancy in the frequency of smooth muscle and macrophage death during regression does not imply that an excess of smooth muscle cells cannot be reduced. Instead, the finding indicates that with our high-cholesterol diet a greater number of macrophages than smooth muscle cells was produced. A build-up of smooth muscle cells rather than of macrophages can be induced in the intima by various experimental means, and it has been established that these smooth muscle cells can again disappear [12, 25].

References

1 ANITSCHKOW, N.N.: Über die Rückbildungsvorgänge bei der experimentellen Atherosklerose. Verh. dt. path. Ges. *23:* 473–478. Zentbl. allg. Path. Anat. *43:* suppl. (1928).

2 BUCK, R.C.: Lesions in the rabbit aorta produced by feeding a high cholesterol diet followed by a normal diet. An electron microscopic study. Br. J. exp. Path. *43:* 236–240 (1962).

3 ERICSSON, J.L.E.; TRUMP, B.F., and WEIBEL, J.: Electron microscopic studies of the proximal tubule of the rat kidney. Lab. Invest. *14:* 1341–1365 (1965).

4 GERRITY, R.G. and CLIFF, W.J.: The aortic tunica intima in young and aging rats. Expl molec. Path. *16:* 382–402 (1972).

5 HOFF, H.F.; McDONALD, L.W., and HAYES, T.L.: An electron microscope study of the rabbit aortic intima after occlusion by brief exposure to a single ligature. Br. J. exp. Path. *49:* 68–73 (1968).

6 IMAI, H. and THOMAS, W.A.: Cerebral atherosclerosis in swine: role of necrosis in progression of diet-induced lesions from proliferative to atheromatous stage. Expl molec. Path. *8:* 330–357 (1968).

7 JORIS, I. and MAJNO, G.: Cellular breakdown within the arterial wall. An ultrastructural study of the coronary artery in young and aging rats. Virchows Arch. Abt. A *364:* 111–127 (1974).

8 JORIS, I.; UNDERWOOD, J.M., and MAJNO, G.: Cell-to-cell herniae in the vascular wall. Am. J. Path. *78:* 21 (1976).

9 ROSSI, M.A.; FERREIRA, A.L., and PAIVA, S.M.: Fine structures of pulmonary changes induced by Brazilian scorpion venom. Archs Path. *97:* 284–288 (1974).

10 SCOTT, R.E.: Plasma membrane vesiculation. A new technique for isolation of plasma membranes. Science *194:* 743–745 (1976).

11 SCOTT, R.F.; JONES, R.; DAOUD, A.S.; ZUMBO, O.; COULSTON, F., and THOMAS, W.A.: Experimental atherosclerosis in rhesus monkeys. II. Cellular elements of proliferative lesions and possible role of cytoplasmic degeneration in pathogenesis as studied by electron microscopy. Expl molec. Path. *7:* 34–57 (1967).

12 SPAET, T.H.; STEMERMAN, M.B.; FRIEDMAN, R.J., and BURNS, E.R.: Arteriosclerosis in the rabbit aorta. Long-term response to a single balloon injury. Ann. N.Y. Acad. Sci. *275:* 76–77 (1976).

13 STARY, H.C.: Cell proliferation and ultrastructural changes in regressing atherosclerotic lesions after reduction of serum cholesterol; in SCHETTLER and WEIZEL Atherosclerosis III, pp. 178–190 (Springer, Berlin 1974).

14 STARY, H.C.: Ultrastructural changes in the lipid inclusions of arterial smooth muscle cells after reduction of high serum cholesterol levels. Progr. biochem. Pharmacol. (this volume).

15 STARY, H.C.: Unpublished.

16 STARY, H.C. and McMILLAN, G.C.: Kinetics of cellular proliferation in experimental atherosclerosis. Archs Path. 89: 173–183 (1970).

17 STARY, H.C. and STRONG, J.P.: Coronary artery fine structure in rhesus monkeys. Nonatherosclerotic intimal thickening. Prim. Med., vol. 9, pp. 321–358 (Karger, Basel 1976).

18 STARY, H.C.; EGGEN, D.A., and STRONG, J.P.: The mechanism of atherosclerosis regression; in Atherosclerosis IV. Proc. 4th Int. Symp. on Atherosclerosis, Tokyo 1976 (Springer, Berlin, in press).

19 STEHBENS, W.E. and LUDATSCHER, R.M.: Ultrastructure of the renal arterial bifurcation of rabbits. Expl molec. Path. 18: 50–67 (1973).

20 TRUMP, B.F. and MERGNER, W.J.: Cell injury; in ZWEIFACH, GRANT and McCLUSKEY The inflammatory process, vol. I, pp. 115–257 (Academic Press, New York 1974).

21 TRUMP, B.F. and ARSTILA, A.U.: Cellular to injury; in LaVIA and HILL Principles of pathobiology, pp. 9–96 (Oxford University Press, New York 1975).

22 TUCKER, C.F.; CATSULIS, C.; STRONG, J.P., and EGGEN, D.A.: Regression of early cholesterol-induced aortic lesions in rhesus monkeys. Am. J. Path. 65: 493–514 (1971).

23 VELTMANN, E.; BACKWINKEL, K.-P.; THEMANN, H. und HAUSS, W.H.: Elektronenmikroskopische Untersuchungen zur Entstehung von «ghost bodies» in Aorten. Virchows Arch. Abt. A Path. Anat. Histol. 367: 281–288 (1975).

24 WEIDENBACH, H. and MASSMANN, J.: Electron microscopic study on the 'ghost bodies' in experimental arteriosclerotic lesions of the vascular wall. Expl Path. 10: 251–257 (1975).

25 ZAHN, F.W.: Untersuchung über die Vernarbung von Querrissen der Arterienintima und Media nach vorheriger Umschnürung. Virchows Arch. path. Anat. Physiol. 96: 1–15 (1884).

H.C. STARY, MD, Professor of Pathology, Louisiana State University School of Medicine, 1542 Tulane Avenue, New Orleans, LA 70112 (USA)

Prog. biochem. Pharmacol., vol. 14, pp. 248–252 (Karger, Basel 1977)

Forms of Lesions in the Smooth Muscles Cells of the Vascular Wall in Experimental Atherosclerosis

H. Weidenbach, J. Massmann and G. Holle

Institute of Pathology, Karl Marx University, Leipzig

Introduction

Depending upon kind, intensity, and duration of action, atherogenic noxae can produce lesions of the vascular wall both in rabbits and in pigs. These lesions may lead to the necrosis of smooth muscle cells; in other cases, they may, however, be compensated by cellular regenerating processes setting in. The existence of catabolic and anabolic processes side by side is reflected in characteristic findings, two of which will be discussed here.

Materials and Methods

Immunologic lesions in rabbits: Three subcutaneous injections of 1 ml of horse's serum at intervals of 1 week; subsequently up to two intravenous injections of 3 ml horse's serum at an interval of 1 week. Atherogenic diet in domestic pigs: Feeding over a period of 7 months with a standard diet containing 15 % butter and 1.5 % cholesterol.

Results

In myogenic foam cells in lipofibrous plaques of the aorta of pigs we were able to see that these cells, after complete foam cell transformation, develop a – at first incomplete – demarcation of the lipid-storing cytoplasm components by the formation of membrane structures. The formation of membranes sets in in the vicinity of the nucleus and demarcates

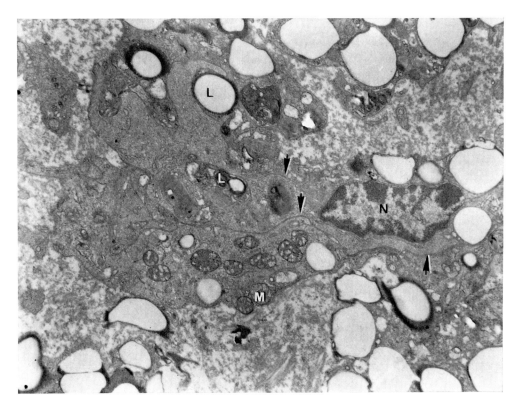

Fig. 1. Lipid-laden smooth muscle cell with membranous demarcation of lipid-containing cell areas. N = Nucleus, L = lipid droplets, M = mitochondria. × 11,000.

in an unsystematic manner cell compartments of different sizes. After complete membranous demarcation, cells with a large ovoid nucleus and a narrow cytoplasmic seam are formed. These cells remind one of myoblasts (fig. 1).

Both in the rabbit aorta and in the pig aorta of our experimental animals, we could find so-called 'ghost bodies'. These are extracellular, mainly ovoid vesicular structures demarcated by membranes, with a granular-filamentous content. Occasionally one finds residues of the endoplasmic reticulum in them. They are found in the vicinity of modified smooth muscle cells (fig. 2a) and are obviously produced by a constriction of hernia-like cytoplasmic protrusions of the smooth muscle cells (fig. 2b). In the vicinity of the ghost bodies there are an increased number of

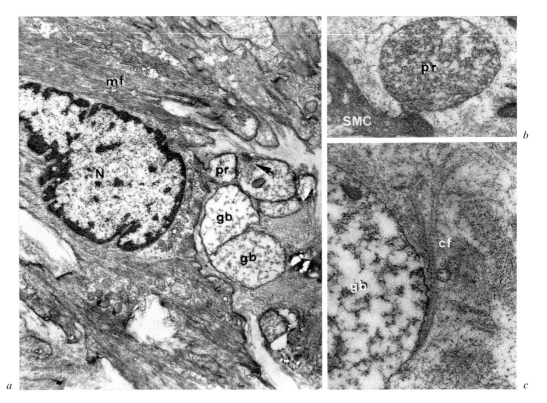

Fig. 2. a Modified smooth muscle cell with protrusions and extracellular ghost bodies. Arrow = disruption gf ghost body membrane with appearance of fibrillar structures, N = nucleus, mf = myofilaments, pr = protrusions, gb = ghost body. × 10,800. *b* Protrusion (pr) of smooth muscle cell (SMC) with constriction. × 18,400. *c* Ghost body (gb) with formation of collagen fibrils (cf) on its membrane. × 24,500.

collagenous fibrils which partly enclose the ghost bodies concentrically. At some points one finds an extrusion of collagenic fibrils from the ghost body membranes (fig. 2c).

Discussion

Lipid storing is a characteristic feature of arteriosclerotic changes in which mainly smooth muscle cells are participating. The foam cell transformation may progress to such an extent that the cells will perish. In part of these cells we found a membranous demarcation and subsequent rejection of lipid-storing cell areas. The cells thus produced have the aspect of embryonal myoblasts. This process in interpreted by us as an attempt to survive the lesion by a kind of self-cleaning in order to be able to take over subsequent functions by a respective differentiation. According to publications in the literature, ghost bodies are not individual structures [1, 2, 5] and are mainly interpreted as degenerative changes. TAKEBAYASHI [4] reported on findings in arterioles after a hypertension had persisted over a prolonged period of time which he describes as a moth-eaten pattern of smooth muscle cells. It is said that occasional rejection of non-necrotic cytoplasmic components into the extracellular space occurs according to the mechanism of apocrinic secretion. This mechanism, which is called microaprocriny, establishes the connection with a secretory process. According to our findings, we hold that the ghost bodies are an expression of secretory processes which proceed under the special conditions of a vascular wall lesion. One can imagine that cisterns of the endoplasmic reticulum protrude in a hernia-like manner and get constricted. They would thus represent the morphologic correlate of an extruding mechanism of the components produced by the cells and required for extracellular fiber synthesis. This assumption is supported by the close structural relations between ghost bodies and collagenic fibrils [6] and the ruthenium red-positive reaction of the ghost body content, which speaks for the existence of glycosaminoglycans [3].

It is one of the special peculiaritis of the modified smooth muscle cell that it compensates for severe catabolic changes by reactive-repairing anabolic processes.

References

1   CAVALLERO, C.; DI TONDO, U.; MINGAZZINI, P.L.; PESANO, P.C., and SPAGNOLI, L.G.: Cell proliferation in the atherosclerotic lesions of cholesterol fed rabbits. Part 2. Atherosclerosis *17:* 49–62 (1973).

2   HOFF, H.F. and GOTTLOB, R.: Ultrastructural changes of large rabbit blood vessels following mild mechanical trauma. Virchows Arch. Abt. A. path. Anat. *345:* 93–106 (1968).

3   MERKER, H.J. und STRUWE, K.: Elektronenmikroskopische Untersuchungen zum Problem der Sekretion der bindegewebigen Interzellularsubstanz. Z. Zellforsch. mikrosk. Anat. *115:* 212–225 (1971).

4   TAKEBAYASHI, S.: Ultrastructural studies on arteriolar lesions in experimental hypertension. J. Electronmicrosc. *19:* 17–31 (1970).

5   TUCKER, C.F.; CATSULIS, C.; STRONG, J.K., and EGGEN, D.A.: Regression of early cholesterol induced lesions in rhesus monkeys. Am. J. Path. *65:* 493–502 (1971).

6   WEIDENBACH, H. und MASSMANN, J.: Zur Frage der «ghost bodies» bei experimenteller Gefässwandschädigung. Expl. Path. *10:* 251–257 (1975).

Dr. med. H. WEIDENBACH, Institute of Pathology, Karl Marx University Leipzig, Liebigstrasse 26, *DDR-701 Leipzig* (DDR)

Prog. biochem. Pharmacol., vol. 14, pp. 253–256 (Karger, Basel 1977)

Is Plasma Lipoprotein Destroyed by Lysosomal Cathepsin in Intima?[1]

ELSPETH B. SMITH and ISOBEL B. MASSIE

Department of Chemical Pathology, University of Aberdeen,
Foresterhill, Aberdeen

Introduction

A high proportion of the cholesterol ester that accumulates in fibrous plaques is extracellular, and appears to be derived directly from plasma low density lipoprotein (LP) [3, 7]. Many workers have demonstrated LP and other plasma proteins in lesions by immunofluorescent microscopy [e.g. 6]; on quantitative assay the concentration of LP in normal intima is about the same as the concentration in the patient's plasma, and in the gelatinous precursor lesions of fibrous plaques it may be two or three times higher [7]. Thus there is a large pool of LP in intima, but very little information on the irreversible deposition of cholesterol and cholesterol esters from it. In this paper we examine some of the factors influencing the loss of electrophoretically mobile and immunologically intact LP on incubation of samples of normal intima and lesions.

Material and Methods

Intima tissue samples. Aortas were obtained from 8 patients within 5 h after death, and from 6 patients 7–10 h after death. Dissection of samples of normal intima and lesions, and preparation of histological control sections, was performed as described previously [8, 9]. Tissue samples were finely minced with scissors after application of 10–20 μl 0.9 % NaCl or 0.2 % EDTA.

1 This work was supported by a grant from the Medical Research Council.

Incubation of tissue. Small aliquots (0.5–1.0 mg dry weight) of the freshly minced tissue were wrapped in thin paper and placed on microscope slides coated with parafilm® [8, 9] in humidifying boxes. They were treated with saline, buffer or inhibitor solutions, and either held at 4° C (controls) or incubated at 37° C [10].

Measurement of LP. LP was measured by electrophoresis directly from the tissue into an antibody-containing gel; after the initial electrophoresis to remove and measure mobile LP the tissue was incubated with plasmin to release immobilized LP which was measured on fresh immunoelectrophoresis plates [9, 10].

Results

There was a decrease in total LP on incubation of all tissue samples. The rate of destruction was increased in samples minced with EDTA compared with aliquots minced with saline and measured in adjacent positions on the same immunoelectrophoresis plate (table I). In EDTA-treated samples, rate of destruction was proportional to LP concentration for both mobile and immobilized LP fractions; for total LP (mobile + immobilized) the correlation between rate of destruction of LP and the total LP concentration in control (4° C) samples was $r = 0.832$ ($p \ll 0.001$). Regression lines for rate of destruction against LP concentration for normal intima, fibrous plaques and fatty streaks containing numerous fat-filled cells are compared in figure 1. In the absence of EDTA the correlation with LP concentration was not significant, and we do not understand the mechanism of the EDTA effect.

Table I. Effect of EDTA on LP in fibro/gelatinous lesions (18 pairs of samples)

	With EDTA	No EDTA	p
Total LP recovered (controls at 4° C), mg/100 mg tissue	8.31	7.48	<0.005
% of LP immobilized	39.2	45.5	0.02
Rate of destruction, mg/100 mg tissue/h			
Mobile LP	0.56	0.13	0.02
Immobilized LP	0.33	0.11	0.05
Total LP	0.89	0.24	0.005

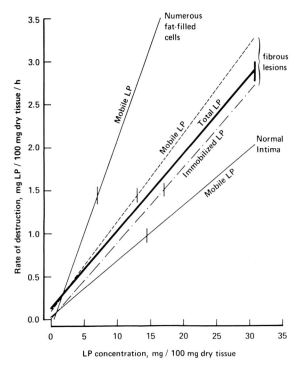

Fig. 1. Relation between the rate of destruction of LP and LP concentration in intimal samples in tissues treated with EDTA. Vertical bars indicate the maximum LP concentration found in each tissue group.

Table II. Effect of pH on rate of destruction of LP

| | Rate of destruction of LP, mg/100 mg tissue/h | | |
	pH 5.1–5.5	pH 5.5–6.1	p
With EDTA (12)[1]	0.98	0.70 (71 %)	<0.001
No EDTA (9)	0.80	0.46 (57 %)	<0.001
	pH <5.1	pH >6.4	p
With EDTA (9)	0.68	0.06 (10 %)	0.001

[1] Number of pairs of samples.

There was no inhibition by trypsin inhibitor, ε-amino-N-caproic acid or DFP, and only slight inhibition (0–20 %) by iodoacetamide and iodoacetic acid. However, destruction was almost completely inhibited (90 %) above pH 6.4, and maximum activity was obtained below pH 5.5 (table II).

References

1 ARNQVIST, H.J. and LUNDHOLM, L.: Influence of oxygen tension on the metabolism of vascular smooth muscle. Demonstration of a Pasteur effect. Atherosclerosis 25: 245 (1976).

2 BERNFELD, P. and KELLEY, T.F.: Proteolysis of human serum β-lipoproteins. J. biol. Chem. 239: 3341 (1964).

3 DAYTON, S. and HASHIMOTO, S.: Cholesterol flux and metabolism in arterial tissue and in atheromata. Expl molec. Path. 13: 253 (1970).

4 HILL, A.V.: The diffusion of oxygen and lactic acid through tissues. Proc. R. Soc., B 104: 39 (1928–29).

5 KIRK, J.E.: The cathepsin activity of arterial tissue in individuals of various ages. J. Geront. 17: 158 (1962).

6 MORE, R.H. and HAUST, M.D.: Atherogenesis and plasma constituents. Am. J. Path. 38: 572 (1961).

7 SMITH, E.B.: The relation between plasma and tissue lipids in human atherosclerosis. Adv. Lipid Res. 12: 1 (1974).

8 SMITH, E.B.; ALEXANDER, K.A., and MASSIE, I.B.: Insoluble 'fibrin' in human aortic intima. Quantitative studies on the relationship between insoluble 'fibrin', soluble fibrinogen and low density lipoprotein. Atherosclerosis 23: 19 (1976).

9 SMITH, E.B.; MASSIE, I.B., and ALEXANDER, K.M.: The release of an immobilized lipoprotein fraction from atherosclerotic lesions by incubation with plasmin. Atherosclerosis 25: 71 (1976).

10 SMITH, E.B. and MASSIE, I.B.: Destruction of endogenous low density lipoprotein in incubated intima. Atherosclerosis 26: 427 (1977).

Dr. E.B. SMITH, Department of Chemical Pathology, University of Aberdeen, *Foresterhill, Aberdeen* (Scotland)

Prog. biochem. Pharmacol., vol. 14, pp. 257–261 (Karger, Basel 1977)

Atherosclerosis and Plasma Lipoprotein Retention in the Human Aorta[1]

H.F. Hoff, C.L. Heideman and J.W. Gaubatz[2]

Department of Neurology and Pathology, Baylor College of Medicine, Houston, Tex.

Plasma lipoproteins, especially the low-density lipoprotein fractions (LDL), have been linked to the atherosclerotic process by clinical and experimental studies. The aim of our studies has been to determine the amount and localization of plasma LDL in human arteries and to correlate these parameters with the estimated degree of atherosclerotic involvement and plasma LDL profile. We have utilized immunofluorescence techniques directed against apolipoprotein B (apoB), the major protein of both the LDL and VLDL fractions to localize this antigen in normal and plaque areas [1, 2]. Since this procedure gives only qualitative results, we now use a more quantitative procedure, namely an electroimmuno-assay (EIA) directed against apoB [3, 5].

Samples of human aortas were obtained at autopsy primarily from accident victims within 12 h after death. The aortic intima was subdivided by gross appearance into normal and plaque regions. Microscopically, the normal areas from adult cases were characterized by a thickened intima filled with smooth muscle cells, collagen fibers, and some glycosamino-glycans. ApoB was usually localized diffusely throughout the intima, together with oil red O-positive lipids, but not in the underlining media [1, 5]. Atherosclerotic plaques were characterized by the presence of a fibrotic or fibromuscular region usually adjacent to the lumen, and by the

[1] Supported by the National Heart and Blood Vessel Research and Demonstration Center, Baylor College of Medicine (NIH Grant HL 17269), NIH Grant NS 09287, and a grant from the Texas Affiliate, American Heart Association. Dr. Hoff is an Established Investigator of the American Heart Association.

[2] We wish to acknowledge the help of the staff of the Harris County Medical Examiner's Office for assisting in the procurement of arterial specimens.

presence of a necrotic core underlining this fibrotic region usually deeper within the plaque and often penetrating into the medial layer. ApoB was localized predominantly to this core region, but some bands of collagen in the fibrotic zone were also positive [1]. At the ultrastructural level using an immunoperoxidase procedure we have localized apoB on the surface of spheres in the size range of LDL and VLDL primarily within the lipid core of plaques [3, 4]. These spheres, believed to represent intact lipoproteins, were found unassociated or in close apposition to collagen and elastic fibers.

In order to quantitate apoB by EIA from normal and plaque regions, the intimal lining was stripped from the underlining media, finely minced, and homogenized in 0.13M Tris-0.1 % EDTA buffer pH 7.4 with a Polytron homogenizer [5]. Samples of supernatants of extracts were applied to the EIA and the peak heights obtained were converted to apoB concentrations using a linear standard curve of peak height vs. apoB concentration in a standard LDL preparation [5].

A statistically significant positive correlation was obtained between buffer-extractable apoB from grossly normal aortic intima and both postmortem plasma cholesterol and triglyceride levels [6]. The positive correlation between apoB in normal intima and plasma cholesterol is consistent with the results of SMITH et al. [7] who used a more semiquantitative technique to measure apoB in the aorta. Poorer correlations in this study were found in the plaques.

We have recently demonstrated that when buffer extracts of normal intima were subjected to differential ultracentrifugation, the d 1.006–1.063 or LDL density range contained most of the immunological reactivity to apoB in the extract [5]. Negatively-stained preparations of this fraction demonstrated spherical particles of the same size range as native LDL [5]. These results suggest that buffer-extractable apoB in the grossly normal intima is almost entirely intact LDL, further suggesting that plasma and intimal apoB are in equilibrium. Since no VLDL-sized particles could be detected in the normal intima [5], the positive correlation between plasma triglyceride levels (estimating plasma VLDL levels) and buffer-extractable apoB in the normal intima could be explained by a recent hypothesis made by ZILVERSMIT [8]. He states that VLDL may be broken down to an apoB-rich remnant particle by the action of a lipoprotein lipase on the endothelial surface. The smaller remnant could then enter the arterial wall, thereby contributing to the total tissue pool of apoB.

When the buffer-extractable apoB content (μg/mg tissue dry weight) of grossly normal and adjacent plaques were compared in 25 cases, surprisingly the values in the normal intima were statistically significantly higher (7.13 $\pm$ 4.38 SD in the normal compared to 4.72 $\pm$ 2.82 in the plaques) [5]. In part, this may be due to the diffuse localization of apoB in the normal intima as compared to the structurally more heterogeneous plaque in which localization is focal, and areas devoid of apoB may contribute to the total weight of the plaque. The lower value of plaque apoB was most likely due to the fact that buffer extraction, although removing essentially all apoB from normal intima, did not remove all apoB from plaques. After buffer-extraction pellets from plaques were still positive for apoB as shown by our immunofluorescence staining procedure [5].

To quantitatively remove this remaining fraction of tightly bound apoB, we extracted the buffer pellets of both normal regions and plaques with the detergent Triton X-100 (3 % in 0.13M Tris buffer pH 7.4). ApoB values of this detergent fraction were obtained from EIA by comparing peak heights of the extracts to a standard LDL (treated with Triton in an identical manner as the extract) which gave a linear curve [1]. Normal intima contained predominantly buffer-extracted apoB whereas in plaques nearly half of the total plaque apoB remained tightly bound after buffer extraction, consistent with the immunofluorescence monitoring of pellets from normal and plaque homogenates.

We have recently found that there is marked variability in total apoB content, that is, the sum of buffer- and Triton-extracted apoB, within different plaques from the same aorta. This is consistent with observed heterogeneity of plaques and is consistent with the findings of immuno-fluorescence localization studies [1]. However, the variability from case to case was found to be even greater than from plaque to plaque within each case. To reduce the heterogeneity of plaques, we have microdissected each fatty-fibrous plaque into a fibrotic and necrotic fraction. The former consisted primarily of the tactually hard fibrous or fibromuscular cap usually adjacent to the lumen and consisting predominantly of collagen fibers. The latter consisted of the tactually soft core regions, predominantly lipid at the base of plaques and usually underlining the fibrotic cap. The fibrotic regions contained primarily apoB extracted with a standard buffer, whereas the necrotic or core regions contained primarily apoB so tightly bound that the detergent Triton X-100 had to be used for extraction.

These overall results suggest that plasma lipoproteins, in particular LDL, enter and are specifically retained by the intimal lining of the human aorta. The grossly normal aortic intima contains apoB which is extractable primarily by standard buffers and may represent loosely bound LDL. The atherosclerotic lesion contains both this loosely bound fraction of apoB, primarily in its fibrotic regions, as well as a tightly bound fraction, primarily in the necrotic region or lipid core. This second fraction contains either tightly bound intact or possibly delipidated lipoprotein. The superposed localization of apoB and lipid [1] is indirect evidence that plaque apoB is not delipidated. It will be of interest to determine if there is a shift from loosely to tightly bound apoB in the aorta with progression of the atherosclerotic process. It will also be of interest to see if a strong positive correlation is found between total plasma apoB as found in LDL and VLDL or plasma cholesterol and triglyceride levels, and total plaque apoB as extracted with both standard buffer and detergent. If these changes are established, it is conceivable that removal of plaque cholesterol could be achieved both by reducing plasma LDL and VLDL levels, and by breaking the bond between lipoproteins and plaque components. This might eventually result in lesion regression to stages of severity below those with clinical implications.

References

1 HOFF, H.F.; JACKSON, R.L.; MAO, J.T., and GOTTO, A.M.: Localization of low density lipoproteins in arterial lesions from normolipemics employing a purified fluorescent-labeled antibody. Biochim. biophys. Acta 351: 407–415 (1974).

2 HOFF, H.F.; LIE, J.T.; TITUS, J.L.; JACKSON, R.L.; DEBAKEY, M.E.; BAYARDO, R.J., and GOTTO, A.M.: Localization of apo-low-density lipoproteins (apoLDL) in atherosclerotic lesions of human normo- and hyperlipemics. Archs Path. 99: 253–258 (1975).

3 HOFF, H.F. and GAUBATZ, J.W.: Ultrastructural localization of plasma lipoproteins in human intracranial arteries. Virchows Arch. path. Anat. 369: 111–122 (1976).

4 HOFF, H.F. and GAUBATZ, J.W.: Ultrastructural localization of apolipoprotein B in human aortic and coronary atherosclerotic plaques. Expl molec Path. 26: 214–227 (1977).

5 HOFF, H.F.; HEIDEMAN, C.L.; GAUBATZ, J.W.; GOTTO, A.M.; ERICKSON, E.E., and JACKSON, R.L.: Quantitation of apolipoprotein B (apoB) in grossly normal human aorta. Circulation Res. 40: 56–64 (1977).

6   HOFF, H.F.; HEIDEMAN, C.L.; GOTTO, A.M., and GAUBATZ, J.W.: Apolipo-
     protein B (apoB) retention in the grossly normal and atherosclerotic human
     aorta. Circulation Res. (in press, 1977).
7   SMITH, E.B.; MASSIE, I.B., and ALEXANDER, K.M.: The release of an immobilized
     lipoprotein fraction from atherosclerotic lesions by incubation with plasmin.
     Atherosclerosis 25: 71–84 (1972).
8   ZILVERSMIT, D.: A proposal linking atherogenesis to the interaction of endo-
     thelial lipoprotein lipase with triglyceride-rich lipoproteins. Circulation Res. 33:
     633–638 (1973).

Dr. H.F. HOFF, Department of Neurology and Pathology, Baylor College of
Medicine, Houston, TX 77030 (USA)

Prog. biochem. Pharmacol., vol. 14, pp. 262–267 (Karger, Basel 1977)

Histochemistry of Free and Esterified Cholesterol in Human Atherosclerotic Arteries

C.M. VAN GENT and J.J. EMEIS

Gaubius Institute, Health Research Organization TNO, Leiden

The intra- and extracellular accumulation of lipid deposits is one of the characteristic features of the atherosclerotic lesion. Chemical analysis of these lesions has demonstrated that cholesterol (free and esterified) is quantitatively the most important component of the accumulating lipid. On the other hand, detailed analyses of small samples of lesions [reviewed by SMITH, 1974] have shown that the lipid composition may be markedly different in the various parts of the lesions, e.g. in the relative and absolute amounts of free and esterified cholesterol present. In order to be able to compare these chemical data with some histochemical observations on the distribution pattern of lipids in atherosclerotic lesions, sensitive, specific and accurate techniques for the histochemical localization of the various classes of lipids are required. These methods exist for most lipid classes [reviewed by ADAMS and BAYLISS, 1975], but methods for free and esterified cholesterol have been unsatisfactory yet.

For some time past, two enzymes (cholesterol hydrolase and cholesterol oxidase) have become commercially available for the enzymatic determination of serum cholesterol. We have used these enzymes for the histochemical localization of both free and esterified cholesterol [EMEIS et al., 1977]. The method is outlined in figure 1, showing the procedure for the demonstration of both free and esterified cholesterol simultaneously.

Free cholesterol is selectively demonstrated by omitting the cholesterol hydrolase from the incubation medium, whereas esterified cholesterol is visualized by preincubating sections with cholesterol oxidase in the

$$\text{Cholesterol ester} \xrightarrow[\text{EC 3.1.1.13}]{\substack{\text{Cholesterol ester} \\ \text{hydrolase}}} \text{Cholesterol} + \text{fatty acid}$$

$$\text{Cholesterol} + O_2 \xrightarrow[\text{EC 1.1.3.6}]{\substack{\text{Cholesterol} \\ \text{oxidase}}} \text{Cholest -4-en-3-on} + H_2O_2$$

$$H_2O_2 + 3,3'\text{-diaminobenzidine} \xrightarrow[\text{EC 1.11.1.7}]{\substack{\text{Horseradish} \\ \text{peroxidase}}} \text{Brown insoluble polymer}$$

Fig. 1.

absence of diaminobenzidine and peroxidase, followed by incubation in complete medium as outlined in figure 1 [for details, see EMEIS *et al.*, 1977].

We applied this method to formaldehyde-fixed, frozen sections of human atherosclerotic arteries. For comparison, serial sections were stained with oil red O; also both methods were used on the same section.

Fig. 2. Fibrous plaque stained for esterified (a) and free (b) cholesterol. Free cholesterol is mainly found in the lipid core, especially near the (unstained) media. In the foam cells in the fibrous cap only cholesterol esters can be demonstrated. Lipid analysis (mg/g dry weight): total lipids 190; free cholesterol 60, cholesterol esters 50, triglycerides 30, phospholipids 45, free fatty acids 5. $\times$ 50.

Fig. 3. Serial sections of the lower part of a fatty streak in a coronary artery, stained for total cholesterol (a), and for total cholesterol followed by oil red O staining (b). Although no cholesterol-negative, oil red O-positive material is present, the combined staining procedure gives enhanced contrast. Lipid analysis (mg/g dry weight): total lipids 380; free cholesterol 45, cholesterol esters 145, triglycerides 130, phospholipids 40, free fatty acids 20. $\times$ 250.

Fig. 4. Intimal-medial area of an intercostal artery. Free cholesterol (a) has a diffuse localization, and is not found in lipid droplets (e.g. at arrow), in contrast to the staining of droplets in figure 4b (cholesterol esters) and figure 4c (oil red O staining). Combined staining for cholesterol esters and neutral lipids gives enhanced contrast (d), compared to either method alone. Lipid analysis (mg/g dry weight): total lipids 150; free cholesterol 30, cholesterol esters 50, triglycerides 30, phospholipids 35, free fatty acids 5. $\times$ 250.

Fig. 2–4 see pages 264 and 265.

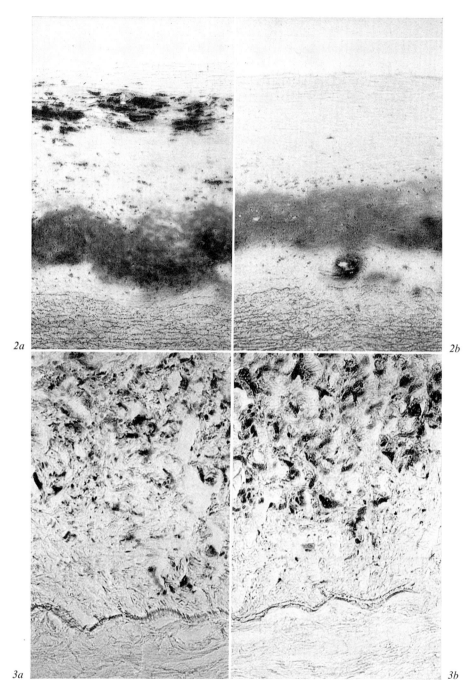

2a

2b

3a

3b

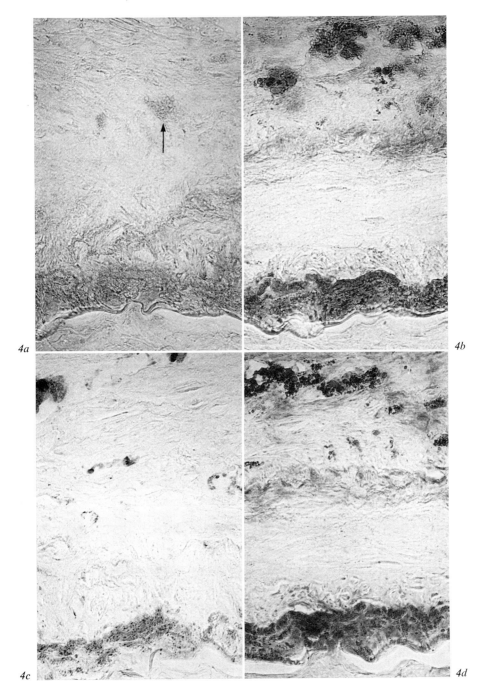

4a

4b

4c

4d

Lipid analyses were performed on serial sections from the same lesion by quantitative thin-layer chromatography [VAN GENT, 1967].

Generally, three staining patterns were observed: diffuse, crystalline and in droplets. Diffuse staining was found in and around the lipid core in the center of plaques, and occasionally in small scattered areas of fibrous caps, as well as in the tunica media. In these diffusely-stained areas, free as well as esterified cholesterol was found, the staining for esterified cholesterol being more intense. Occasionally, staining of free cholesterol was pronounced, especially at the base of the lipid core of lesions (fig. 2).

Crystals present in the lipid core occasionally stained as free cholesterol, but were predominantly cholesterol esters, as could also be shown by the disappearance of birefringence after incubation in the presence of cholesterol hydrolase.

In the lipid droplets of fatty streaks and fibrous plaques merely the presence of cholesterol ester could be demonstrated (fig. 2, 3). This was so for extracellular, as well as for intracellular lipid droplets, both of intimal and endothelial cells.

Poststaining with oil red O of sections incubated for total cholesterol only very occasionally showed oil red O-positive, cholesterol-negative cells. These cells were generally found at the shoulders of plaques. However, combined cholesterol-oil red O staining resulted in a more intense staining than either technique by itself, although the staining pattern was identical (fig. 3, 4).

In conclusion, our technique provides a sensitive, specific and accurate method for the nondestructive localization of cholesterol in tissues. The staining patterns observed closely correspond to those obtained with oil red O, but allow discrimination between sites where free and esterified cholesterol is present. A more detailed description of the cholesterol staining of lesions will be published elsewhere.

Summary

The described technique provides a sensitive, specific and accurate method for the nondestructive localization of cholesterol in tissues. The staining patterns observed closely correspond to those obtained with oil red O, but allow discrimination between sites where free and esterified cholesterol is present.

References

ADAMS, C.W.M. and BAYLISS, O.B.: Lipid histochemistry; in GLICK and ROSENBAUM Techniques of biochemical and biophysical morphology, vol. 2, pp. 99–156 (Wiley, New York 1975).

EMEIS, J.J.; GENT, C.M. VAN, and SABBEN, C.M. VAN: An enzymatic method for the histochemical localization of free and esterified cholesterol separately. Histochem. J. *9:* 197–204 (1977).

GENT, C.M. VAN: Separation and microdetermination of lipids by thin-layer chromatography followed by densitometry. Z. analyt. Chem. *236:* 344–350 (1967).

SMITH, E.B.: The relationship between plasma and tissue lipids in human atherosclerosis. Adv. Lipid Res. *12:* 1–49 (1974).

Dr. C.M. VAN GENT, Gaubius Institute, Health Research Organization TNO, Herenstraat 5d, *Leiden* (The Netherlands)

Prog. biochem. Pharmacol., vol. 14, pp. 268–270 (Karger, Basel 1977)

Cyclic Adenosine Monophosphate System in Rat Experimental Atherosclerosis

Z. JURUKOVA and B. BOSHKOV

Institute of Cardiovascular Diseases, Medical Academy, Sofia

The metabolism of adenosine 3′,5′-monophosphate (cAMP) in vascular tissue has become of great interest in connection with recent studies establishing the capability of endothelial cells to contract [2] and the role of cAMP as a relaxant of arterial endothelial cells [3]. The studies reported here relate to alterations in the arterial cAMP system in experimental atherosclerosis which might influence the permeability of arterial endothelium and play a role in the initiation and progression of atherosclerotic lesions.

Material and Methods

Experimental atherosclerosis was induced in 13 male Wistar rats which were given for 6 months an atherogenic diet. 6 Wistar rats, fed on standard food, served as controls. The experimental animals were sacrificed by decapitation. One segment of the aorta was taken for histological study. The remaining part of the vessel was frozen in liquid nitrogen and used for the preparation of three types of homogenates: (1) for determination of the content of cAMP by the radioimmunoassay method and (2) for the assays of (a) adenylate cyclase (AC) and (b) phosphodiesterase (PDE) activity by the method of DELAAGE et al. [1]. The cAMP content was expressed as pmol per gram tissue (wet weight); the AC activity as pmol cAMP formed/mg protein/10 min; the PDE activity as pmol cAMP hydrolized/mg protein/min.

Results and Discussion

Gross atherosclerosis was established in the aorta of rats kept on atherogenic diet. Microscopically atherosclerotic lesions at different stages were observed – from fatty streaks to complicated fibrous plaques. The results from the biochemical estimation of the cAMP content and the activity of the enzyme controlling its intracellular level indicate a general decline of cAMP metabolism in the aortic wall of animals with experimental atherosclerosis. The level of the intracellular cAMP is significantly lower as compared to control aortas. The activities of AC and PDE (total) are also decreased in atherosclerotic aortas. PDE activity decrease is not significant, but that of AC activity is very pronounced. After β-adrenergic stimulation with hydrocortisone the activity of AC in atherosclerotic aortas shows a threefold rise, whereas in the aortas of control animals its activity increases 10 times. The decrease in the activity and the lowering of the AC reactivity are most probably the cause for the low level of arterial intracellular cAMP in atherosclerosis.

The factors causing the decline of cAMP metabolism in the arterial wall in atherosclerosis are still unknown. However, the lowering of the intracellular level of cAMP may accelerate the initiation and progression of atherosclerotic lesions. Taking into consideration the relaxing effect of cAMP on the microfilamentous system of endothelial cells [3], it may be assumed that a decrease in the cAMP content of the arterial wall would induce an enhanced reactivity of endothelial cells and their contraction under the influence of a variety of subthreshold stimuli. Endothelial contraction, associated with transient openings of interendothelial junctions, allows the passage of plasma macromolecules like lipoproteins into the subendothelial space. It is also accompanied by exposure of endothelial basement membrane collagen to circulating platelets, which release vasoactive and mitogenic factors into the arterial wall. The penetration of circulating macromolecules and platelet factors in the arterial wall stimulates both the migration of medial SMC into the intima and their further proliferation. On the other hand, one of the important physiological effects of cAMP in the animal organism is its capacity to inhibit cell multiplication. It is suggested, therefore, that the reduction of the intracellular level of cAMP in the arterial wall may favor the proliferation of SMC in the subendothelial space, induced by the plasma macromolecules and mitogenic platelet factors. Experiments establishing the prevention of experimental atherosclerosis in rabbits by inhibition of cAMP phosphodiesterase with pyridinolcarbamate [3] lend support to the conception about a role of the lowered cAMP level in atherogenesis.

Cyclic AMP metabolism disturbances in the arterial wall seems to be an important mechanism, whose interaction with other injurious factors results in arterial lesions, leading to focal proliferation of SMC.

References

1   DELAAGE, B.; BELLON, N., and CAILLA, H.L.: Rapid assays for adenylate cyclase and 3′,5′ cyclic AMP phosphodiesterase activities. Simultaneous measurements of other pathways of ATP catabolism. Analyt. Biochem. *62:* 417–425 (1974).
2   MAJNO, G.; SHEA, S.M., and LEVENTHAL, M.: Endothelial contraction induced by histamine-type mediators. An electron microscopic study. J. Cell Biol. *42:* 647–672 (1969).
3   SHIMAMOTO, T.: Hyperreactive arterial endothelial cells in atherogenesis and cyclic AMP phosphodiesterase inhibition in prevention and treatment of atherosclerotic disorders. Jap. Heart J. *16:* 76–97 (1975).

Dr. Z. JURUKOVA, Institute of Cardiovascular Diseases, Medical Academy, *Sofia* (Bulgaria)

Prog. biochem. Pharmacol., vol. 14, pp. 271–275 (Karger, Basel 1977)

Distribution of DNA Template Activity in Artery Wall Cells

R. Lehmann, R. Dénes and T. Kerényi

Institute for Arteriosclerosis Research, University of Münster, Münster, and 3rd Department of Medicine and 2nd Department of Pathology, Semmelweis University, Budapest

It is the attempt of this paper (1) to demonstrate how DNA template activity can be visualized within nuclei of artery wall cells, (2) to give an example for the distribution pattern of DNA template activity within the artery wall, and (3) to discuss briefly the significance of this method to study early alterations of normal and diseased artery wall cells.

In one or the other way all processes in a living system are related to nucleic acids and proteins (fig. 1). From concepts of molecular biology it is generally known that the sequence of amino acids of proteins is determined by the sequence of base pairs of the DNA macromolecule. Those DNA sites which are available for RNA synthesis are considered as active templates. From this relation follows that an altered DNA activity may result in an altered protein synthesis, or in other words,

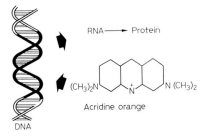

Fig. 1. General concept of expression of DNA templates (black part of the double helix) through RNA intermediaries, which in turn act as templates for the synthesis of proteins. Acridine orange preferentially binds to these active DNA templates.

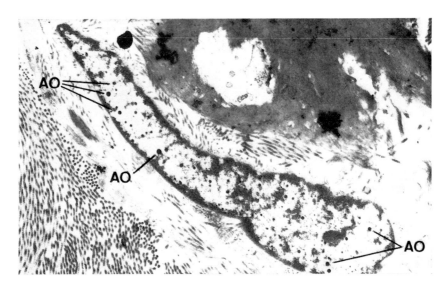

Fig. 2. Abundant acridine orange chromatin reaction products (AO) within the euchromatin portion of a nucleus of an aortic wall cell localized at the border region media/adventitia of a hypertensive rabbit. × 19,000.

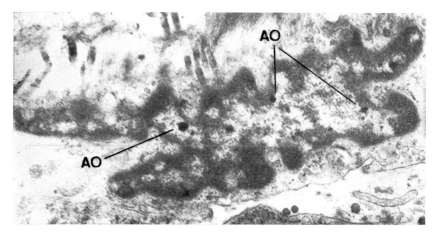

Fig. 3. Relatively less acridine orange chromatin reaction products within the nucleus of a medial smooth muscle cell of the thoracal aortic wall. × 54,000.

if we notice an altered protein synthesis it may be preceded by an altered DNA template activity.

How can DNA template activity be visualized? For this purpose an ultracytochemical method has been employed using acridine orange (AO) as an ultracytochemical probe [1, 4]. Numerous studies on the binding mechanisms and binding capacity of AO to DNA [e.g. 3] have shown that AO interacts with those DNA sites which are available for RNA synthesis. The treatment with AO results in electron-dense particles (fig. 2) confined to the euchromatin portion of the nucleus as previously reported [1, 2].

Survey ultrastructural examinations of the thoracal aortic wall revealed a characteristic distribution pattern of nuclei containing AO chromatin reaction products (fig. 2, 3). Nuclei with a relatively high number of AO chromatin reaction products were routinely found in the endothelial and in the border region media/adventitia of the hypertensive aortic wall. Cells with active nuclei appeared either as small cell groups or as individual cells in those specific regions. Other nuclei throughout the aortic wall demonstrated appreciably less AO chromatin reaction products per single section of the nucleus in the same tissue sections (fig. 3).

If in the aortic wall of normotensive animals any AO chromatin reaction products could be detected it was always a relatively low number of reaction products per single section of a nucleus. Supposed that the DNA template activity in an individual nuclei is relatively low it may not be expected that active sites could be demonstrated in each one of the sections. This might explain the lack of any AO chromatin reaction products in many sections of nuclei of artery wall cells in hypertensive as well as in normotensive animals. From the representative distribution pattern of nuclei containing AO chromatin reaction products the conclusion can be drawn that experimental renal hypertension compared to normotensive animals results in an increased DNA template activity in specific populations of aortic wall cells. Similar results were obtained in rats following renal hypertension and experimental diabetes produced by streptozotocin.

The significance of this ultracytochemical method critically depends on the interpretation of the AO chromatin reaction products. With high resolution electron microscopy we lately have discovered in our laboratory that the AO chromatin reaction products are composed of spherical subunits resembling recently described nucleosomes or nu-bodies [see OLINS et al., 4, for further references]. This observations suggest that transcriptively active nucleosomes are assembled into a higher organized particle which is visualized after AO treatment (fig. 4). Since many

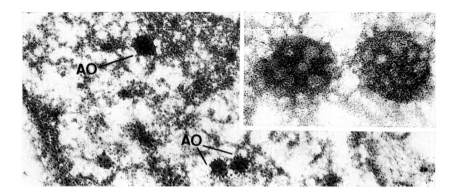

Fig. 4. Fine structure of acridine orange chromatin reaction products. × 95,000. *Inset* Two of the acridine orange reaction products at higher magnification. It is clearly seen that the reaction products are composed of chromatin subunits within a granulated electron-dense matrix. × 380,000.

nucleosomes are associated in such a particle it has been defined as polynucleosome.

Activation of DNA template sites after stimulation by extrinsic factors like experimentally derived hypertension is part of a general concept on differential distribution of gene activity occurring in embryo-genesis, regeneration, neoplastic transformation, as response to hormones, or in activated lymphocytes. Visualization of DNA template activity enable us to ask a number of important questions, e.g. where are activated cells localized, which cell types are involved, when does activation occur? We are convinced that this technique may become a useful tool to identify earlier than with other methods those cells within the artery wall which have been stimulated to switch from one to another functional state.

References

1   FRENSTER, J.H.: Electron microscopic localization of acridine orange binding to DNA within human leukemic bone marrow cells. Cancer Res. *31:* 1128–1136 (1971).
2   LEHMANN, R. and SLAVKIN, H.C.: Localization of 'transcriptively active' cells during odontogenesis using acridine orange ultrastructural cytochemistry. Devl. Biol. *49:* 438–456 (1976).

3 LIEDEMAN, R. and BOLUND, L.: Acridine orange binding to chromatin of individual cells and nuclei under different staining conditions. Expl Cell Res. *101:* 164–174 (1976).

4 OLINS, A.L.; CARLSON, R.D.; WRIGHT, E.B., and OLINS, D.E.: Chromatin γ bodies: isolation, subfractionation and physical characterization. Nucleic Acids Res. *3:* 3271–3291 (1976).

Dr. R. LEHMANN, Institute for Arteriosclerosis Research at the University of Münster, *D-4400 Münster* (FRG)

Prog. biochem. Pharmacol., vol. 14, pp. 276–282 (Karger, Basel 1977)

Endothelial Regeneration: the Role of Smooth Muscle Cells, Blood Cells and Histiocytes

R. Gottlob

Department of Experimental Surgery, Ist Surgical Clinic, Vienna University, Vienna

In a study of the endothelial regeneration after various lesions the following modes of regeneration were seen in en face full thickness or 'Häutchen' preparations.

Regeneration from Adjacent Endothelial Cells

Hard traumatization [7]. In jugular veins of rabbits a circular zone of desquamation was produced by a temporary ligature. The defect was first covered by blood cells. Later a new endothelium grew over the parietal thrombus. After silver staining the new cells displayed weakly stained endothelial silver lines. The regenerated endothelium was permeable to the silver nitrate solution so that underlaying structures were stained as well. In some instances also a layer of smooth muscle cells was seen between the parietal thrombus and the regenerated endothelium. The new endothelium cells became less permeable a few days later but in these cells staining of the cytoplasm occurred, sparing the nuclear region. Normal permeability was restored 2–3 weeks after injury.

Soft traumatization. Mild mechanical injury was induced by compressing the veins with a clamp which was covered by rubber tubing. No changes were seen immediately thereafter (fig. 1A). A few hours later some damaged cells were covered by thrombocytes and erythrocytes. The next days these cells displayed cytoplasm staining sparing out the nuclear region (fig. 1B). The same cells became considerably narrower while their normally stained neighbor cells rather widened. Regions with narrow cells and broad cells sometimes alternated quite regularly so that the

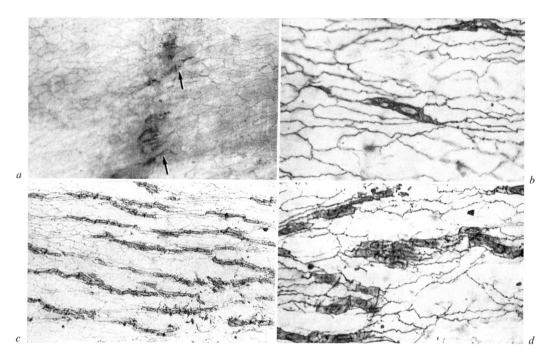

Fig. 1. Soft traumatization. *A* After releasing the rubber-covered clamp the endothelia appear normal. Only at the edge of the mildly compressed tissue a few lesions are visible (↑). *B* Narrow dark cells, loaded with blood cells (thrombocytes) alternating with broad cells displaying delicately stained silver lines. *C* Regeneration waves. *D* The same as in C at a higher magnification.

endothelial lining presented a wave-like appearance (fig. 1C, D). Occasionally the dark cells protruded into the lumen, suggesting an incipient desquamation. Other narrow cells were covered by their less damaged or regenerated neighbor cells. Again the silver lines were stained less in regenerating cells. After about 10 days the endothelium again appeared normal with the exception that a great number of multinucleated cells was found. In ultrastructural investigations two layers of endothelia were found frequently [8]. Sometimes normal cells overlapped cells with an abnormally electron-translucent ground cytoplasm. Little is known about the provenience of the new cells; an origin by division of adjacent endothelia or by metaplasia of smooth muscle cells seems possible.

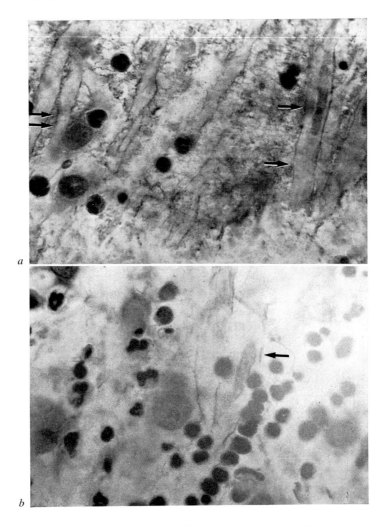

Fig. 2. Top: Smooth muscle cells, covering an endothelial defect in a grafted vessel. Bottom: Transition from smooth muscle cell to endothelium-like cell (←).

Regeneration from Smooth Muscle Cells

Jugular veins of dogs were grafted into the carotid arteries of the same animals. After conventional dissection of the graft great parts of the endothelial lining were destroyed. Most of the defects were overgrown by new cells originating from adjacent preserved endothelia. In some instances, however, long thin cells with fusiform nuclei, situated transversely to the axis of the vessel, were found covering the inner vascular surface. Undoubtedly these were smooth muscle cells. There were, however, many transitions between these muscle cells and similar cells with more round nuclei (fig. 2). At later stages regions were found where the endothelial cells were still situated in a direction transverse to the axis of the vein. It was felt that these findings could be explained by metaplasia of smooth muscle cells [2, 3], normally in contact with the endothelial cells through the fenestrae of the elastic membrane [4].

Blood-Borne Cells

Thromboses were induced in the jugular veins of rabbits by a modified Wessler technique [11]. 3–4 days later the thrombi were covered by endothelial cells. These cells were scattered loosely at the surface of the thrombi and a continuous layer formed at later stages.

Human emboli obtained by surgery shortly after embolization were examined in conventional sections by HE staining. Again the emboli were covered by a more or less continuous layer of endothelial cells [5]. In addition, in the majority of emboli clefts were seen, some of them communicating with the exterior space. The clefts were covered by a discontinuous endothelial lining.

It is most unlikely that all these endothelia had grown in continuity from the endocardium into the emboli. If this would have been the case, the embolus would have been attached so firmly to the heart that embolization would be impossible. These findings and the experiments of O'NEAL *et al.* [9] favor the assumption that blood-borne cells might have the capacity to replace endothelia.

Connective Tissue Cells

BORNEMISZA [1] and later SPARKS [10] designed implantable devices for the growth of autogenous reinforced artery grafts. It consists of a smooth plastic mandril surrounded by a porous textile. After subcutaneous implantation connective tissue grows through the pores of the textile until it contacts the mandril. The so formed new vessel may be inserted

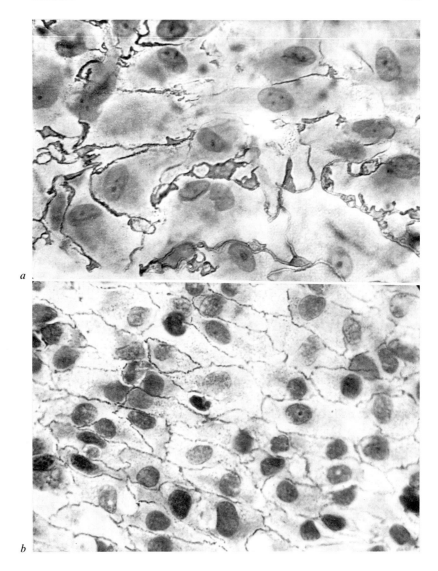

Fig. 3. Endothelium-like linings of Sparks prosthesis, not connected to the vascular system. Top: More dissociated cells as frequently observed in regenerating endothelia. Bottom: Endothelium-like structures from the same prosthesis.

into the vascular system after 8 weeks or later. In our investigations we examined häutchen preparations from the surface of the Sparks prostheses facing the mandril. The knitted dacron textile was cut open so that the mandril could be removed without damaging the inner surface of the newly formed vessel. In the microscope fibers of the textile coating, surrounded by histiocytes and fibroblasts, were found to form the greatest part of the surface. There were, however, patches, consisting of round cells, containing vesiculous nuclei, forming an endothelium-like lining. The cells were separated by silver lines not distinguishable from endothelial silver lines or from silver lines from serous membranes [6] (fig. 3). We have no information about the ultrastructure of these cells. It is a matter of personal preference whether we call them endothelia or endothelium-like cells. Our investigations, however, stress the great capacity of cells of mesenchymal origin to transform to endothelium-like structures when growing on surfaces.

References

1   BORNEMISZA, G.: Gewebeersatz mit Hilfe der auto-alloplastischen Methode; in SALZER und DENCK 13. Tag. Öster. Ges. Chirurgie, Krems 1972 (Egermann, Wien 1973).

2   GOTTLOB, R.; DONAS, P., und EL NASHEF, B.: Untersuchungen am Endothel arterialisierter Venen. Die Wirkung einer «Atraumatischen Präparation». Vasa *4:* 243 (1975).

3   GOTTLOB, R.; DONAS, P.; EL NASHEF, B., und SAGHIR, F.: Untersuchungen am Endothel arterialisierter Venen. II. Morphologische Befunde bei autologen Venentransplantaten bei Hunden. Vasa *5:* 111 (1976).

4   GOTTLOB, R. and HOFF, H.F.: A study of the relations between endothelial silver lines, medial transverse lines and the ultrastructural morphology of blood vessels. Vasc. Surg. *1:* 92 (1967).

5   GOTTLOB, R. und KLOS, I.: Morphologie und Lysierbarkeit von Emboli. Vasa *3:* 169 (1974).

6   GOTTLOB, R. und PIZA, F.: Die Bildung endothelialer Formationen in einer Sparks-Prothese vor Herstellung des Gefässanschlusses. Acta chir. austriaca *6:* 130 (1974).

7   GOTTLOB, R. und ZINNER, G.: Über die Regeneration geschädigter Endothelien nach hartem und weichem Trauma. Virchows Arch. path. Anat. Physiol. *336:* 16 (1962).

8   HOFF, H.F. and GOTTLOB, R.: Ultrastructural changes of large rabbit blood vessels following mild mechanical trauma. Virchows Arch. path. Anat. Physiol. *345:* 93 (1968).

9   O'NEAL, R.M.; JORDAN, G.J.; RABIN, E.R.; BAKEY, M.E., and HALPERT, B.:
     Cells grown on isolated intravascular dacron hub. An electron microscopic
     study. Expl molec. Path. *3:* 403 (1964).

10   SPARKS, C.H.: Silicone mandril method for growing reinforced autogenous
     femoro-popliteal artery grafts *in situ*. Ann. Surg. *177:* 293 (1973).

11   WESSLER, S.; WARD, K., and HO, C.: Studies on intravascular coagulation.
     J. clin. Invest. *34:* 647 (1955).

R. GOTTLOB, M.D., Department of Experimental Surgery, Ist Surgical Clinic,
Vienna University, Alserstrasse 4, *A-1097 Vienna* (Austria)

Prog. biochem. Pharmacol., vol. 14, pp. 283–286 (Karger, Basel 1977)

Immunological Factors in Vascular Diseases

S. Gerö, E. Szondy, G. Füst, M. Horváth, and J. Székely

Arteriosclerosis Research Group (Head: Prof. S. Gerö), Ministry of Health, Budapest

The presence of antibodies against homologous arterial tissues in the sera of arteriosclerotic patients has been shown in our previous investigations [3].

In our present study an extraction with calcium chloride-Tris-citrate buffer (CTC) was applied to human aortic and venous tissue. Figure 1 shows the immunoelectrophoretic pattern of aorta and vena CTC extracts. On the left side, developed with anti-CTC immune sera absorbed with normal human serum, two arcs (with α_2 and β_1 mobility) can be seen. The arcs with α mobility seem to be tissue specific [4].

Table I summarizes the results of the assays for the demonstration of antibodies against the CTC extracts containing water-soluble proteins and proteoglycans of the vessel wall. Antibodies were found in the sera of about 50 % of the patients with various manifestations of arteriosclerosis and in 75 % of patients with phlebothrombosis [2].

At various intervals after immunization partly with aortic and partly with venous CTC extracts, *in vivo* intracutaneous skin test, *in vitro* migration inhibition, lymphocyte DNA synthesis assay and immunodiffusion tests were carried out in guinea pigs with both antigens.

In the immunized groups the antigens induced a cell-mediated immune response by all three techniques. By the skin test and migration inhibition, cross-reactions were observed with both antigens. However the induction of DNA synthesis was found to be a specific reaction, since in this case no cross-reactivity could be observed.

Recently migration inhibition and lymphocyte DNA synthesis were tested with human aortic and venous CTC extracts in patients with arterial and venous diseases.

Table 1. Immunological tests with aortic and venous CTC extracts

Diagnosis	Aortic extract							Venous extracts						
	linear		immuno-diffusion		passive		hemagglu-tination		linear		immuno-diffusion		passive		hemagglu-tination
	n		pos		n		pos		n		pos		n		pos
Coronary sclerosis	31		15		17		14		31		0		17		0
Myocardial infarction	18		4		18		12		18		0		18		0
Cerebral artery sclerosis	22		10		29		21		22		0		29		0
Arteriosclerosis obliterans	11		0		11		0		11		0		11		0
Phlebothrombosis	61		1		45		2		61		47		39		29
Control	22		0		22		0		22		0		22		0

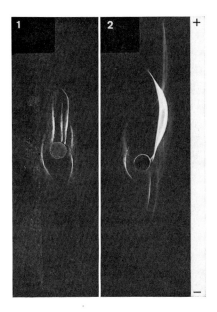

Fig. 1. Immunoelectrophoretic pattern of aortic and venous CTC extracts. Wells: (1) CTC extract obtained from aorta, (2) CTC extract obtained from vein. Right side: Rabbit antiserum against CTC extract of aorta (1) and vein (2). Left side: Absorbed anti-aorta (1) and anti-vein (2) immune sera.

Table II. Immune complexes in sera of patients with various vascular diseases

Diagnosis	Number of patients	Positive results
Myocardial infarction	51	19
Coronary sclerosis	51	10
Cerebral artery sclerosis	26	8
Cerebral thrombosis	12	6
Arteriosclerosis obliterans	11	7
Pulmonary infarction	3	3
Thrombophlebitis	15	4
Total	169	57 (34 %)

In the patient groups a significant inhibition of the leukocyte migration was observed and similarly to the animal experiments a cross-reactivity was seen between the two antigens. With the DNA synthesis test an increased ^{3}H-thymidine incorporation, without any cross-reactivity, was detected.

Next we have investigated immune complexes in sera of patients with various atherosclerotic diseases and in thrombophlebitis by an anti-complementary (anti-C) assay and a Clq solubility (Clq-s) test [1]. Table II shows that circulating immune complexes were found in 34 % of the patients investigated until now.

References

1   FÜST, G.; SZÉKELY, J., and GERÖ, S.: Circulating immune complexes in vascular diseases. Lancet *i:* 193–194 (1977).

2   GERÖ, S.; SZÉKELY, J.; SZONDY, E., and SEREGÉLYI, E.: Immunological studies with aortic and venous tissue antigens. II. Antibodies to vascular antigens. Paroi artérielle/Arterial Wall *3:* 89–92 (1975).

3   SZÉKELY, J.; DOBIÁS, G., and SZÉCSEY, G.: Homolog antigénnel reagáló szérumfaktor elöfordulása arteriosclerotikus betegeken. Orv.Hetil. *110:* 1365–1367 (1969).

4   SZONDY, E.; JOBBÁGY, A.; LINK, E., and GERÖ, S.: Immunological studies with aortic and venous tissue antigens. I. The antigen structure of vascular tissues. Paroi artérielle/Arterial Wall *3:* 81–87 (1975)

S. GERÖ, MD, DSc, Arteriosclerosis Research Group, Ministry of Health, Mezö Imre út 17, *1081 Budapest* (Hungary)

Prog. biochem. Pharmacol., vol. 14, pp. 287–291 (Karger, Basel 1977)

Histological Investigation of Aortic Wall in Experimental Sclerosis of Rabbits

F. Schneider, A. Hesz, and G. Lusztig

Pathological Institute and Research Laboratory, County Hospital, Kecskemét

Introduction

Quantitative and qualitative changes of mucopolysaccharides (acid glycosaminoglycans) in aortic histological preparations were analyzed after different sclerogenic diets on rabbits.

Material and Methods

50 male LATI rabbits, weighing 2–3 kg, were split into three groups. Group 1, containing 20 rabbits, got normal food and 1 g cholesterol/day. Group 2, 20 rabbits, got normal food and in addition 1 g cholesterol + 3,000 IU vitamin D_3 + 15 ml sour cream daily. Group 3, 10 rabbits, control group, got normal food. 5 rabbits of groups 1 and 2 were killed at the end of the 1st, 2nd and 3 rd month. 5 rabbits of group 3 were killed at the end of the 1st week and 3rd month.

First, 3–4 mm wide parts of ascending aortas were fixed in Ca-formol during 24 h. Slides obtained by freezing microtome were stained with oil red O. Second, 3–4 mm wide parts of ascending aortas were fixed in a alcohol:formol 4:1 mixture during 24 h, and embedded in paraffin. Slides were stained with 0.1 % toluidine blue solution at pH 1, 3 and 5. Slides were stained with toluidine blue and different molar concentrations of $MgCl_2$ to estimate the 'critical electrolyte concentration' (CEC) value of different metachromatic stained chromotropes [2, 3]. Other slides were digested with testicular hyaluronidase at 37° C for 16 h and stained with

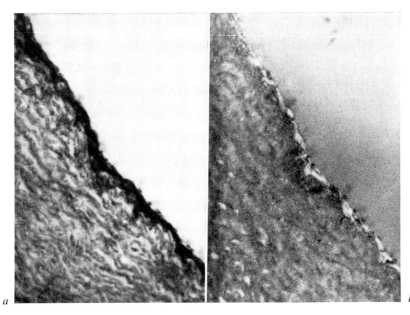

Fig. 1. Aortic wall. Subintimally metachromatic stained layer. Topooptical reaction with toluidine blue at pH 3. *a* Ordinary light photomicrograph. *b* Polarization photomicrograph.

0.1 % toluidine blue solution. Kossa silver impregnation was carried out with other slides.

The preparations were examined under a Zeiss Amplival-pol microscope in normal and in polarized light.

Results

Plaques could be observed after the 3rd week in group 1 and after the 2nd week in group 2.

In normal control animals and plaque-free parts of treated rabbit aortas, subintimally with toluidine blue at pH 1 and 3, a strong metachromatic stained layer could be observed (fig. 1): this layer is hyaluronidase sensitive and can be followed to the plaque area where it is interrupted. CEC value expressed in $MgCl_2$ concentration: 0.4M.

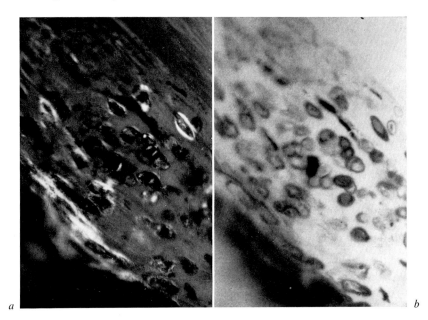

Fig. 2. Chondroid metaplasia in aortic wall. Metachromatic staining and strong birefringence due to chondrocyte capsules. Hyaluronidase digestion and toluidine blue staining at pH 3. *a* Ordinary light photomicrograph. *b* Polarization photomicrograph.

In the media as subintimally as in deeper parts of it, necrotic, calcified areas and sometimes small foci scattered over a large area, can be observed. The latter were observed mainly in animals of group 2 after the 3rd month. Some necroses were in group 1 after 3 weeks (2 from 5), and in group 2 (4 from 5). In the control group thre was one small necrosis each in media both after the 1st week and after 3 months.

In other preparations of aortas among the remaining degenerated elastic lamellas separated from fibers, small round or oval shaped chondroid-like cells were seen. With toluidine blue at pH 3 there was metachromatic stained material in plasma and around the cells. With crossed polars strong birefringence can be seen. Somewhere around chondrones, with toluidine blue at pH 3, there is metachromatic stained ground substance which is partly hyaluronidase sensitive (fig. 2). CEC value in $MgCl_2$ concentration: 0.8м.

Discussion

Two different sclerogenic diets were used in our experiment. Aortic changes were similar in both groups. Plaques in animals fed three components containing sclerogenic diet were seen earlier. Necrosis and chondroid metaplasia were more widely spaced out in this group.

The metachromatic stained subintimal layer is held to be chondroitin sulfate. This layer was not observed anywhere as being continuous on the basis of foam plaque, and was valued as a sign of structural change of the vessel wall accompanying plaque formation. Medial necrosis observed by us is known in the literature as spontaneous calcifying medial sclerosis of rabbits. MASSMANN and WEIDENBACH [1] demonstrated by electronmicroscopical examination that cells in the necrotic area showing chondroid metaplasia proved to be modified smooth muscle cells. In our experiment, mucopolysaccharide secretion of these cells was observed. This material proved to be partly chondroitin sulfate and partly keratosulfate.

Summary

Rabbit aortic changes were investigated after different sclerogenic diets. A subintimal chondroitin sulfate layer was characterized by toluidine blue metachromatic staining at pH 1–3, CEC value expressed in $MgCl_2$ concentration: 0.4M, hyaluronidase sensitivity. This layer becomes disorganized during plaque formation and partly disappears. A long-lasting sclerogenic diet, as well as a diet containing several sclerogenic factors, produced an increase of frequency and extension of the media necrosis, calcification, and chondroid metaplasia of the aortic wall. In these lesions, an increase of mucopolysaccharide secretion of modified smooth muscle cells was observed.

References

1   MASSMANN, J. und WEIDENBACH, H.: Lichtmikroskopische und elektronenoptische Untersuchungen zur spontanen kalzifizierenden Mediasklerose des Kaninchens. Zentbl. allg. Path. path. Anat. *119:* 179–188 (1975).
2   MÓDIS, L.: Topo-optical investigations of mucopolysaccharides (acid glycosaminoglycans); in GRAUMANN und NEUMANN Handbuch der Histochemie, vol. II/4, pp. 1–170 (Fischer, Stuttgart 1974).

3   SCOTT, J.E.: Critical electrolyte concentration (CEC) effects in interactions between acid glycosaminoglycans and organic cations and polycations; in BALAZS Chemistry and molecular biology of the intercellular matrix, vol. 2, pp. 1105–1119 (Academic Press, London 1970).

F. SCHNEIDER, MD, Pathology Institute of County Hospital, *H-6001 Kecskemét* (Hungary)

Prog. biochem. Pharmacol., vol. 14, pp. 292–297 (Karger, Basel 1977)

Is the Sclerotic Vessel Wall Really More Rigid than the Normal One?

G. Márk, A.G. Hudetz, T. Kerényi, E. Monos and A.G.B. Kovách

Experimental Research Department and II. Pathology Institute,
Semmelweis Medical University, Budapest

Introduction

During the past decade increasing attention has been paid to the hemodynamic forces in pathogenesis of arteriosclerosis [7]. The reason is that arteriosclerotic processes are localized to the ramifications and curvatures of vessels where the mechanical load is increased.

It is generally accepted that arteriosclerosis is accompanied by thickening and stiffening of the vessel wall. However, we have not found any quantitative information in the literature concerning the changes in elastic properties of vessels in arteriosclerotic diseases.

The present work concerns the study of biomechanical properties of the human anterior cerebral artery. Mechanical properties of vessels with relaxed smooth muscle have been characterized by incremental elastic modulus, strain energy density and incremental distensibility [1]. The importance of this study is underlined by the fact that the frequent and serious cerebral diseases are mostly of vascular origin. The anterior cerebral artery is often damaged by arteriosclerotic lesions and is often involved in cerebral arterial spasm.

Methods

The arteries were excised not later than 2 days after death from 20 cadavers. A relatively straight 10–15 mm long segment was dissected and tied to cylindrical plastic plugs in a temperature-controlled tissue bath containing oxygenated (95 % O_2, 5 % CO_2) Krebs-Ringer solution [2]. Considering that the cerebral arteries are embedded in the soft media of a mechanically closed system it was assumed that the *in situ* and the excised lengths of these arteries were nearly equal. Therefore the segments were stretched axially just to be straightened, the extending force was always below 5 g. We continuously monitored the pressure and the outer diameter of the arteries, at constant axial length, while the intraluminal pressure has been changed (between 20 and 250 mm Hg). For obtaining wall thickness of the artery, net weight of the segment was determined. After measurements the arteries were examined histologically under a light microscope. The specimens were classified into fibrosclerotic (F) and normal (N) groups estimating the increase in collagen content in the media and considering other histological evidences of fibrosclerosis (e.g. intimal proliferation, smooth muscle damage). After digitalizing the diameter versus pressure curves the average tangential stress, average strain energy density, overall incremental elastic modulus, incremental distensibility and other related quantities were computed by R 20 computer. For F and N groups statistical averaging was performed. The various quantities were computed for 10 mm Hg steps in the range of 20–250 mm Hg internal pressure.

Results

Fibrotic arteries were found to be more elastic than the normal ones at the same pressure levels since the incremental modulus (B) is by 34–45 % smaller in the fibrosclerotic group (fig. 1). The relative difference slightly decreases with increasing pressure but it is significant in the whole pressure range ($p < 0.01$–0.02). The internal radius to wall thickness ratio (R_i/h) is by 25–30 % smaller in the fibrotic group than in the normal one ($p < 0.05$ up to 150 mm Hg, $p < 0.05$ above) which may be the consequence of intimal proliferation (fig. 2). Incremental distensibility (D) of the arteries seems to be by 28–35 % higher in group F than in N, however, this difference is significant only at a few pressure values above 120 mm Hg (fig. 3). It can be easily shown that for thin-walled vessels D can be expressed by

$$D = \frac{2}{B} \cdot \frac{R_1}{h} \cdot$$

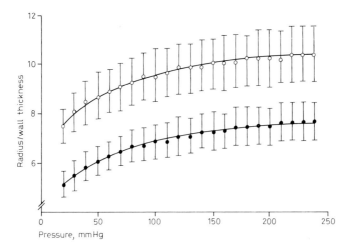

Fig. 1. The dependence of the incremental elastic modulus ($\pm$ SE) on the internal pressure ● = Fibrotic, ○ = normal.

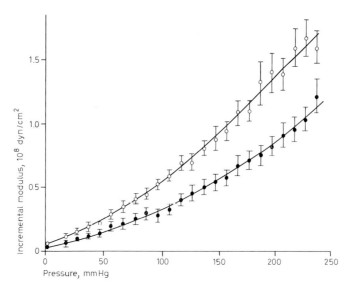

Fig. 2. Internal radius to wall thickness ratio ($\pm$ SE) versus internal pressure. ● = Fibrotic, ○ = normal.

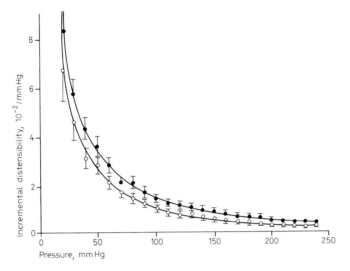

Fig. 3. The dependence of incremental distensibility ($\pm$ SE) on the intraluminal pressure. ● = Fibrotic, ○ = normal.

Since both R_i/h and B are smaller in F than in N, their deviations partly compensate each other leading to the relative constancy of the incremental distensibility.

Discussion

It has been shown that fibrotic alterations of anterior cerebral arteries are accompanied by significant increase in passive tangential-radial elasticity. This is surprising because the normal and fibrotic groups were formed on the basis of the medial collagen content. It is supposed that collagen fibers appearing during the fibrosclerotic process are arranged in an altered structure which does not increase the rigidity of the vessel wall. The new collagen may also have different elastic properties than the normal one. Nevertheless it can be concluded that the greater content of collagen fibers does not cause greater rigidity of the arterial wall.

Furthermore, the passive distensibility of fibrotic arteries is not smaller than that of normal ones, because of the decreased elastic modulus in the fibrosclerotic group. Smooth muscle activity may change however the obtained relationship since the incremental modulus of the vessel decreases when smooth muscle contracts at a given internal pressure [3, 6]. According to the histological examinations, no or only few intact smooth muscle cells could be identified in most of the fibrotic arterial segments. Therefore, incremental modulus of the fibrosclerotic cerebral arteries may be higher than that of the arteries with normal smooth muscle tone *in vivo*.

Changes in structure of the vessels are usually considered as pathological processes but they may also have compensatory character [4, 5]. We hypothesize that the observed elevated elasticity (the low modulus) of the fibrosclerotic arterial wall is the consequence of a local compensatory process tending to prevent pathological alterations in the incremental distensibility. Indeed, incremental distensibility is the main factor in determining the blood flow configuration and the damping function of the vessel wall, which protects the arteries from rupture, as well as protects the microcirculation from fast pressure and flow transients.

Summary

Quasistatic passive mechanical properties of fibrosclerotic and normal human anterior cerebral arteries were studied *in vitro*. Mechanical properties were characterized by incremental elastic modulus, strain energy density and incremental distensibility for a 20–250 mm Hg intraluminal pressure range. Fibrotic arteries were found to have a 34–45 % lower elastic modulus at the same pressure levels than normal ones ($p < 0.01$–0.02). Distensibility however proved to be only 28–35 % higher in the fibrotic group, this difference was significant just at a few pressure values above 120 mm Hg. This was due to the opposite changes in elastic properties and radius to wall thickness ratio. It is supposed that higher elasticity of the fibrotic arterial wall is the consequence of a local compensatory process tending to prevent pathological alterations in distensibility of the arteries.

References

1   BERGEL, D.H.: The static elastic properties of the arterial wall. J. Physiol., Lond. *156:* 445–454 (1961).

2   COX, R.H.: Three-dimensional mechanics of arterial segments *in vitro*. Methods. J. appl. Physiol. *36:* 380–384 (1974).

3   Cox, R.H.: Arterial wall mechanics and composition and the effects of smooth muscle activation. Am. J. Physiol. *299:* 807–812 (1975).
4   Fry, D.L.: Responses of the arterial wall to certain physical factors; in Athero-genesis initiating factors. CIBA Found Symp. 12 (new series), pp. 127–164 (Assoc. Sci. Publ., Amsterdam 1973).
5   Jellinek, H.: Arterial lesions and arteriosclerosis (Publ. House Hung., Acad. Sci., Budapest 1974).
6   Monos, E.; Cox, R.H., and Peterson, L.H.: Effects of hypophysectomy and vasopressin on canine arterial mechanical properties *in vivo*. Circulation *7,8:* suppl. IV, p. 29 (1973).
7   Patel, D.J.; Vaishnav, R.N.; Gow, B.S., and Kot, P.A.: Haemodynamics. A. Rev. Physiol. *36:* 125–154 (1976).

G. Márk, MD, Experimental Research Department, Semmelweis Medical University, Üllöi ut 78/a, *H-1082 Budapest* (Hungary)

Prog. biochem. Pharmacol., vol. 14, pp. 298–305 (Karger, Basel 1977)

Genetic Factors in the Development of Atheroma and on Serum Total Cholesterol Levels in Inbred Mice and Their Hybrids[1]

A. ROBERTS and J.S. THOMPSON

Department of Anatomy, University of Toronto, Toronto, Ont.

Introduction

Members of an inbred strain of the same sex are more than 99.44 % homozygous for the same genome or combination of gene pairs [4]. These members show similar characteristics that are inherited such as coat colour in mice, while other characteristics, such as life span, are not absolutely uniform because they are functions of both heredity and environment.

As previously reported [2], male mice of 13 inbred strains were fed a special diet that contained 9 parts of a diet containing 5 % cholesterol, 30 % cocoa butter and 30 % casein mixed with 1 part Purina laboratory chow. The C57BR/cdJ and CBA/J strains were selected from the 13 strains as the two strains that showed the most marked differences in the development of atheromatous lesions in the wall of the aortic sinus.

Material and Methods

The C57BR/cdJ (designated the P_1 parent strain) and the CBA/J (designated the P_2 parent strain) were reciprocally crossbred to produce two groups of F_1 offspring. The two groups of F_1 hybrids were reciprocal-

[1] Supported by grants from the Ontario (Canada) Heart Foundation and the Physicians Services Incorporated Foundation (Ontario, Canada).

ly crossbred to produce four groups of F_2 offspring and backcrossed reciprocally with each parent strain to produce four groups of B_1 and four groups of B_2 backcross mice.

The following experiments involved a total of 1,536 male mice that were used in the calculations. At 10 weeks of age, mice of each parent strain and of the F_1, F_2, B_1 and B_2 generations were identified by coded ear punches, weighed and divided into experimental groups that were started on the high-fat, high-cholesterol diet and corresponding control groups that were maintained on the regular Purina laboratory chow. Experimental animals, in sample sizes of 15–20 mice, with corresponding controls, were identified, weighed and sacrificed at intervals of 3, 5, 10 and 15 weeks after being on the high-fat, high-cholesterol diet. The backcross generations were only continued to the 10-week interval because of the difficulty of breeding sufficient male mice for the 15-week interval. Under intraperitoneal sodium pentobarbital anaesthesia, blood was removed from the inferior vena cava for serum total cholesterol determination using the Technicon Auto-Analyser method N-24a at the Wellesley Hospital Laboratory, Toronto. Immediately following removal of the blood from the inferior vena cava, the heart and ascending aorta were removed for sectioning through the area of the attachment of the aortic valve to the sinus wall. The sections were cut with a freezing microtome and stained with oil red 0 and counterstained with haematoxylin and light green.

Fortran computer programs determined the significant differences between groups for three parameters: total number of foam cells and size of the largest single lesion in the aortic sinus wall and mean serum total cholesterol levels. Only sections that contained a portion of the attachments of the aortic valves to the sinus wall were examined and from these, one section was selected for each animal that showed the highest total number of foam cells and the largest single lesion. The total number of foam cells in each section was classified into one of four categories: no foam cells, 1–4, 5–15, and more than 15 foam cells. The size of the largest single lesion in each section was classified into one of four categories: no lesion, a lesion occupying less than one eighth of the aortic sinus wall between the attachment of two adjacent valve cusps, occupying one eighth to one fourth, and occupying more than one fourth. A Fortran computer program determined the value of chi square in comparing any two groups for the size of the largest single lesion or for the total number of foam cells. Another Fortran computer program determined the mean serum total cholesterol of a sample group in mg/100 ml, the standard error of the mean, the variance and the significance of the difference between any two means, as given by the t prime (t^1) test [5], at the 0.05 and 0.01 levels of confidence. For serum total cholesterol determinations, the vast majority were obtained from individual mice. Pooled samples and samples obtained from individual mice were combined for each of the experimental and control mice for the two parent strains and the F_1, F_2, B_1 and B_2 generations at the different weekly intervals and used in the calculations.

Results and Discussion

The mother and father exert an equal influence on the development of fatty deposits in the aortic sinus wall (the parameters of total number of foam cells and size of the largest single lesions) and on mean serum total cholesterol levels. There are no statistically significant differences at the 0.05 level of confidence for the three parameters between the two groups of F_1, between the four groups of F_2, between the four groups of B_1 and between the four groups of B_2 (experimental vs. experimental and control vs. control), except for the parameter of mean serum total cholesterol levels when 6 of 24 experimental pairs and 4 of 24 control pairs of F_2 mice and one experimental pair of B_2 mice are significantly different.

When the two parent strains and the F_1, F_2, B_1 and B_2 generations on the high-fat, high-cholesterol diet are compared with each other by pairs, the C57BR/cdJ (P_1) strain always has the highest values for the three parameters at the 3, 5, 10 and 15-week intervals. The CBA/J (P_2) strain has the lowest values for the parameters of total number of foam cells and mean serum total cholesterol levels, but has a value above the B_2 and F_1 generations for the parameter of the size of the largest single lesion. The F_1 generation is always closer in value to the CBA/J (P_2) strain than to the C57BR/cdJ (P_1) strain. For the two parameters of total number of foam cells and mean serum total cholesterol levels the order is $P_1 > B_1 > F_2 > B_2 > F_1 > P_2$, but for the parameter of largest single lesion the order is $P_1 > B_1 > F_2 > P_2 > B_2 > F_1$. The latter order being different from the order of the first two parameters may be due to the fact that only the size of the largest single lesion is estimated lengthwise in the section and other smaller lesions are ignored because it is extremely

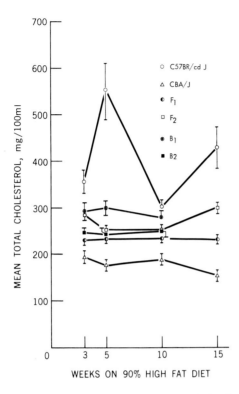

Fig. 1. Mean serum total cholesterol levels (combining pooled samples and samples from individual mice) of the C57BR/cdJ (P_1), CBA/J (P_2), F_1, F_2, B_1 and B_2 mice on the high-fat, high-cholesterol diet (mean $\pm$ 1 SE).

difficult to calculate accurately the total area and volume occupied by all lesions in a section.

Figure 1 represents the mean serum total cholesterol levels ($\pm$ 1 SE) of the two parent strains and the F_1, F_2, B_1 and B_2 generations on the high-fat, high-cholesterol diet. The C57BR/cdJ (P_1) has significantly higher ($p < 0.05$) mean total cholesterol levels than the other five populations except at 3 weeks when the P_1 strain has higher values, though not significantly higher than the B_1 generation. The CBA/J (P_2) has significantly lower ($p < 0.01$) values than the other populations at all weeks.

Figure 2 is a photograph of the cross-section of the aortic sinus wall with the attachment of the valve cusps of a C57BR/cdJ male mouse after

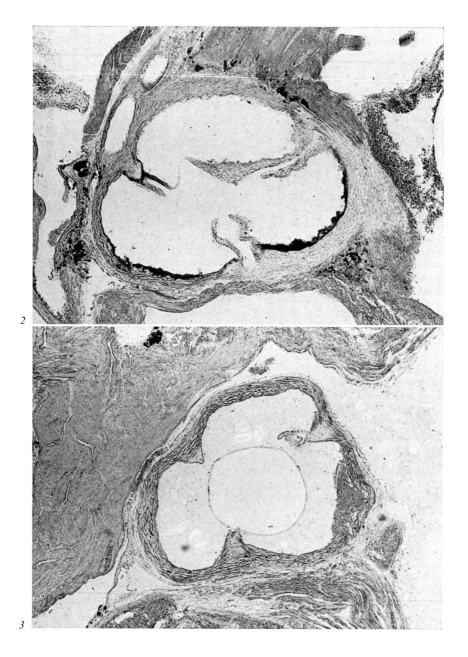

Fig. 2. Cross-section of the wall of the aortic sinus of a C57BR/cdJ (P$_1$) mouse after 3 weeks on the high-fat, high-cholesterol diet.

Fig. 3. Cross-section of the wall of the aortic sinus of a CBA/J (P$_2$) mouse after 3 weeks on the high-fat, high-cholesterol diet.

3 weeks on the high-fat, high-cholesterol diet. Extensive lesions which have raised the lining endothelium occupy most of the left and right lower aortic sinus walls with involvement of the valve cusp at 9.30 o'clock. These are classified as large lesions since they occupy more than one fourth of the aortic sinus wall between the attachment of two adjacent valve cusps and there are more than 15 total foam cells in the section. Figure 3 is a cross-section of the aortic sinus wall of a CBA/J male mouse after 3 weeks on the high-fat, high-cholesterol diet. There are faint deposits of fat in the attachments of the aortic valve cusps to the sinus wall which are difficult to see in the photograph. Deposits of fat are usually first seen in the attachments of the aortic valve cusps to the sinus wall and/or at the openings of the coronary arteries when present in the section.

On the high-fat, high-cholesterol diet representative sections of the C57BR/cdJ (P_1) strain at 5, 10 and 15-week intervals show large lesions with numerous foam cells. The endothelium is raised and, by the 15-week interval, the lesions have extended through the media into the adventitia. The CBA/J (P_2) strain shows lesions gradually increasing in size mainly affecting the intima and adjacent media. There are usually one to four foam cells in moderate sized lesions occupying one eighth to one fourth of the aortic sinus wall by the 15-week interval.

On comparing the control P_1, P_2, F_1, F_2, B_1 and B_2 mice with each other by pairs, only rarely is a foam cell seen and there are no significant differences for the parameter of the total number of foam cells. For the parameters of the size of the largest single lesion and mean serum total cholesterol levels, the CBA/J (P_2) strain usually has lower values than the other five groups when there are any significant differences. The experimental P_1, P_2, F_1, F_2, B_1 and B_2 populations nearly always have significantly higher values than their corresponding control populations for the three parameters at the different weekly intervals.

The experimental results indicate a multifactorial (polygenic) system of inheritance since the F_1 generation is closer to the P_2 strain and has values below the B_1 and B_2 generations for all three parameters. Also the variance of the F_2 generation is larger than the variance of the F_1 generation for mean serum total cholesterol levels and there are a wide range of values with no discernible ratios within each of the two groups of the F_1, within each of the four groups of the F_2, within each of the four groups of the B_1 and within each of the four groups of the B_2.

On the high-fat, high-cholesterol diet, the average minimum number of loci or the minimum number of independently segregating pairs of alleles affecting serum total cholesterol levels is two at the 3, 5, 10 and 15-week intervals, employing the following equation [3, 7]:

$$n = \frac{(m_1 - m_2)^2}{8 \, (V_{F2} - V_{F1})}$$

where n is the minimum number of loci affecting serum total cholesterol levels, m_1 and m_2 are the means of the C57BR/cdJ and CBA/J strains, respectively, and V_{F2} and V_{F1} are the computed variances of the F_2 and F_1 generations. This equation is based on five assumptions [7], the violation of any one will tend to underestimate n. The average minimum number of loci for the control mice is zero for the 3, 5, 10 and 15-week intervals, indicating that the five assumptions are only slightly applicable to the control mice.

The serum total cholesterol levels do not appear to follow a simple additive-dominance model since the order of the populations was P_1–B_1–B_2–F_1–P_2 instead of the expected order in a simple model of P_1–B_1–F_1–B_2–P_2. Also scaling tests [1] based on two assumptions [6] indicate an additive-dominance model for the C57BR/cdJ strain at the 3- and 10-week intervals on the high-fat, high-cholesterol diet and for the control CBA/J strain at the 5- and 10-week intervals and the control C57BR/cdJ strain at the 10-week interval.

In conclusion, the inbred strains of mice have proven reliable animal models that produce consistent results within each of the parent strains and their F_1, F_2, B_1 and B_2 generations. These results depend on a multifactorial (polygenic) type of inheritance that appears to be more complicated than a simple additive-dominance model. The mother and father exert an equal influence on the development of fatty deposits in the aortic sinus wall and on serum total cholesterol levels.

Summary

There is a consistent genetic relationship between the development of atheromata in the aortic sinus wall and serum total cholesterol levels using inbred strains of male mice. This relationship is dependent on a multifactorial (polygenic) type of inheritance that is more complicated than the simple additive-dominance model. There is no special maternal or paternal influence on serum total cholesterol levels or on the development of atheromata.

References

1   MATHER, K. and JINKS, J.L.: Biometrical genetics, pp. 71–75 (Chapman & Hall, London 1971).
2   ROBERTS, A. and THOMPSON, J.S.: Inbred mice and their hybrids as an animal model for atherosclerosis research; in DAY Atherosclerosis drug discovery, pp. 313–327 (Plenum Press, New York 1976).
3   RODERICK, T.H. and SCHLAGER, G.: Multiple factor inheritance; in GREEN Biology of the laboratory mouse; 2nd ed., pp. 151–152 (McGraw-Hill, Toronto 1966).
4   RUSSELL, E.S.: The importance of animal genetics in biomedical research. National Academy of Sciences Publication 1679, Washington (1969).
5   SOKAL, R.R. and ROHLUF, F.J.: Biometry, pp. 374–376 (Freeman, San Francisco 1969).
6   WIMER, R.E. and FULLER, J.L.: Patterns of behaviour; in GREEN Biology of the laboratory mouse; 2nd ed., p. 643 (McGraw-Hill, Toronto 1966).
7   WRIGHT, S.: Evolution and the genetics of populations, vol. 1: Genetic and biometric foundations, pp. 381–383 (University of Chicago Press, Chicago 1968).

A. ROBERTS, MD, PhD, Department of Anatomy, University of Toronto, Toronto M5S 1A8 (Canada)

Prog. biochem. Pharmacol., vol. 14, pp. 306–311 (Karger, Basel 1977)

Some Aspects of Scanning Electron Microscopy Techniques Applied to the Study of Large Arteries

Ross G. Gerrity

Department of Atherosclerosis and Thrombosis Research,
The Cleveland Clinic Foundation, Cleveland, Ohio

It is obvious that there are a wide variety of techniques being used for the preservation of arterial tissue for scanning electron microscopy in the field of vascular research. It is probably not feasible to produce standardized techniques which everyone can use, since the techniques which one uses most, of necessity, vary according to the experimental protocol and the tissue used. We have found in our experience that the following points are of considerable importance in terms of the quality of preservation of the artery to be studied. The preparation procedure can be broken down into five major categories beginning with fixation, proceeding through dehydration, critical point drying, specimen coating, and viewing the specimen in the electron microscope. We would like to consider these five major categories in some detail.

Fixation

While it is obviously not possible for everyone to use perfusion fixation, particularly if one is working with human material such as surgical biopsy or autopsy specimens, in terms of experimental animals there is no question that perfusion fixation yields optimal ultrastructural preservation, particularly of the endothelium and intima. It is important that the animal be alive when the perfusion is begun. We have noticed considerable ultrastructural change if the animal is killed prior to the initiation of perfusion. Secondly, blood should be flushed out of the arterial or venous system prior to the perfusion of fixative. The system which we have found works satisfactorily for both large arteries and small vessels is that we flush initially with nontoxic buffer. Sodium cacodylate buffer, which is an arsenate compound, is cytotoxic and should be avoided in the viable state. We have found that an oxygenated-Krebs-Ringer-bicarbonate solution is a very fine flushing agent, and we perfuse this into the animal at a temperature of 37° C. With small vessels or with small animals, the addition of heparin to the flushing solution in physiological concentrations aids perfusion, in that it prevents clotting and it does not, in our experience, appear to alter endothelial structure.

The pressure at which one perfuses the flushing solution and the fixative should be measured in each animal separately, rather than having a mean blood pressure (say 110 mm) used in general aid for all animals. Our most successful perfusions are done directly into the aortic arch by cannulation of the carotid artery. A blood pressure monitoring device, either a pressure transducer or a small manometer on a side branch of the cannula immediately above the carotid artery, serves very well to monitor the blood pressure of the animal. The perfusion system is then set at a pressure equal to the blood pressure, the flushing solution is perfused, and at the same time the femoral arteries on both sides are cut. This allows the blood to drain from the system very quickly, and at the same time it is being replaced by a flushing solution. The flushing solution is oxygenated at 37° C. With this procedure, heart beat and respiration will continue, even in a pig up to 150–200 pounds. Adequate flushing of the blood from the system occurs within 5–10 min. The fixative solution is then perfused, and the animal is killed by the fixative itself, rather than being killed beforehand.

The rate at which the fixative is perfused is very important, and it is therefore essential to clamp off femoral arteries once the fixative has begun to drain from them. This provides a back pressure onto the fixative which maintains the perfusion pressure and also allows the arteries to fill with fixative. Particularly with large animals such as the pig, dog, or monkey, where the aorta can be up to 1 inch in diameter, the rate of perfusion must be fairly slow, and there must be a back pressure on it in order to fill the whole vessel, otherwise the fixative just effectively runs down the vessel like it would down a drainpipe. The time of perfusion is variable depending on the animal. With large animals we perfuse 1–2 liters of fixative over the course of 1 h. Following perfusion the tissue is removed immediately and diced as quickly as possible, with a fresh razor blade. The endothelial surface is never touched, and the tissue is handled with forceps from the adventitial side. The diced tissue is then immersed in the same fixative that is used for perfusion, for periods of 6 h in the case of a large aorta, such as that from the pig, and for 3–4 h in the case of small aortas, such as rats, rabbits, and mice. Failure to do immersion fixation following perfusion fixation, results, in our opinion, in inadequate fixation of the middle media of the vessel, with subsequent collapse of the tissue at later stages of SEM processing, or inadequate penetration of resins for TEM. The tissue is then washed in a wash buffer, and immersed in 1 % osmium tetroxide for periods of 1.5–2 h at 4° C.

The choice of fixative used for perfusion is limited to the aldehydes. Our best results have been with Karnovsky's half-strength paraformaldehyde-glutaraldehyde in sodium cacodylate buffer. Glutaraldehyde at 1–2 % in the same buffer is also good. In general, arterial preservation appears to be superior if a hyperosmotic fixative is used, with the osmolality of the buffer being the critical component. We have also used acrolein with excellent results in perfusing rats and mice, but this noxious compound is extremely difficult to work with for this purpose. Above all, the commonly used histopathology fixatives such as formal-saline and other formalin fixatives should be avoided for all electron microscopy. They yield poor ultrastructural preservation with coarse precipitation of proteins and generally, osmotically-induced artifact. If autopsy or surgical biopsy material is to be studied, it is usually feasible to have glutaraldehyde available. Autopsy is performed immediately after death.

Dehydration

Because of the density of collagen and elastin in the aortic media, longer dehydration times are necessary than one would normally use for most tissues. We prefer alcohol as a dehydrant for scanning electron microscopy, and obtain better dehydration and less shrinkage artifact if we use a graded series, beginning with 10 % ethanol, and advancing by stages of 10 % up to absolute ethanol. We have also experienced difficulties with water contamination of ethanol, which is a very serious problem when one comes to critical point dry the tissue. In our experience, most large organizations order absolute ethanol in 50- to 100-gallon drums, and there is undoubtedly water uptake in these drums, particularly as the drum empties. This problem can be effectively overcome by keeping the absolute ethanol over molecular sieve, which absorbs the water. The same problem and remedy are true for acetone. One is faced with the choice of dehydrating solvent in scanning electron microscopy, the choice being at least partly dependent on the type of critical point drying used.

Critical Point Drying

It has been our experience that the freons are inferior to CO_2 for arterial endothelium, and particularly for endothelium and arterial smooth muscle grown in tissue culture. In the latter cases, neither freon TF, acetone or amyl acetate can be used in the processing if plastic culture dishes are used. In addition, the freons are so volatile that surface drying of the tissue easily occurs in simply transferring the sample from the freon to the critical point dryer. This speed of transferring the sample to the critical point dryer from the dehydrant or transitional fluid is extremely important, in that it is possible, even with ethanol, to get surface drying of the specimen. The use of ethanol as a dehydrating fluid allows samples to be placed directly into the bomb of the critical point dryer without using amyl acetate as a transitional fluid. Use of this technique has the benefit, in our laboratory at least, of allowing us to standardize on one technique – that is, ethanol-CO_2 – for both arterial samples and tissue culture samples. However, when one uses ethanol as an intermediate fluid, the length of time necessary to leave the specimen in the critical point dryer becomes longer, and it is necessary to flush specimens three or four times in the critical point dryer prior to heating. Another thing which we have recently had some success with is using 2,2-dimethoxypropane as a chemical dehydrant, as opposed to solvent dehydration [MULLER, I.L. and JACKS, T.J., J. Histochem. Cytochem. *23:* 107, 1975]. At this point our initial results with it have been quite successful.

Following critical point drying it is essential for optimal preservation to coat the specimen immediately, as there is degeneration with time after critical point drying and prior to coating, or even after coating. Preferably a specimen should be dehydrated, critical point dried, coated and viewed at all in 1 day. If it is impossible to view a specimen immediately after coating, it is advisable to put it in a vacuum desiccator and evacuate it over a desiccant until such time as it can be viewed.

Coating

There are, of course, two possible types of coating that one can do for scanning electron microscopy – vacuum evaporation or sputter coating. We now have considerable experience with both techniques, and we find that with vacuum evaporation, the best results are obtained using gold as the metal for coating, with the second choice being gold:palladium in the 60:40 ratio. The gold seems to give a much finer grain size and much better resolution than either gold:palladium, platinum:palladium, or pure platinum. We have also found with certain samples which tend to charge that a short burst of carbon coating followed by gold coating is helpful. It is advisable with vacuum evaporation for scanning electron microscope preparations to have the sample rotated while the evaporation is being carried out, in order to insure an even deposition of metal on all aspects of the cells to be viewed. Vacuum evaporation has the one possible advantage in that it does not appear to heat up the specimen as much, and one can place the specimen farther away from the source, such that heating is not such a problem and can be carried out over a fair length of time. In our experience, vacuum evaporation can be carried out with rotation at a distance of about 20 cm for a time of 3–4 min.

With gold sputter coating, the coating is much more even and uniform, and it tends to be particularly good for cells which have a lot of surface detail, in that all aspects of cellular projections etc. are coated evenly. Its one possible great disadvantage is in terms of specimen heating, where with sputter coating it is necessary to keep the specimen fairly close to the source, which tends to cause heating in the specimen. It has been suggested by several people that some form of temperature monitoring of the stub on which the specimen is placed be carried out during the process. In our experience and after talking with others we find that this gives an unrealistic value of the temperature which is actually found at the surface of the specimen, and we can only say that it is essential to keep the time of specimen sputtering to a minimum of 1–2 min, and to keep the voltage as low as possible. Despite this problem we find in general that our sputtering techniques are far superior to our vacuum coating techniques. We also use rotation of the specimen during sputtering and we find that this does again aid in the even coating of the specimen.

Viewing the Specimen

About the only point that we can consider with respect to viewing of biological specimens in the scanning electron microscope is to consider the aspects of beam damage to the specimen. There is no question that biological specimens do not stand up well to the beam of the electron microscope and that surface deterioration can occur within seconds under certain circumstances. Very recently there have been a number of papers given at SEM conferences in which low accelerating voltages have been used to view biological specimens with very good results, and we are now in the process of experimenting with this technique ourselves. To date, we have used 5–10 kV with very good results. Depth of focus and resolution appears to be excellent. Another aspect of viewing specimens of particular interest to those of us who are interested in the arterial wall and the accumulation of lipid, is that if one has a backscatter detector on their machine it is possible to use the affinity that osmium has for certain lipids to visualize lipid droplets in the cytoplasm of cells by collecting backscattered electrons. Usually this would involve slight over-osmification of the sample to make sure that the lipid is well osmified, and then viewing the sample using backscattered electrons. This procedure allows visualization of lipid droplets beneath the plasma membrane. The image obtained is rather like a three-dimensional image of a transmission electron micrograph, and can provide much useful information when used in conjunction with the standard secondary electron image.

I would say in conclusion that I feel it is impossible to standardize techniques among all workers in this field, since we all have various applications and various constraints imposed upon us by our experimental protocols and the type of tissue we are working with. It is possible, however, for each laboratory to maintain rigid technical excellence in this field. It cannot be stressed enough that there are no short cuts in electron microscopy. Within any given laboratory it is essential that various processing techniques and methods be carried out until one is satisfied with the quality of preservation obtained with their system. Once having achieved that, strict standardization and adherence to that technique from one animal, or one experiment, to the next is essential in order to fairly interpret the results one gets from one experiment to the next. Failure to adhere rigidly to the experimental protocol decided upon can lead to significant differences in the ultrastructural appearance to the tissue, and thus make it difficult to arrive at adequate interpretations and comparisons over the time course of a study. I feel that the best type of standardization that we can hope for in this field is basically, that everyone is maintaining excellent techniques and is adhering rigidly to their standardized techniques within their own laboratory.

R.G. GERRITY, PhD, Department of Atherosclerosis and Thrombosis Research, The Cleveland Clinic Foundation, *Cleveland, OH 44106* (USA)

Prog. biochem. Pharmacol., vol. 14, pp. 312–325 (Karger, Basel 1977)

Platelets, Thrombosis and Atherosclerosis

J.F. Mustard, S. Moore, M.A. Packham, and
R.L. Kinlough-Rathbone

Faculty of Health Sciences, McMaster University, Hamilton, Ont., and
Department of Biochemistry, University of Toronto, Toronto, Ont.

Platelets play an important part in the development of atherosclerosis and its complications by their involvement in at least three fundamental aspects of the problem [1–3]. First, the platelets, together with other blood cells, may cause vessel injury, particularly alterations in the endothelium. Second, platelets have a major role in the development of thrombi during the response of blood to vessel wall injury. Third, platelets release a material which stimulates smooth muscle cell proliferation as a result of endothelial cell injury. In order to understand these relationships it is useful to review the mechanisms whereby platelets can interact with the vessel wall and with each other.

Response of Blood to Vessel Injury

When the endothelium is lost, platelets interact with the subendo-thelial structures, particularly collagen, basement membrane and micro-fibrils [4]. Only collagen has been specifically shown to cause the platelets to discharge their granule contents [5–7] and to form aggregates through the release of formation of material from the platelets. Collagen causes the discharge of the contents of the storage granules of platelets [7] and also activates a membrane phospholipase A_2 which catalyses the hydrolysis of the ester bond at C2 of phosphatidylcholine and phosphatidylinositol. The arachidonate that is freed by this reaction is converted by platelet cyclo-oxygenase to the intermediate prostaglandin endoperoxides PGH_2 and PGG_2 and to thromboxane A_2 [8, 9]. These unstable substances, particularly thromboxane A_2, cause platelet aggregation and the platelet release reaction. The arachidonic acid pathway can be completely inhibited by the use of non-steroidal anti-inflammatory drugs such as aspirin and indomethacin which block the cyclo-oxygenase necessary to form the prostaglandin endoperoxides [10–13]. When platelets are induced to change shape by agents such as thromboxane A_2 and ADP, the normally non-adhesive platelets can adhere to each other and to platelets that have adhered to the vessel wall. When platelets adhere to each other, membrane phospholipoprotein (platelet factor 3) becomes available for the clotting reaction [14]. There are also a number of clotting factors closely associated with the platelet surface [15]. It appears that the platelet aggregate serves as a focus for the local acceleration of the coagulation mechanism. In addition, when the subendothelial structures are exposed, collagen can activate factor XII [16], and when the platelets interact with collagen, factor XI can be activated [17]. Therefore, the injury site is not only a focus for the formation of platelet aggregates but is also a site for the local generation of thrombin. The thrombin which forms can also induce the platelets to change shape and discharge their granule contents [7]. It appears to do this through at least three mechanisms; (i) the release of ADP; (ii) activation of the arachidonate pathway with the formation of prostaglandin endoperoxides and thromboxane A_2; (iii) a third pathway which is strong and independent of the first two pathways [18]. In addition, thrombin causes the polymerization of fibrinogen to fibrin and polymerizing fibrin sticks to platelets [19]. Indeed, because platelets rapidly deaggregate after they are aggregated by most aggregating agents, it is the polymerization of fibrin and its binding to the aggregated platelets which holds the platelet aggregates together. Injury to the endothelium can lead to release of activators of the fibrinolytic system that can digest the fibrin which forms.

There are also factors released or formed by platelets during the response of blood to vessel wall injury which can affect the vessel wall. The prostaglandin endoperoxides and thromboxane A_2 can cause contraction of arterial smooth muscle [20] while prostaglandins such as PGE_1 and PGI_2 inhibit smooth muscle contraction [21, 22]. Although there is no evidence at the present moment, it is possible that some of these intermediates of arachidonic acid metabolism have direct effects on the endothelium. The platelets release enzymes including lysosomal enzymes which can affect the vessel wall. In particular there is an elastase and a collagenase formed which can digest the elastin and collagen in the vessel wall [23, 24]. The platelets release a cationic protein which can cause mast

interaction with the subendothelium, release of the mitogenic factor, and resulting smooth muscle cell proliferation could be a major cause of intimal thickening. There is good evidence from animal studies that this can occur. Several years ago MOORE [44] found that if cannulae were left in the aortas of rabbits to cause repeated endothelial injury, the full spectrum of atherosclerotic lesions developed including atheroma with cholesterol clefts. These animals were given a normal low-fat rabbit diet and had normal serum cholesterol levels. TYSON et al. [45] have recently shown that indwelling catheters in the aortas of high risk, newborn infants produce similar lesions. Many studies have now demonstrated that endothelial injury produced by a variety of methods (endothelial antibodies, balloon catheters, homocystinemia, hypercholesterolemia), can lead to intimal thickening in which the platelet-vessel wall reactions are involved [1, 46–49].

The most substantial proof of platelet involvement comes from the work of MOORE et al. [50] in which it was found that an indwelling catheter in the aorta caused very little atherosclerosis to develop in thrombocytopenic rabbits. It has also been shown that thrombocytopenia prevents the intimal thickening which develops following balloon injury to the rabbit aorta. It has also been reported that drugs which inhibit the platelet-vessel wall interactions also inhibit the development of intimal thickening following injury to the endothelium by mechanical means or by homocystinemia [47].

Of considerable importance is the observation that repeated injury to the endothelium in rabbits causes the formation of lipid-rich lesions, many of which resemble atheroma. MOORE [51] has recently found that six balloon injuries to the aortas of rabbits at 2-week intervals produced lipid-rich lesions around the orifices of vessels at points where there has been regeneration of endothelium from the orifices over the denuded wall. The areas that do not have endothelium do not show lipid accumulation. These observations are, to some extent, analogous to those of MINICK et al. [52] in hypercholesterolemic rabbits subjected to a single balloon injury to the aorta. If the rabbits are hypercholesterolemic before the balloon injury, only one injury is required to produce extensive lipid accumulation around the intercostal vessel orifices where there has been endothelial regeneration. It is of considerable interest that the same type of lesion can be produced by six mechanical injuries or by one mechanical injury plus hypercholesterolemia. This may mean that the hypercholesterolemia acts as an injury stimulus. In contrast to what might have been expected, the sites where there is no endothelium (where one would predict maximum permeability to plasma protein including serum lipids) do not show much lipid accumulation. In the repeated injury experiments, the source of the lipid may be from increased turnover and changes in metabolism of smooth muscle cells in the intima. Smooth muscle cells that die may also be a major source of the lipid.

A key to understanding atherosclerosis, as ROSS and GLOMSET [53] have emphasized, is to determine the factors that cause endothelial injury. As well as the hemodynamic effects, it has been shown that endothelial antibodies, homocystinemia, and hypercholesterolemia can damage the endothelium in animals [47–49]. Viruses, bacteria and bacterial products such as endotoxins, and smoking are other possible factors [1]. The antigen-antibody complexes that occur in serum sickness cause arterial injury through a mechanism that appears to involve the platelets [49]. It has been found that serum sickness together with hypercholesterolemia can cause extensive atherosclerosis.

Platelet Survival, Thrombosis and Atherosclerosis

There appears to be a relationship between platelet survival and turnover in man and clinical evidence of atherosclerosis [1, 54]. Subjects with clinical manifestations of the complications of atherosclerosis tend to have a shortened platelet survival when compared with control subjects. A number of drugs that may be useful in the management of atherosclerosis and its complications are known to prolong platelet survival in man. There is therefore considerable interest in the factors that influence platelet survival. It has been shown [54] that exposure of platelets to ADP and thrombin does not lead to irreversible damage and that platelets that have been exposed to these agents show a normal platelet survival when they return to the circulation. Removal of platelet sialic acid with neuraminidase and treatment of platelets with viruses such as influenza viruses that have neuraminidase activity, also shortens platelet survival [54, 55]. Thus, alterations of platelet surface glycoproteins may be important in their being recognized as old platelets and removed from the circulation. ROSS and HARKER [48] have reported evidence that endothelial injury shortens platelet survival. If endothelial injury is a major cause of shortened platelet survival, platelet survival measurements could be a way of monitoring the extent of endothelial injury in man.

We have recently found that with a single balloon injury to the rabbit aorta from the arch to the femoral artery, there is no detectable change in platelet survival [56]. Examination of the vessel surface by scanning electronmicroscopy showed the surface of the injured aorta to be covered by a monolayer of platelets immediately after the injury. Sections examined 2 days later showed very few platelets on the injured surface. The morphological evidence indicates that there is an initial platelet reaction with the surface following the injury but that there is little subsequent platelet interaction. The difference between these results and those of HARKER et al. [47] and ROSS and HARKER [48] could be due to repeated endothelial injury in their experiments and also more diffuse injury, particularly in the homocystinemia and hypercholesterolemia experiments. However, it is clear that in the rabbit, after the initial platelet interaction, the denuded vessel surface tends to become non-reactive to platelets.

Thrombosis and Complications of Atherosclerosis

The early work of VON ROKITANSKY [57], subsequent studies by CLARK et al. [58] and DUGUID [59], and more recent work by MORE and HAUST [60] and CHANDLER [61], have demonstrated that the organization of mural thrombi is important in the development of the large complicated atherosclerotic lesion in man.

Mural thrombi are probably also involved in causing many of the clinical complications of atherosclerosis. As implied in the earlier part of this paper, thrombi can repeatedly form and break up for a period of time following an initial injury. The mechanisms involved in this have been reviewed elsewhere. The platelet emboli and platelet-fibrin emboli from these mural thrombi will embolize the distal microcirculation. In addition to temporarily blocking flow in some of these vessels, if the platelets in the emboli are also forming thromboxane A_2, this material could cause vasoconstriction in the microcirculation with further impairment of flow. (If this occurs and is of clinical significance, aspirin would be an effective inhibitor.) Platelet-fibrin emboli appear to be involved in transient attacks of retinal and cerebral ischemia [1, 62]. This mechanism has been shown to cause sudden death through ventricular fibrillation in animals and to produce areas of focal myocarditis such as are seen in some humans who die suddenly. Such a mechanism may also be responsible for some forms of chronic renal disease in older humans when thromboemboli arise from mural thrombi in the atherosclerotic aorta above the renal arteries [1, 63]. In contrast to observations obtained from individuals who die suddenly, patients who live for a day after the onset of chest pain usually have full thickness infarcts and the lesions subtend from an occluding thrombus [1]. This may indicate that the mechanisms for sudden death in coronary artery disease differ from those involved in myocardial infarction in which death occurs hours or days later.

Prevention of Atherosclerosis and Its Complications

There is considerable interest in the possibility that drugs which modify platelet function may inhibit the development of atherosclerosis and prevent the clinical complications [64]. Most of the drugs that are presently being tested in man arose from the observation in man that they tend to prolong platelet survival, particularly if it is shortened (i.e. sulfinpyrazone, dipyridamole, clofibrate) [54, 64]. Aspirin is the exception. After the observation that the pyrazole drugs (sulfinpyrazone, phenyl-butazone) inhibited the platelet-collagen reactions, it was quickly found that other non-steroidal anti-inflammatory drugs such as aspirin had this effect. Aspirin, however, in the doses usually administered, has no effect on platelet survival in man although it will inhibit collagen-induced platelet aggregation. The results of the use of these drugs (sulfinpyrazone, dipyridamole and aspirin) in extensive trials for the prevention of death in subjects who have had a myocardial infarct and in the prevention of strokes in subjects who have had transient attacks of cerebral ischemia, will be available in the near future. Sulfinpyrazone has been shown to prevent thrombi in the arterial venous shunts of patients undergoing chronic renal dialysis [65]. If drugs which correct shortened platelet survival towards normal are effective, then other methods of influencing platelet survival should be explored.

If human subjects stop smoking, their platelet survival is prolonged [66]. Some of the materials in smoke are believed to damage the endothelium; removal of this source of injurious substances may account for the prolongation of platelet survival when the subjects stop smoking. The high risk of myocardial infarction in subjects who smoke [67] and the apparent benefits when individuals stop smoking indicate that changing smoking habits or modifying cigarettes so that the smoke does not damage the vessel, may be an important public health measure.

Diet also affects platelet survival [68]. A change of diet from one rich in dairy fats and eggs to one rich in vegetable fat caused a lengthening of platelet survival greater than that produced by sulfinpyrazone in similar subjects. Furthermore, when the subjects were changed to a low-fat diet there was a further lengthening of platelet survival. This effect of dietary fat seems important in view of the effect of linoleic acid [69] in the diet on platelet function in man and experimental animals and on experimental thrombosis. In animals, saturated fats such as those in butter enhance platelet aggregation whereas fats containing unsaturated fatty acids make platelets less sensitive to aggregation and prevent thrombosis [70]. Human subjects given linoleic acid show a diminished sensitivity to platelet aggregation [71]. It has recently been shown in monkeys that hyper-cholesterolemia causes endothelial injury and shortened platelet survival and that this is because of endothelial injury and is not due to an effect on platelets [48]. Thus, dietary fat may have two effects, one on the platelets and one on the vessel wall. Again, modification of dietary fat, if it can be shown in man to affect the mechanisms that lead to vessel wall injury, may be a more important public health measure than the use of drugs where there are the problems of patient compliance and cost.

Summary

The interaction of platelets with the vessel wall can contribute to the early stages in the development of atherosclerosis through effects on smooth muscle cell proliferation, endothelial permeability, and possibly by causing vessel wall injury. Platelets are involved in the development of thrombi in response to vessel injury, and the repeated formation of platelet emboli and platelet-fibrin emboli from the mural thrombi may be one of the factors that cause clinical complications of atherosclerosis. Drugs which inhibit platelet function, particularly those that prolong shortened platelet survival (sulfinpyrazone and dipyridamole) may prove to be important in inhibiting the response of blood to vessel injury and thereby modifying the extent of atherosclerosis and its complications.

References

1   MUSTARD, J.F.: Function of blood platelets and their role in thrombosis. Trans. Am. clin. clim. Ass. *87:* 104–127 (1976).

2   MUSTARD, J.F. and PACKHAM, M.A.: The role of blood and platelets in atherosclerosis and the complications of atherosclerosis. Thromb. Diath. haemorrh. *33:* 445–456 (1975).

3   RUTHERFORD, R.B. and ROSS, R.: Platelet factors stimulate fibroblasts and smooth muscle cells quiescent in plasma serum to proliferate. J. Cell Biol. *69:* 196–203 (1976).

4   BAUMGARTNER, H.R.; MUGGLI, R.; TSCHOPP, T.B., and TURITTO, V.T.: Platelet adhesion, release and aggregation in flowing blood: effects of surface properties and platelet function. Thrombos. Haemostas. *35:* 124–138 (1976).

5   HOVIG, T.: Release of a platelet aggregating substance (adenosine diphosphate) from rabbit blood platelets induced by saline 'extract' of tendons. Thromb. Diath. haemorrh. *9:* 264–278 (1963).

6   ZUCKER, M.B. and BORRELLI, J.: Platelet clumping produced by connective tissue suspensions and by collagen. Proc. Soc. exp. Biol. Med. *109:* 779–787 (1962).

7   HOLMSEN, H.: Biochemistry of the platelet release reaction; in Biochemistry and pharmacology of platelets. Ciba Foundation Symposium 35 (new series), pp. 175–196 (Elsevier, New York 1975).

8   HAMBERG, M.; SVENSSON, J., and SAMUELSSON, B.: Thromboxanes. A new group of biologically active compounds derived from prostaglandin endoperoxides. Proc. natn. Acad. Sci. USA *72:* 2994–2998 (1975).

9   BILLS, T.K.; SMITH, J.B., and SILVER, M.J.: Metabolism of [^{14}C] arachidonic acid by human platelets. Biochim. biophys. Acta *424:* 303–314 (1976).

10 SILVER, M.J.; SMITH, J.B.; INGERMAN, C.M., and KOCSIS, J.J.: Arachidonic acid-induced human platelet aggregation and prostaglandin formation. Prostaglandins *4:* 863–875 (1973).

11 WILLIS, A.L. and KUHN, D.C.: A new potential mediator of arterial thrombosis whose biosynthesis is inhibited by aspirin. Prostaglandins *4:* 127–129 (1973).

12 ROME, L.H.; LANDS, W.E.M.; ROTH, G.J., and MAJERUS, P.W.: Aspirin as a quantitative acetylating reagent for the fatty acid oxygenase that forms prostaglandins. Prostaglandins *11:* 23–30 (1976).

13 HAMBERG, M. and SAMUELSSON, B.: Prostaglandin endoperoxides. Novel transformation of arachidonic acid in human platelets. Proc. natn. Acad. Sci. USA *71:* 3400–3404 (1974).

14 JOIST, J.H.; DOLEZEL, G.; LLOYD, J.V.; KINLOUGH-RATHBONE, R.L., and MUSTARD, J.F.: Platelet factor-3 availability and the platelet release reaction. J. Lab. clin. Med. *84:* 474–482 (1974).

15 WALSH, P.N.: The possible role of platelet coagulant activities in the pathogenesis of venous thrombosis. Thromb. Diath. haemorrh. *33:* 435–443 (1975).

16 NIEWIAROWSKI, S.; STUART, R.K., and THOMAS, D.P.: Activation of intravascular coagulation by collagen. Proc. Soc. exp. Biol. Med. *123:* 196–200 (1966).

17 WALSH, P.N.: The role of platelets in the contact phase of blood coagulation. Br. J. Haemat. *22:* 237–254 (1972).

18 PACKHAM, M.A.; KINLOUGH-RATHBONE, R.L.; REIMERS, H.-J.; SCOTT, S., and MUSTARD, J.F.: Mechanisms of platelet aggregation independent of adenosine diphosphate; in SILVER, SMITH and KOCSIS Prostaglandins in hematology (Spectrum Publications, New York, in press 1977).

19 Niewiarowski, S.; Regoeczi, E.; Stewart, G.J.; Senyi, A., and Mustard, J.F.: Platelet interaction with polymerizing fibrin. J. clin. Invest. *51:* 685–700 (1972).

20 Nilsson, I.M. and Pandolfi, M.: Fibrinolysis and vessel wall. Thromb. Diath. haemorrh., suppl. *40,* pp. 231–242 (1970).

21 Needleman, P.; Kulkarni, P.S., and Raz, A.: Coronary tone modulation: formation and actions of prostaglandins, endoperoxides and thromboxanes. Science *195:* 409–412 (1977).

22 Dusting, G.J.; Moncada, S., and Vane, J.R.: Prostacyclin (PGX) is the endogenous metabolite responsible for relaxation of coronary arteries induced by arachidonic acid. Prostaglandins *13:* 3–15 (1977).

23 Chesney, C.M.; Harper, E., and Colman, R.W.: Human platelet collagenase. J. clin. Invest. *53:* 1647–1654 (1974).

24 Robert, B.; Robert, L.; Legrand, Y.; Pignaud, G., and Caen, J.: Elastolytic protease in blood platelets. Ser. haematol. *4:* 175–185 (1971).

25 Nachman, R.L.; Weksler, B., and Ferris, B.: Characterization of human platelet vascular permeability enhancing activity. J. clin. Invest. *51:* 549–556 (1972).

26 Packham, M.A.: Nishizawa, E.E., and Mustard, J.F.: Response of platelets to tissue injury. Biochem. Pharmac., suppl., pp. 171–184 (1968).

27 Weksler, B.B. and Coupal, C.E.: Platelet-dependent generation of chemotactic activity in serum. J. exp. Med. *137:* 1419–1430 (1973).

28 Turner, S.R.; Tainer, J.A., and Lynn, W.S.: Biogenesis of chemotactic molecules by the arachidonate lipoxygenase system of platelets. Nature, Lond. *257:* 680–681 (1975).

29 Cazenave, J.-P.; Packham, M.A.; Davies, J.A.; Kinlough-Rathbone, R.L., and Mustard, J.F.: Studies of platelet adherence to collagen and the subendothelium; in Day, Zucker and Holmsen The significance of platelet function tests in the evaluation of hemostatic and thrombotic tendencies (Workshop on Platelets, Philadelphia, in press 1976).

30 Bunting, S.; Gryglewski, R.; Moncada, S., and Vane, J.R.: Arterial walls generate from prostaglandin endoperoxides a substance (prostaglandin X) which relaxes strips of mesenteric and coeliac arteries and inhibits platelet aggregation. Prostaglandins *12:* 897–913 (1976).

31 Gryglewski, R.J.; Bunting, S.; Moncada, S.; Flower, R.J., and Vane, J.R.: Arterial walls are protected against deposition of platelet thrombi by a substance (prostaglandin X) which they make from prostaglandin endoperoxides. Prostaglandins *12:* 685–713 (1976).

32 Cazenave, J.-P.; Packham, M.A.; Guccione, M.A., and Mustard, J.F.: Inhibition of platelet adherence to damaged surface of rabbit aorta. J. Lab. clin. Med. *86:* 551–563 (1975).

33 Cazenave, J.-P.; Davies, J.A.; Senyi, A.F.; Blajchman, M.A.; Hirsh, J., and Mustard, J.F.: Effects of methylprednisolone on platelet adhesion to damaged aorta, bleeding time and platelet survival. Blood *48:* 1009 (1976).

34 Lewis, G.P. and Piper, P.J.: Inhibition of release of prostaglandins as an explanation of some of the actions of anti-inflammatory corticosteroids. Nature, Lond. *254:* 308–311 (1975).

35 ESSIEN, E.M.; CAZENAVE, J.-P.; MOORE, S., and MUSTARD, J.F.: Effect of heparin and thrombin on platelet adherence to the surface of the rabbit aorta (submitted for publication, 1977).

36 JØRGENSEN, L.; PACKHAM, M.A.; ROWSELL, H.C., and MUSTARD, J.F.: Deposition of formed elements of blood on the intima and signs of intimal injury in the aorta of rabbit, pig, and man. Lab. Invest. 27: 341–350 (1972).

37 REIDY, M.A. and BOWYER, D.E.: Scanning electron microscopy of arteries. The morphology of aortic endothelium in haemodynamically stressed areas associated with branches. Atherosclerosis 26: 181–194 (1977).

38 WRIGHT, H.P.: Endothelial mitosis around aortic branches in normal guinea-pigs. Nature, Lond. 220: 78–79 (1968).

39 STARY, H.C. and MCMILLAN, G.C.: Kinetics of cellular proliferation in experimental atherosclerosis. Radioautography with grain counts in cholesterol-fed rabbits. Archs Path. 89: 173–183 (1970).

40 CAPLAN, B.A. and SCHWARTZ, C.J.: Increased endothelial cell turnover in areas of in vivo Evans blue uptake in the pig aorta. Atherosclerosis 17: 401–417 (1973).

41 FRY, D.L.: Response of the arterial wall to certain physical factors; in Atherogenesis: initiating factors. Ciba Foundation Symposium 12 (new series), pp. 93–125 (Elsevier, Excerpta Medica, North-Holland, Associated Scientific Publishers, New York 1973).

42 GOLDSMITH, H.L.: Blood flow and thrombosis. Thromb. Diath. haemorrh. 32: 35–48 (1974).

43 ROSS, R.; GLOMSET, J.; KARIYA, B., and HARKER, L.: A platelet-dependent serum factor that stimulates the proliferation of arterial smooth muscle cells in vitro. Proc. natn. Acad. Sci. USA 71: 1207–1210 (1974).

44 MOORE, S.: Thromboatherosclerosis in normolipemic rabbits: a result of continued endothelial damage. Lab. Invest. 29: 478–487 (1973).

45 TYSON, J.E.; DESA, D.J., and MOORE, S.: Thromboatheromatous complications of umbilical arterial catheterization in the newborn period. Archs Dis. Childh. 51: 744–754 (1976).

46 LEE, W.M. and LEE, K.T.: Advanced coronary atherosclerosis in swine produced by combination of balloon-catheter injury and cholesterol feeding. Expl molec. Path. 23: 491–499 (1975).

47 HARKER, L.A.; ROSS, R.; SLICHTER, S.J., and SCOTT, C.R.: Homocystine-induced arteriosclerosis. The role of endothelial cell injury and platelet response in its genesis. J. clin. Invest. 58: 731–741 (1976).

48 ROSS, R. and HARKER, L.: Hyperlipidemia and atherosclerosis. Chronic hyperlipidemia initiates and maintains lesions by endothelial cell desquamation and lipid accumulation. Science 193: 1094–1100 (1976).

49 MINICK, C.R.: Immunologic arterial injury in atherogenesis. Ann. N.Y. Acad. Sci. 275: 210–227 (1976).

50 MOORE, S.; FRIEDMAN, R.J.; SINGAL, D.P.; GAULDIE, J.; BLAJCHMAN, M.A., and ROBERTS, R.S.: Inhibition of injury induced thromboatherosclerotic lesions by anti-platelet serum in rabbits. Thrombos. Haemostas. 35: 70–81 (1976).

51 MOORE, S.: Unpublished observations.

52 MINICK, C.R.; LITRENTA, M.M.; ALONSO, D.R.; SILANE, M.F., and STEMERMAN, M.B.: Effect of regenerated endothelium on intimal lipid accumulation. Fed. Proc. Fed. Am. Socs exp. Biol. *36:* 392 (1977).

53 ROSS, R. and GLOMSET, J.A.: The pathogenesis of atherosclerosis. New Engl. J. Med. *295:* 369–377 (1976).

54 MUSTARD, J.F.; PACKHAM, M.A., and KINLOUGH-RATHBONE, R.L.: Platelet survival; in DAY, ZUCKER and HOLMSEN The significance of platelet function tests in the evaluation of hemostatic and thrombotic tendencies (Workshop on Platelets. Philadelphia, in press 1976).

55 SCOTT, S.; REIMERS, H.-J.; CHERNESKY, M.; GREENBERG, J.P.; KINLOUGH-RATHBONE, R.L.; PACKHAM, M.A., and MUSTARD, J.F.: The effect of viruses on platelet aggregation and platelet survival in rabbits. Circulation *54:* 199 (1976).

56 GROVES, H.M.; KINLOUGH-RATHBONE, R.L.; MOORE, S., and MUSTARD, J.F.: Unpublished observations.

57 ROKITANSKY, C. VON: Handbuch der Pathologischen Anatomie (Braumüller & Seidel, Vienna 1841–1846).

58 CLARK, E.; GRAEF, T., and CHASIS, H.: Thrombosis of the aorta and coronary arteries with special reference to the 'fibrinoid' lesions. Archs Path. *22:* 183–212 (1936).

59 DUGUID, J.B.: Thrombosis as a factor in the pathogenesis of aortic atherosclerosis. J. Path. Bact. *60:* 57–61 (1948).

60 MORE, R.H. and HAUST, M.D.: Atherogenesis and plasma constituents. Am. J. Path. *38:* 527–537 (1961).

61 CHANDLER, A.B.: Thrombosis and the development of atherosclerotic lesions; in JONES Atherosclerosis, pp. 88–93 (Springer, New York 1970).

62 GUNNING, A.J.; PICKERING, G.W.; ROBB-SMITH, A.H.T., and RUSSELL, R.R.: Mural thrombosis of the internal carotid artery and subsequent embolism. Jl Med. *33:* 155–195 (1964).

63 MOORE, S.: Hypertension and renal ischemia. Geriatrics *24:* 81–90 (1969).

64 MUSTARD, J.F. and PACKHAM, M.A.: Platelets, thrombosis and drugs; in Current drug reviews: cardiology, vol. 3 (Adis Press, Sydney, in press).

65 KAEGI, A.; PINEO, G.F.; SHIMIZU, A.; TRIVEDI, H.; HIRSH, J., and GENT, M.: Arteriovenous-shunt thrombosis; prevention by sulfinpyrazone. New Engl. J. Med. *290:* 304–306 (1974).

66 MUSTARD, J.F. and MURPHY, E.A.: Effect of smoking on blood coagulation and platelet survival in man. Br. med. J. *i:* 846–849 (1963).

67 STRONG, J.P. and RICHARDS, M.L.: Cigarette smoking and atherosclerosis in autopsied men. Atherosclerosis *23:* 451–476 (1976).

68 MUSTARD, J.F. and MURPHY, E.A.: Effect of different dietary fats on blood coagulation, platelet economy, and blood lipids. Br. med. J. *i:* 1651–1655 (1962).

69 HORNSTRA, G. and LUSSENBURG, R.N.: Relationship between the type of dietary fatty acid and arterial thrombosis tendency in rats. Atherosclerosis *22:* 499–516 (1975).

70 RENAUD, S.; KINLOUGH-RATHBONE, R.L., and MUSTARD, J.F.: Relationship between platelet aggregation and the thrombotic tendency in rats fed hyperlipemic diets. Lab. Invest. *22:* 339–343 (1970).

71 HORNSTRA, G.; CHAIT, A.; KARVONEN, M.J.; LEWIS, B.; TURPEINEN, O., and VERGROESEN, A.J.: Influence of dietary fat on platelet function in men. Lancet *i:* 1155–1157 (1973).

J.F. MUSTARD, Faculty of Health Sciences, McMaster University, *Hamilton, Ontario* (Canada)

Prog. biochem. Pharmacol., vol. 14, pp. 326–338 (Karger, Basel 1977)

Dietary Fats and Arterial Thrombosis:
Effects and Mechanism of Action

Gerard Hornstra

Unilever Research, Vlaardingen

Introduction

The influence of the type of dietary fat on experimental athero-sclerosis in animals has been known for a long time [11, 33, 45]. Investigations in man [17, 31, 34] have also shown that dietary fats affect athero-genesis.

Atherosclerosis is a multi-factorial disease. This implies that the fat effects can be mediated by different pathways. Arterial thrombosis is the main lethal complication of atherosclerosis [13, 16, 40] and most probably contributes to the atherogenetic process [3, 37, 44]. The effects of dietary fats on arterial thrombosis are therefore of great interest.

In the present paper, these effects will be briefly described. Moreover, some investigations we performed to elucidate the underlying mechanisms of action will be discussed.

Basic Experiments in Rats

The arterial thrombosis model we used is based on the introduction of a loop-shaped polyethylene cannula – the aorta loop – into the abdominal aorta of male rats [26]. Endothelial damage at the tips of the cannula, regional flow disturbances and local fibrin formation cause the growth of a mural thrombus which, in comparative phases of development, very much resembles the structure of a human arterial thrombus. At a given moment the growing thrombus obstructs the cannula completely. The time between insertion and complete obstruction of the loop – the obstruction

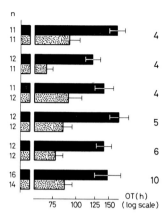

Fig. 1. Arterial thrombosis tendency (OT) of rats fed diets containing SO (■) or HCO (□) for 4–10 weeks (n=12, mean ± SEM).

time (OT) – is dependent on the thrombosis tendency of the animal: the lower the tendency, the longer the OT. Using this device, we found [24] that fats containing a large amount of long-chain saturated fatty acids promote arterial thrombosis, whereas dietary linoleic acid has a specific, anti-thrombotic effect. Oleic acid on its own does not seem to act as an anti-thrombotic substance. However, replacement of thrombogenic fatty acids in the diet by oleic acid decreases the dietary thrombogenic potency independent of whether oleic acid has the *cis* or the *trans* configuration. Moreover, the results indicated that the thrombogenicity of saturated fatty acids increases with the chain length.

Effects of Dietary Linoleic Acid in Man

Unfortunately, suitable laboratory techniques to quantity actual thrombus formation in man are not available. When it became evident that a high thrombosis tendency in rats is associated with a high tendency of platelets to aggregate, we constructed a device to measure 'spontaneous' platelet aggregation in venous blood in man: the filtragometer [25]. The principle of the method is based on the continuous measurement of the pressure difference across a filter with pores of 20 μm in diameter, through which blood from a forearm vein is drawn. When platelet aggregates obstruct the filter, they change the pressure difference proportional to the degree of platelet aggregation. The filtragometer response is inhibited by ingestion of aspirin and by infusion of prostaglandin E_1, and is enhanced in coronary artery disease [22]. With this device platelet aggregation was measured in two groups of male subjects receiving diets with a high or low linoleic acid content (12 and 4 % of total dietary energy, respectively) over a 6-year period. MIETTINEN et al. [34] found that in the population from which the subjects were randomly sampled, the use of the high-linoleic-acid diet was associated with a significantly reduced mortality from coronary heart disease, while we showed [21] that in the high-linoleic-acid group platelet aggregation is significantly reduced compared with the low-linoleic-acid group. The anti-aggregatory effect of dietary linoleic acid has been confirmed by FLEISCHMAN et al. [5, 6]. Moreover, O'BRIEN et al. [39] have recently shown that dietary linoleate inhibits platelet activation.

Mechanism of Action of Dietary Fat Effects

In arterial thrombosis, platelet function is of primary importance, whereas coagulation definitely contributes to thrombogenesis. Recent findings indicate that vessel well has thromboregulatory potency. These three factors are, therefore, included in our search for the mechanism(s) underlying the dietary fat effects on arterial thrombosis. Most of the experiments were performed with sunflowerseed oil (SO) and hydrogenated coconut oil (HCO), the fatty acid compositions of which are given in table I. These fats, when constituting 50 % of the dietary energy, induce

Table I. Fatty acid composition (%) of SO and HCO

Fatty acid	SO	HCO
≤C10:0		14
C12:0	–	44
C14:0	–	19
C16:0	6	10
C18:0	5	10
C18:1	25	2
C18:2	63	1
C22:0	1	–

significantly different OT's, even after 4 weeks of feeding, which is probably due to their different amounts of linoleic acid (anti-thrombotic) and long-chain saturated fatty acids (pro-thrombotic).

Platelet Function

Since platelets are of major importance in our thrombosis model, we speculated that dietary fats exert their effect on arterial thrombosis by affecting platelet function. We, indeed, repeatedly found (fig. 2) that the platelet count in the thrombogenic group (HCO) is significantly higher than that in the SO group. It has not yet been investigated whether this coincides with alterations in platelet life span.

Platelet aggregation was investigated by the conventional turbidometric technique in citrated platelet-rich plasma (cPRP) and by the 'filter-loop technique' which measures platelet aggregation in circulating blood [20]. In cPRP (fig. 3) aggregation induced by thrombin and adenosine diphosphate (ADP) was not different in the two groups. The collagen-induced aggregation, however, was somewhat depressed in the thrombogenic (HCO) group. On the other hand, platelet shape change induced by collagen is significantly enhanced on HCO feeding, which indicates that HCO platelets are more activated by collagen contact than are SO platelets. Since platelet factor 3 (PF-3) availability, triggered by collagen, was also lower in the HCO group, we assume that the platelet-collagen interaction is disturbed in HCO-fed animals in a way which is not in line with the thrombogenic effect of HCO. This is, therefore, a subject for further investigation.

With the 'filter-loop technique', only the ADP-induced aggregation has been measured. In general, a good correlation exists between this parameter and the arterial thrombosis tendency induced by different dietary fats (fig. 4). Moreover, this platelet function is invariably increased in the thrombogenic HCO group as compared with the SO-fed animals, while in the thrombogenic group the frequency and degree of 'spontaneous' aggregation (transient aggregation without ADP administration) is invariably higher than in the animals of the anti-throbotic SO group (fig. 5). Finally, in man, dietary linoleic acid decreases platelet aggregation. All these findings indicate that thrombosis tendency and platelet aggregability are, indeed, related phenomena and that the effect of dietary fats may be mediated by changes in the activation level of the blood platelets, leading to increased platelet aggregability.

Under normal conditions platelet arachidonic acid is assumed to

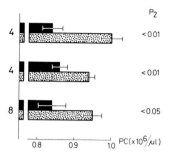

Fig. 2. Platelet concentration (PC) in blood of rats fed diets containing SO (■) or HCO (□) for 4 and 8 weeks (n=12, mean ± SEM).

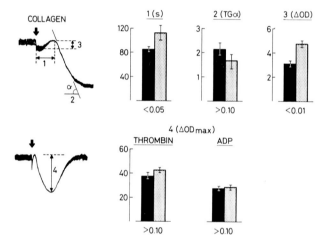

Fig. 3. Platelet aggregation (1, 2 and 4) and shape change (3) in cPRP of rats fed diets containing SO (■) or HCO (□) for 8 weeks (n=16, mean ± SEM).

play a key role in platelet aggregation and thrombogenesis via its conversion into the endoperoxides PGG_2 and PGH_2, thromboxane A_2, prostaglandins and prostacyclin (fig. 6) [14, 15, 36, 42, 49]. Any substance affecting this metabolic pathway may influence thrombogenesis by shifting the balance between thromboxane A_2, prostaglandins and prostacyclin. As far as dietary fats are concerned, two substances are likely to have such an effect: vitamin E and linoleic acid.

Vitamin E inhibits the oxidative metabolism of arachidonic acid and therefore interferes with the production of thromboregulatory metabolites

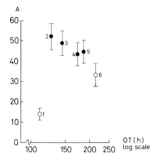

Fig. 4. Relationship between ADP-induced platelet aggregation in circulating blood (A ± SEM) and arterial thrombosis tendency (OT) in rats fed diets containing 50 % of total energy from: (1) whale oil; (2) hydrogenated soybean oil; (3) olive oil; (4) sunflowerseed oil; (5) linseed oil; (6) rapeseed oil (n=12). Aggregation values indicated by open circles differ significantly from the other values.

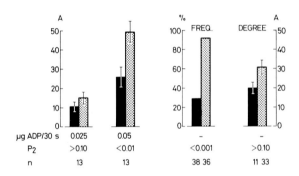

Fig. 5. ADP-induced (left n=13, A ± SEM) and frequency (%) and degree (A) of 'spontaneous' aggregation (right) in circulating blood of rats, fed diets containing SO (■) or HCO (□) for 4–8 weeks.

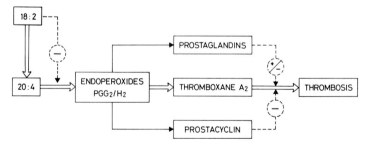

Fig. 6. Simplified pathway of thromboregulation by dietary, platelet and vessel wall fatty acids [derived from 14, 15, 36, 42, 49].

Table II. Effect of varying amounts of additional vitamin E (D-α-tocopherol acetate) on arterial thrombosis tendency in rats (log OT ± SEM, n=16)

Vitamin E		Thrombosis tendency	
mg/1000 cal = mg/4,200 J	equivalent to dietary energy from SO, %	log OT ± SEM	OT/h
0	5	2.05 ± 0.04	112
23	30	1.94 ± 0.03	87
61	60	2.06 ± 0.03	114
173	100	1.97 ± 005	93

of arachidonic acid [19, 30]. Although the evidence is conflicting [10], platelet aggregation has been reported to be inhibited by vitamin E [7, 18, 32, 43]. Since the platelet vitamin E level can be influenced by the dietary intake [43] – although this has also been disputed [38] – and, in general, the vitamin E content of vegetable oils and fats increases with the degree of unsaturation [27], it may be assumed that the dietary fat effects on arterial thrombogenesis are mediated by differences in the vitamin E intake. However, no effect of varying amounts of vitamin E on the arterial thrombosis tendency in rats (table II) could be observed.

Linoleic acid also inhibits the enzymatic conversion of arachidonic acid into endoperoxides [9, 30, 41] and it also inhibits platelet aggregation [9, 23].

For the thromboregulatory role of endogenous platelet fatty acids, phosphatidylcholine may be of key importance, since this phospholipid has been suggested as the main source of these fatty acids [1]. Whe therefore postulated that the anti-thrombotic effect of dietary linoleate can be mediated by a decrease in the arachidonic/linoleic acid ratio in platelet phosphatidylcholine. We tested this hypothesis in rats which had been fed diets containing 10 or 50 % of long-chain saturated fatty acids and varying amounts of oleic and linoleic acid. For both saturated fat levels the dietary linoleic acid content was found to be negatively related to the arachidonic/linoleic acid ratio in platelet phosphatidylcholine, while in similar experiments thrombosis tendency (OT measurements) was likewise negatively related to the dietary linoleic acid content (fig. 7). These findings support our hypothesis that the anti-thrombotic effect of dietary linoleate is mediated by its lowering effect on the arachidonic/linoleic acid ratio in platelet phosphatidylcholine. However, the results

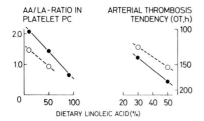

Fig. 7. Effect of dietary linoleic acid content on the arachidonic acid (AA)/ linoleic acid (LA) ratio in rat platelet phosphatidylcholine (PC, left) and arterial thrombosis tendency (OT, right). ● = 10 % saturated fat, ○ = 50 % saturated fat.

shown in figure 7 also indicate that the thrombosis-promoting effect of dietary saturated fats is not mediated by an increase in this ratio, since a higher saturated fat content causes it to decrease, whereas the thrombosis tendency is enhanced.

Blood Coagulation

Although it is generally agreed that in arterial thrombosis coagulation is of less importance than platelet adhesion, platelet release and platelet aggregation, the strands of fibrin found in the experimentally induced arterial thrombi indicate that the dietary fat effect may have been mediated, at least in part, by changes in blood coagulability. With CHANDLER's [2] rotating loop, no differences were observed in the thrombus formation time in native blood, which indicates that both HCO and SO do not induce differences in thrombin generation [4].

GAUTHERON and RENAUD [8], applying a model that resembles venous thrombosis, observed a close correlation between thrombosis tendency, modified by different dietary fats, and the clotting time of platelet-rich plasma on recalcification. This dietary fat effect was thought to be mediated by a change in PF-3 activity. However, using the same clotting test, we could not find differences between HCO- and SO-fed groups after 4–15 weeks of feeding.

PF-3 activity and content were measured with Russel's viper venom in citrated whole blood or in cPRP, the latter before and after three times freezing and thawing. No significant differences between the groups were observed.

PF-3 availability was investigated by measuring the shortening of the Stypven time on incubation of citrated whole blood with either saline or

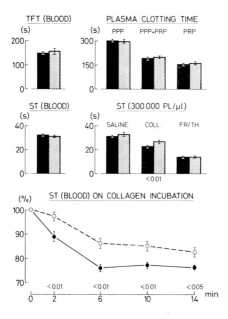

Fig. 8. Some coagulation parameters determined in rats fed diets containing SO (●) or HCO (○) for 4–15 weeks. TFT = Thrombus formation time in Chandler's rotating loop; ST = Stypven time (n=12–16, mean ± SEM).

a collagen suspension in saline. PF-3 availability in the thrombogenic HCO group was found to be significantly lower than in the anti-thrombotic SO group. The prothrombin time (Quick) was the same in both groups. All this evidence, summarized in figure 8, makes it highly probable that differences in systemic blood coagulability cannot have contributed to a large extent to the differences in arterial thrombosis tendency induced by dietary fats. It should be realized, however, that the clot-promoting activities of blood platelets different from PF-3 [28, 46] have not yet been measured. Since these platelet properties seem to be of importance in thrombogenesis [29, 47, 48], a contribution of local fibrin formation cannot yet be excluded.

Vessel Wall

Since the discovery that vascular tissue generates a highly active anti-aggregatory substance – prostacyclin – from the endoperoxides PGG_2/PGH_2 [12, 35, 36], the vessel wall may also be involved in the mechanism by which dietary fats affect arterial thrombosis tendency. To start the

Table III. Prostacyclin formation by aortic tissue, incubated in This-buffered saline at room temperature

Activity of prostacyclin is expressed in equivalents of ng PGE_1/min (n=8, mean ± SEM).

Part of aorta	SO	HCO	P_2
Thoracic	20.6±3.33	20.7±3.03	>0.10
Abdominal	22.1±3.41	18.5±2.57	>0.10

investigations into this very intriguing possibility, we measured the prostacyclin generation by incubating a standardized amount of aortic tissue with Tris-buffered saline at room temperature. Prostacyclin formation was quantified by its aggregation inhibiting potency, the activities being expressed as equivalents of prostaglandin E_1. Results, given in table III, indicate no difference between the HCO and SO groups. Experiments are in progress to further explore the importance of this possible thromboregulatory mechanism.

Summary

Dietary fats have a pronounced effect on arterial thrombosis: in rats, long-chain saturated fatty acids are thrombogenic, oleic acid is neutral, and linoleic acid is anti-thrombotic. These effects are likely to be mediated, at least in part, by changes in platelet fatty acid composition and – consequently – platelet function. Blood coagulability and differences in vitamin E intake seem of no (or minor) importance. In man, dietary linoleic acid inhibits platelet aggregation and other parameters of platelet activation. Dietary fat effects on vascular prostacyclin formation have not yet been found.

References

1   BILLS, T.K.; SMITH, J.B., and SILVER, M.J.: Metablism of ^{14}C-arachidonic acid by human platelets. Biochim. biophys. Acta *424:* 303–314 (1976).

2   CHANDLER, A.B.: *In vitro* thrombotic coagulation of blood. Lab. Invest. *7:* 110–115 (1958).

3 DUGUID, J.B.: Thrombosis as a factor in the pathogenesis of coronary atherosclerosis. Am. J. Path. Bact. *58:* 207–212 (1946).

4 ENGELBERG, H.: Studies with the Chandler rotating loop. Evidence that thrombin generation is responsible for the formation of the artificial *in vitro* thrombi. Thromb. Diath. haemorrh. *22:* 344–350 (1969).

5 FLEISCHMAN, A.I.; BIERENBAUM, M.L., and JUSTICE, D.: Titrating dietary linoleate to *in vivo* platelet function in man. Am. J. clin. Nutr. *28:* 601–605 (1975).

6 FLEISCHMAN, A.I.; JUSTICE, D.; BIERENBAUM, M.L., and STIER, A.: Beneficial effect of increased dietary linoleate upon *in vivo* platelet function in man. J. Nutr. *105:* 1286–1290 (1975).

7 FONG, J.S.C.: Alpha tocopherol: its inhibition of human platelet aggregation. Experientia *32:* 639–641 (1976).

8 GAUTHERON, P. and RENAUD, S.: Hyperlipemia induced hypercoagulable state in rat. Role of increased activity of platelet phosphatidyl serine in response to certain dietary fatty acids. Thromb. Res. *1:* 353–370 (1972).

9 GERRARD, J.M.; WHITE, J.G., and KRIVITT, W.: Labile aggregation stimulating substance, free fatty acids and platelet aggregation. J. Lab. clin. Med. *87:* 73–82 (1976).

10 GOMES, J.A.; VENKATACHALAPATHY, D., and HAFT, J.I.: Effect of vitamin E on platelet aggregation. Abstract. Circulation *50:* 278 (1974).

11 GOTTENBOS, J.J. and THOMASSON, H.J.: Aorta atheromatosis in rabbits on feeding cholesterol or fats. Coll. Int. Cent. Nat. Rech., No 99, pp. 221–239 (1961).

12 GRYGLEWSKI, R.J.; BUNTING, S.; MONCADA, S.; FLOWER, R.J., and VANE, J.R.: Arterial walls are protected against deposition of platelet thrombi by an substance (prostaglandin X) which they make from prostaglandin endoperoxides. Prostaglandins *12:* 685–713 (1976).

13 HAEREM, J.W.: Platelet aggregates and mural micro-thrombi in early stages of acute, fatal coronary disease. Thromb. Res. *5:* 243–249 (1974).

14 HAMBERG, M.; SVENSSON, J., and SAMUELSSON, B.: Prostaglandin endoperoxides. A new concept concerning the mode of action and release of prostaglandins. Proc. natn. Acad. Sci. USA *71:* 3824–3828 (1974).

15 HAMBERG, M.; SVENSSON, J., and SAMUELSSON, B.: Thromboxanes, a new group of biologically active compounds derived from prostaglandin endoperoxides. Proc. natn. Acad. Sci. USA *72:* 2994–2998 (1975).

16 HARLAND, W.A. and HOLBURN, A.M.: Coronary thrombosis and myocardial infarction. Lancet *ii:* 1158–1159 (1966).

17 HEYDEN, S.: Epidemiological data on dietary fat intake and atherosclerosis with an appendix on possible side effects; in VERGROESEN The role of fats in human nutrition, pp. 44–113 (Academic Press, London 1975).

18 HIGASHI, O. and KIKUCHI, Y.: Effects of vitamin E on the aggregation and the lipid peroxidation of platelets exposed to hydrogen peroxide. Tohoku J. exp. Med. *112:* 271–278 (1974).

19 HOPE, W.C.; DALTON, C.; MACHLIN, L.J.; FILIPSKI, R.J., and VANE, F.M.: Influence of dietary vitamin E on prostaglandin biosynthesis in rat blood. Prostaglandins *10:* 557–571 (1975).

20 HORNSTRA, G.: Method to determine the degree of ADP-induced platelet aggregation in circulating rat blood ('filter-loop technique'). Br. J. Haemat. *19:* 321–329 (1970).

21 HORNSTRA, G.; LEWIS, B.; CHAIT, A.; TURPEINEN, O.; KARVONEN, M.J., and VERGROESEN, A.J.: Influence of dietary fat on platelet function in men. Lancet *i:* 1155–1157 (1973).

22 HORNSTRA, G.: The filtragometer in thrombosis research; in HOLMSEN Proc. Workshop on Platelets, Philadelphia, 1976 (in press).

23 HORNSTRA, G. and HADDEMAN, E.: Effects of dietary fats on the role of platelets in arterial thromboembolism; in MILLS and PARETI Platelets and thrombosis (Academic Press, London, in press).

24 HORNSTRA, G. and LUSSENBURG, R.N.: Relationship between the type of dietary fatty acid and arterial thrombosis tendency in rats. Atherosclerosis *22:* 499–516 (1975).

25 HORNSTRA, G. and TEN HOOR, F.: The filtragometer: a new-device for measuring platelet aggregation in venous blood of man. Thromb. Diath. haemorrh. *34:* 531–544 (1975).

26 HORNSTRA, G. and VENDELMANS-STARRENBURG, A.: Induction of experimental arterial occlusive thrombi in rats. Atherosclerosis *17:* 369–382 (1973).

27 JAGER, F.: Linoleic intake and vitamin E requirement; in VERGROESEN The role of fats in human nutrition, pp. 381–432 (Academic Press, London 1975).

28 KING, J.B.: The function of the platelet surface in coagulation. Some preliminary observations with two new tests of platelet function. Thromb. Diath. haemorrh. *32:* 492–501 (1974).

29 KING, J.B. and JOFFE, S.M.: The predisposition of post-operative deep vein thrombosis using a newly described test of platelet function. Thromb. Diath. haemorrh. *32:* 502–509 (1974).

30 LANDS, W.E.M.; LETELLIER, P.R.; ROME, L.H., and VANDERHOEK J.Y.: Inhibition of prostaglandin biosynthesis. Adv. Biosci. *9:* 15–28 (1973).

31 LEREN, P.: The Oslo diet-heart study. Circulation *42:* 935–942 (1970).

32 MACHLIN, L.J.; FILIPSKI, R.; WILLIS, A.L.; KUHN, D.C., and BRIN, M.: Influence of vitamin E on platelet aggregation and thrombocythemia in the rat. Proc. Soc. exp. Biol. Med. *149:* 275–277 (1975).

33 MALMROS, H.: Dietary prevention of atherosclerosis. Lancet *ii:* 479–484 (1969).

34 MIETTINEN, M.; TURPEINEN, O.; KARVONEN, M.J.; ELOSUO, R., and PAAVILAINEN, E.: Effect of cholesterol lowering diet on mortality from coronary heart disease and other causes. A twelve year clinical trial in men and women. Lancet *ii:* 835–838 (1972).

35 MONCODA, S.; HIGGS, E.A., and VANE, J.R.: Human arterial and venous tissue generate prostacyclin (prostaglandin X), a potent inhibitor of platelet aggregation. Lancet *i:* 18–20 (1977).

36 MONCADA, S.; GRYGLEWSKI, R.; BUNTING, S., and VANE, J.R.: An enzyme isolated from arteries transforms prostaglandin endoperoxides to an unstable substance that inhibits platelet aggregation. Nature, Lond. *263:* 663–665 (1976).

37 MOORE, S.: Thrombosis and atherosclerosis. Thromb. Diath. haemorrh., suppl. 60, pp. 205–212 (1974).

38 NORDØY, A. and STRØM, E.: Tocophenol in human platelets. J. Lipid Res. *16:* 386–391 (1975).

39 O'BRIEN, J.R.; ETHERINGTON, M.D.; JAMIESON, S.; VERGROESEN, A.J., and TEN HOOR, F.: Effect of a diet of polyunsaturated fats on some platelet function tests. Lancet *ii:* 995–997 (1976).

40 OWREN, P.A.: Nutrition and thrombosing atherosclerosis. Biblthca Nutr. Dieta, vol. 6, pp. 156–182 (1964).

41 PACE-ASCIAK, C. and WOLFE, L.S.: Inhibition of prostaglandin synthesis by oleic, linoleic and linolenic acids. Biochim. biophys. Acta *152:* 784–787 (1968).

42 SILVER, M.J.; SMITH, J.B.; INGERMAN, C., and KOCSIS, J.J.: Arachidonic acid-induced human platelet aggregation and prostaglandin formation. Prostaglandins *4:* 863–875 (1973).

43 STEINER, M. and ANASTASI, J.: Vitamin E, an inhibitor of the platelet release reaction. J. clin. Invest. *57:* 732–737 (1976).

44 SUMIYOSHI, A.; MORE, R.H., and WEIGENSBERG, B.I.: Aortic fibrofatty type atherosclerosis from thrombus in normolipidemic rabbits. Atherosclerosis *18:* 43–57 (1973).

45 VLES, R.O.; BÜLLER, J.; GOTTENBOS, J.J., and THOMASSON, H.J.: Influence of type of dietary fat on cholesterol-induced atherosclerosis in the rabbit. J. Atheroscler. Res. *4:* 170–183 (1964).

46 WALSH, P.N.: Platelet coagulant activities and hemostasis: a hypothesis. Blood *43:* 597–605 (1974).

47 WALSH, P.N.; PARETI, F.I., and CORBETT, J.J.: Platelet coagulant activity and serum lipids in transient cerebral ischemia. New Engl. J. Med. *295:* 854–858 (1976).

48 WALSH, P.N.; ROGERS, P.H.; MARDER, V.J.; GAGNATELLI, G.; ESKOVITZ, E.S., and SHERRY, S.: The relationship of platelet coagulant activities to venous thrombosis following hip surgery. Br. J. Haemat. *32:* 421–437 (1976).

49 WILLIS, A.L.; VANE, F.M.; KUHN, D.C.; SCOTT, C.G., and PETRIN, M.: Endoperoxide aggregator 'LASS' formed in platelets in response to thrombotic stimuli. Purification, identification and unique biological significance. Prostaglandins *8:* 453–508 (1974).

Dr. P.M. BAALMAN, Editorial Department, Unilever Research, P.O. Box 114, *Vlaardingen* (The Netherlands)

Prog. biochem. Pharmacol., vol. 14, pp. 339–343 (Karger, Basel 1977)

Photometric Platelet Aggregation Test III: A New Tool for the Detection of Enhancet Platelet Aggregation

K. BREDDIN and H.J. KRZYWANEK

Department of Angiology, Center of Internal Medicine, University of Frankfurt, Frankfurt a.M.

In recent years we were able to demonstrate enhanced 'spontaneous' platelet aggregation in patients with diabetes mellitus, myocardial infarction and peripheral atherosclerotic occlusions. The data which we collected since 1963 using the microscopic PAT I led to the conclusion that enhanced platelet aggregation may be a risk factor indicating progressive atherosclerosis or impending thrombotic complications either in the venous or in the arterial vascular system. In 1974 we developed a new photometric measuring system for the study of spontaneous platelet aggregation (PAT III), which improved our original method [BREDDIN et al., 1976].

Method

0.6 ml of citrated PRP are rotated in a disc-shaped polystyrol cuvette at 20 rpm and at a constant temperature of 37° C. Inducing substances are not added. Changes of optimal density which follow the formation of platelet aggregates are registered using a chart recorder. The aggregation curves are evaluated as follows: (1) 'primary aggregation' is expressed by the angle α_1 between the flat part of the curve and the horizontal line; (2) angle α_2 between the steepest part of the curve and the horizontal is a measure of the maximum aggregation speed; (3) T_r is the reaction time, measured from the onset of rotation to the steepest part of the aggregation curve. α_2 and T_r are the most important parameters for the evaluation of the aggregation pattern. A great angle α_2 and a short T_r are indicating a strongly enhanced platelet aggregation.

Factors Influencing Spontaneous Platelet Aggregation

Aspirin ingestion inhibits platelet aggregation, and even the incidental intake of one tablet of an aspirin-containing analgesis influences the test for several days. Test results are altered by *plasma turbidity,* e.g. by lipemia or erythrocyte admixture to PRP. Aggregation is reduced or missing if the *platelet count* in PRP is below 200,000/mm^3. Spontaneous aggregation is triggered by the pH *increase* in PRP which is caused by the evaporation of CO_2 from the plasma sample during rotation. Aggregation does not occur if the PRP is superimposed by a layer of CO_2 gas, thus inhibiting the evaporation of CO_2 from the plasma.

There is no correlation between the magnitude of the pH increase and the aggregability of the PRP. Aggregating and nonaggregating PRP samples show the same increase of pH during rotation. This indicates that an increase of pH in PRP is essential but not the cause of spontaneous platelet aggregation.

There are also distinct *time*-dependent changes of the aggregation pattern after blood sampling. 15 min after blood drawing platelet aggregation very rarely occurred. Testing of the same PRP at various time intervals revealed an increase of the maximum aggregability (angle a_2) during the 90 min following blood sampling. From then on test results varied very little for the next 3 h. The spontaneous aggregability of thrombocytes is *temperature* dependent. If PRP is stored at room temperature the steepness of the aggregation curve increases up to 90 min after blood sampling and remains rather constant from then on to the 4th hour. Incubation at 37° C inhibits aggregation in the same PRP completely.

From our experience we suggest the following test conditions for best reproducible results: storage of the blood sample or PRP in a 25° C water bath and performance of the test between 1.5 and 4 h after blood collection.

Clinical Results

Starting in January 1975 more than 4,000 in- and out-clinic patients of the Frankfurt University Medical Center and a number of healthy volunteers were studied using PAT III. The data were collected using the following criteria: no spontaneous aggregation: $T_r > 10$ min, no angle a_2; strongly enhanced aggregation: angle a_2 greater than 60°.

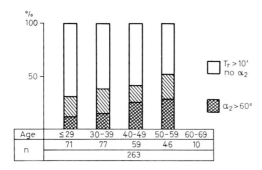

Fig. 1. Angle α of PAT III in healthy subjects.

The test results of 263 *healthy volunteers* are summarized in figure 1. As in our previous studies an age-dependent increase of platelet aggregation can be demonstrated. 70.4 % of the healthy young people below 29 years showed no spontaneous aggregation with a gradual decrease of this percentage to 47.8 % in the 50- to 59-year age group. The incidence of strongly enhanced aggregation increases with age from 11.3 to 28.3 % in the respective age groups.

Spontaneous aggregation was studied in 502 patients with *diabetes mellitus,* a disease which is well known for its vascular complications. In this group the incidence of missing spontaneous aggregation was reduced in all age groups and the percentage of strongly enhanced aggregation was over 40 % in the patient groups above 50 years of age. The most striking differences were observed in young diabetics under 29 years with missing spontaneous aggregation in 40 % (vs. 70 % in the control group) and 38 % enhanced aggregation (vs. 11 % in the control group).

In 345 patients with *intermittent claudication* as the main symptom of peripheral atherosclerosis we found a rather great variation in the mean percentage of nonaggregating PRP with an overall value of 40.3 %. Strongly enhanced platelet aggregation was present in one third to one half of the patients in the various age groups.

The diagnosis of *coronary heart disease* in 274 patients was based either on a history of myocardial infarction (n = 173) or the angiographic proof of coronary artery stenosis and occlusions of various degree. There was no age-dependent increase of enhanced platelet aggregation with a percentage between 40.5 and 46.9 % from 30 to 69 years of age. The high incidence of strongly enhanced aggregation in the 30–39 and 40–49 years

Table I. Incidence of missing spontaneous platelet aggregation (T_r >10 min, no angle a_2) and strongly enhanced aggregation (a_2 >60°) in normals (N), diabetics (D) and patients with intermittent claudication (IC) or coronary heart disease (CHD)

	N		D		IC		CHD	
	n	%	n	%	n	%	n	%
T_r >10 min no angle a_2	162/263	61.6	174/502	34.7	139/345	40.3	100/274	30.5
a_2 >60°	49/263	18.6	206/502	41.0	148/345	42.9	113/274	41.2

age groups (42.9 and 46.9 %, respectively) is again remarkable in comparison with the age-matched healthy controls (14.3 and 25.4 %, respectively). The rather small percentage of patients over 70 years with strongly enhanced aggregation may be due to death selection.

The data are summarized in the table I, disregarding the age distribution. The differences between healthy subjects and patients with diabetes mellitus or complications of atherosclerosis are highly significant (a>0.0001, χ^2-test) both for missing spontaneous aggregation and strongly enhanced aggregation.

Discussion

The number of 'healthy' persons with enhanced platelet aggregation is growing with age. This may be correlated with the progress of atherosclerosis with advancing years. In patients with complications of atherosclerosis like recent myocardial infarction, peripheral occlusive disease, but also in diabetics the incidence of enhanced platelet aggregations was significantly higher than in 'healthy' subjects.

In earlier investigations using PAT I the highest incidence of enhanced aggregation was observed prior to thrombotic incidents in atherosclerotic patients and in patients with diabetes and recent myocardial infarction.

It may be concluded that enhanced spontaneous platelet aggregation, if repeatedly evident in one of the aggregation tests (PAT I or III), by itself represents an independent risk factor for thrombotic complications, especially in patients with advanced atherosclerosis.

Summary

In clinical investigation on enhanced platelet aggregation the changes of the various tests with time after blood sampling must be considered. The photometric PAT III for the evaluation of spontaneous aggregation showed enhanced aggregation in a high percentage of patients with vascular disease, and prospective data obtained so far make it likely that enhanced aggregation is a risk factor for thrombosis. More prospective studies are necessary to prove whether continuously enhanced spontaneous platelet aggregation is indicating progressive atherosclerosis.

Reference

BREDDIN, K.; GRUN, H.; KRZYWANEK, H.J., and SCHREMMER, W.P.: On the measurement of spontaneous platelet aggregation. The platelet aggregation test III. Methods and first clinical results. Thromb. Haemostas. *35:* 669 (1976).

Prof. Dr. K. BREDDIN, Zentrum der Inneren Medizin, Abteilung für Angiologie, Klinikum der J.W. Goethe-Universität, Theodor-Stern-Kai 7, *D-6000 Frankfurt a.M.* (FRG)

Prog. biochem. Pharmacol., vol. 14, pp. 344–348 (Karger, Basel 1977)

Platelet-Mediated Pulmonary Hypertension: Reduction by Platelet Inhibition

J. Mlczoch, J.T. Reeves and R.F. Grover

CVP-Research Laboratory, University of Colorado, Denver, Colo.

The regulation of the pulmonary circulation and of the pressures in the lung is rather complex. Changes in left heart filling pressure, intrathoracic pressure and intraalveolar pressure are involved. In addition to these more or less mechanical influences, the pulmonary arteries themselves are able to contribute to the changes in intravascular pressure in the lung. The mechanisms for this active regulation are not known in detail, although vasoactive substances might be responsible or at least involved.

One of the mediators of this regulation might be the platelet, because platelets are known to contain or to produce a number of vasoactive substances including histamine, serotonin, adenine nucleotides and prostaglandins.

Circulating platelets may also be involved in pulmonary hypertension following pulmonary embolism. This has been suggested by several investigators and for example, serotonin antagonists like methysergide or reserpine strikingly modified the adverse effects of pulmonary embolism on the pulmonary circulation in the dog, again suggesting that a vasoconstrictor substance is involved.

And the question we posed was if circulating platelets were important in the pathogenesis of pulmonary hypertension following pulmonary embolism, then removal of the platelets should reduce the pressor response.

The purpose of the present study was therefore to further investigate the role of the platelet and the effects of platelet-inhibiting drugs in experimental pulmonary embolism with glass beads in the dog.

Methods

Particulate microembolism was produced by rapid injection of 0.15 cm³/kg glass beads with a diameter of 150–250 μm in saline into the right ventricular outflow tract to achieve equal embolization of both lungs. Cardiac output mean pulmonary arterial, mean pulmonary capillary and mean systemic pressure were obtained prior to and at 5, 10, 20 and 30 min post embolization.

The control group consisted of 8 dogs given emboli with no pre-treatment. Thrombocytopenia was induced in a group of 10 dogs by platelet antiserum and the mean platelet count was reduced from 234,000 ± 28,000 to 9,000 ± 4,000 mm³. The platelet antiserum was prepared in rabbits and tested by indirect immunofluorescence, using goat anti-rabbit immunoglobulin. Activity was only demonstrated against platelets but not against red or white cells. The antiserum was administered either the day before the experiment or if on the same day more than 2 h before the embolism to ensure normal vascular reactivity.

To an additional 5 dogs sulfinpyrazone was given in a dose of 7 mg/kg directly into the stomach through an intragastric tube at least 60 min prior to embolization. To another group of 5 dogs 10,000 U of heparin sodium was given intravenously at least 30 min prior to embolization.

Results

Figure 1 shows the effects of pulmonary microembolism on the pulmonary vascular resistance (PVR) in the different groups. The control group shows an almost threefold increase in PVR 5 min post embolization and PVR slowly tended downward during the 30 min of observation. No difference was found in the dogs receiving the antiserum 2 h or 18 h prior to the experiment and the data were combined. In these 10 dogs the increase in PVR was only 41 % of that observed in the control dogs. Microembolization after sulfinpyrazone increased PVR only 44 %, as much as in the control dogs. Pretreatment with heparin also reduced the pressor response to pulmonary microembolization and the increase was only 45 % of that observed with embolism in the control dogs.

The decrease in the pressor response was not due to a changed flow pattern but to a decrease in vasoconstriction, because mean pulmonary artery pressures reflect the observed differences in PVR.

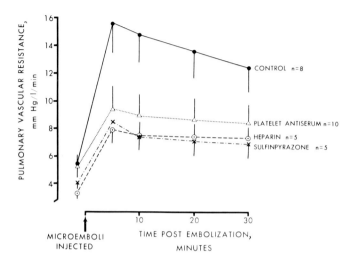

Fig. 1. Effects of pulmonary microembolism on the pulmonary resistance (PVR) in the different groups.

Sulfinpyrazone and heparin *per se* had no effects on the pulmonary vascular bed, neither during normoxia nor alveolar hypoxia. The effects of sulfinpyrazone or heparin on hypoxic response were tested, because we found in a related study that another platelet-inhibiting substance, dipyridamole, had a direct vasodilating effect on pulmonary vascular smooth muscle.

Discussion

The results of previous studies following the induction of thrombocytopenia have not been consistent. In one study, CADE [1] found that thrombocytopenia reduced the pulmonary pressor effects of massive pulmonary embolism with autologous blood clots. On the other hand another study from PUCKETT *et al.* [2] indicated that thrombocytopenia did not protect embolized animals against the increase in PVR or the changes in airway compliance or resistance. Repeated infusions of platelet antiserum protected cats against pulmonary microembolism with barium sulfate, despite rather high platelet counts in some animals. Thus the effects of platelet removal have not been clearly established.

Platelet aggregation in the lung causes an increase in pulmonary pressure and PVR, probably by the release of vasoactive substances [4]. In experiments in the mice it was shown that platelet aggregation followed by release reaction is the mechanism by which platelet antiserum might be acting [5]. In earlier experiments, we could show that acute destruction of circulating platelets increases pulmonary vascular resistance probably by the release of a vasoconstrictor prostaglandin [6]. The results of the present study indicate that thrombocytopenia reduced by more than half the pulmonary hypertension from experimental glass bead pulmonary embolism.

The fact that sulfinpyrazone and heparin ameliorated the pulmonary hypertensive effects of microembolism to the same extent as platelet depletion suggests that the effects of those agents were largely those on platelets.

Leukocytes did not seem to contribute to the pressor response because at least in the dogs receiving the antiserum the day before the experiment, thrombocytopenia was not accompanied by leukopenia.

The mechanism by which sulfinpyrazone affects the platelet is no clear in that its *in vitro* effects on platelets are rather weak [7]. It may act by modifying some plasma or endothelial factors which are important for platelet behavior *in vivo* [7] or by inhibiting the platelet release reaction [8].

Heparin prevents platelet accretion on an embolus through inhibition of thrombin by accelerating the action of antithrombin and inhibits the thrombin-induced platelet release reaction [9].

In conclusion, in the present model of experimental pulmonary embolism with glass beads in the dog, the role of the platelet seems important. Altering platelet behavior with sulfinpyrazone or heparin – probably by inhibiting the platelet release reaction – reduces the emboli-induced pulmonary hypertension to the same extent as platelet depletion. Evaluation of platelet function in human pulmonary microembolism and consideration of substances which minimize or prevent platelet effects seems to be warranted on the basis of these experiments.

Summary

Altering the platelet behavior with sulfinpyrazone or heparin – probably by inhibiting the platelet release reaction – reduces the emboli-induced pulmonary hypertension to the same extent as platelet depletion.

Evaluation of platelet function in human pulmonary microembolism and consideration of substances which minimize or prevent platelet effects seems to be warranted on the basis of these experiments.

References

1   CADE, J.F.: Platelets, pulmonary hypertension and pulmonary embolism. Platelets, Drugs and Thrombosis. Proc. Symp., Hamilton 1972, pp. 191–199 (Karger, Basel 1975).

2   PUCKETT, C.L.; GERVIN, A.S.; RHODES, G.R., and SILVER, D.: Role of platelets and serotonin in acute massive pulmonary embolism. Surgery Gynec. Obstet. *137:* 618–622 (1973).

3   BO, G.; HOGNESTAD, J., and VAAGE, J.: The role of blood platelets in pulmonary responses to microembolization with barium sulphate. Acta physiol. scand. *90:* 244–251 (1974).

4   BO, G. and HOGNESTAD, J.: Pulmonary vascular effects of suddenly induced unilateral blood platelet aggregation. Acta physiol. scand. *90:* 237–243 (1974).

5   MCDONALD, T.P. and CLIFT, R.: Mechanism of thrombocytopenia induced in mice by platelet antiserum. Haemostasis *5:* 38–50 (1976).

6   WEIR, E.H.; MLCZOCH, J.; SEAVY, J.; COHEN, J.J., and GROVER, R.F.: Platelet antiserum inhibits hypoxic pulmonary vasoconstriction in the dog. J. appl. Physiol. *41* (1976).

7   PARETI, F.I. and MANUCCI, P.M.: Drugs affecting platelet behaviour. I. Roll. Coll. Phycns *10:* 194–201 (1976).

8   GENTON, E.; GENT, M.; HIRSH, J., and HARKER, L.A.: Platelet inhibiting drugs in the prevention of clinical thrombotic disease. New Engl. J. Med. *293:* 1174–1178 (1975).

9   THOMAS, D.P.: Therapeutic role of heparin in acute pulmonary embolism. Curr. Ther. Res. *18:* 21–33 (1975).

Dr. J. MLCZOCH, Department of Cardiology, University of Vienna, *Vienna* (Austria)

Prog. biochem. Pharmacol., vol. 14, pp. 349–352 (Karger, Basel 1977)

Relationship between Disturbed Rheological Properties and Cerebral Hemodynamics in Recent Cerebral Infarction

E.O. Ott, G. Ladurner and H. Lechner

University Clinic for Neurology and Psychiatry, University of Graz, Graz

Introduction

Global as well as regional hemodynamic and metabolic alterations take place following severe ischemic anoxia due to cerebral vessel occlusion. Endothelial damage occurs followed by extravasation of the fluid constituents of blood resulting in edema of the brain and further reduction of cerebral blood flow. Increased vascular permeability causes hemoconcentration and stasis and yields clumping of erythrocytes and formation of mural thrombi by agglutinated platelets in the terminal vessels.

The present investigation reports findings in patients with recent cerebral infarction demonstrating that hemodynamic and rheologic alterations of cerebrovascular insufficiency are closely related.

Patients and Methods

Before treatment was started measurements of serum fibrinogen, whole blood viscosity and platelet aggregability have been performed in 75 patients (35 males and 40 females) ranging in age from 54 to 84 years with a mean age of 72, admitted because of neurological symptoms due to recent cerebral infarction (RCI) involving the carotid artery territory.

Blood viscosity was determined at 37° C and four different share rates by means of a cone-plate viscometer [1], and platelet aggregability was tested using a photometrical method [2]. In addition hemispheric cerebral blood flow (HBF) measurements have been performed in 24 of the patients using the intra-arterial ^{133}Xe technique [3] prior to angiographic examination.

Results

In patients with RCI whole blood viscosity was found significantly increased at all shear rates. Increased levels of serum fibrinogen were determined as well when blood viscosity was increased and when there was evidence of enhanced platelet aggregation. In these cases there had been a close relationship between serum fibrinogen and increased blood viscosity (fig. 1) on one hand and enhanced platelet aggregation on the other. Furthermore, at low shear rates increased levels of blood viscosity correlated significantly with reduction of HBF (fig. 2).

Discussion

As previously reported increased blood viscosity has been observed in patients with complete cerebral infarction [4] but may also occur in patients with cerebral transient ischemic attacks [5]. This behavior of blood is due to the content of serum fibrinogen [4, 5] but may also be influenced by other factors, such as enhanced aggregation of blood cells [4]. Furthermore, it has been shown that fibrinogen may enhance platelet aggregability in the case of a certain thrombin-platelet ratio [6].

It can be concluded from the present results that in patients with RCI high levels of serum fibrinogen are contributing to enhanced platelet aggregation and thus increasing blood viscosity predominantly at low shear rates such as exist in small vessels. At the same rate of shear, viscosity contributes significantly to impairment of HBF (fig. 2) and thereby demonstrates the link between hemodynamic and rheologic alterations in cerebral infarction.

Summary

In 75 patients with neurological symptoms due to RCI serum fibrinogen, whole blood viscosity and platelet aggregability have been determined before treatment was started. In addition, in 24 of the patients also

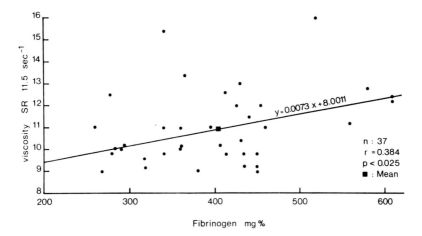

Fig. 1. Correlation fibrinogen-increased viscosity in cerebral infarction.

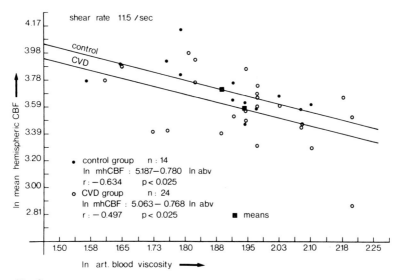

Fig. 2.

HBF has been measured. In patients with RCI viscosity was significantly increased. Serum fibrinogen was higher at increased viscosity levels and when enhanced platelet aggregation was evident. At low shear rates increased blood viscosity correlated significantly with serum fibrinogen as well as with reduction of HBF.

References

1   WELLS, R.E.; DENTON, R., and MERRILL, E.W.: Measurement of viscosity of
     biologic fluid by cone plate viscometer. J. Lab. clin. Med. *57:* 646–656 (1961).
2   BREDDIN, K.; GRUN, H.; KRZYMANEK, H.J., *et al.:* Zur Messung der spontanen
     Thrombozytenaggregation. Plättchenaggregationstest III. Klin. Wschr. *53:*
     81–89 (1975).
3   HØEDT-RASMUSSEN, K.; SVEINSDOTTIR, E., and LASSEN, N.A.: Regional cerebral
     blood flow in man determined by intraarterial injection of radioactive inert gas.
     Circulation Res. *18:* 137–247 (1966).
4   OTT, E.O.; LECHNER, H., and ARANIBAR, A.: High blood viscosity syndrome in
     cerebral infarction. Stroke *5:* 330–333 (1974).
5   LECHNER, H. und OTT, E.: Klinische Bedeutung von Blutviskositätsveränderungen
     im Rahmen der cerebrovasculären Insuffizienz. Münch. med. Wschr. *117:*
     1599–1602 (1975).
6   CHAO, F.C.; TULLIS, J.L.; KENNEDY, D.M., *et al.:* Concentration effects of
     platelets, fibrinogen and thrombin on platelet aggregation and fibrin clotting.
     Thromb. Diath. haemorrh. *32:* 216–231 (1974).

Dr. E.O. OTT, University Clinic for Neurology and Psychiatry, Auenbrugger-
platz 22, *8036 Graz* (Austria)